Anemia

Pathophysiology, Diagnosis, and Management

D1495048

Anemia

Pathophysiology, Diagnosis, and Management

Edited by

Edward J. Benz, Jr., MD

Nancy Berliner, MD

Fred J. Schiffman, MD

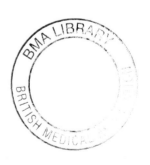
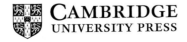
CAMBRIDGE
UNIVERSITY PRESS

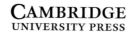

University Printing House, Cambridge CB2 8BS, United Kingdom

One Liberty Plaza, 20th Floor, New York, NY 10006, USA

477 Williamstown Road, Port Melbourne, VIC 3207, Australia

314–321, 3rd Floor, Plot 3, Splendor Forum, Jasola District Centre, New Delhi – 110025, India

79 Anson Road, #06–04/06, Singapore 079906

Cambridge University Press is part of the University of Cambridge.

It furthers the University's mission by disseminating knowledge in the pursuit of education, learning, and research at the highest international levels of excellence.

www.cambridge.org
Information on this title: www.cambridge.org/9780521514262
DOI: 10.1017/9781108586900

First published 2018

Printed in the United Kingdom by Clays, St Ives plc

A catalogue record for this publication is available from the British Library.

Library of Congress Cataloging-in-Publication Data
Names: Benz, Edward J., Jr., editor. | Berliner, Nancy (Hematologist), editor. | Schiffman, Fred J., editor.
Title: Anemia : pathophysiology, diagnosis and management / edited by Edward J. Benz, Jr., Nancy Berliner, Fred J. Schiffman.
Other titles: Anemia (Benz)
Description: Cambridge, United Kingdom ; New York, NY : Cambridge University Press, 2018. | Includes bibliographical references and index.
Identifiers: LCCN 2017038688 | ISBN 9780521514262 (hardback : alk. paper) | ISBN 9781108425209 (pbk. : alk. paper)
Subjects: | MESH: Anemia
Classification: LCC RC641.7.A6 | NLM WH 155 | DDC 616.1/52–dc23
LC record available at https://lccn.loc.gov/2017038688

ISBN 978-0-521-51426-2 Mixed Media
ISBN 978-1-108-42520-9 Paperback
ISBN 978-1-108-58690-0 Cambridge Core

....

Contents

List of Contributors   vii
Preface   xi

Section 1 The Normal Human Red Blood Cell

1   **Anemias, Red Cells, and the Essential Elements of Red Cell Homeostasis**   1
Edward J. Benz, Jr.

2   **Red Cell Production**   14
Anupama Narla and Benjamin L. Ebert

3   **Red Blood Cell Life Span, Senescence, and Destruction**   19
Richard Kaufman

Section 2 The Patient with Anemia

4   **The Clinical Approach to the Patient with Anemia**   23
Matthew Quesenberry, Alina Huang, and Fred J. Schiffman

5   **Anemia in Children**   34
Wendy Wong and Bertil Glader

Section 3 Specific Forms of Anemia

Part A Microcytic Anemias

6   **Iron Deficiency Anemia**   39
Paula Fraenkel

7   **Sideroblastic Anemias**   44
Nathan T. Connell and Edward J. Benz, Jr.

8   **The Thalassemia Syndromes**   48
Madeleine M. Verhovsek and David H. K. Chui

Part B Macrocytic Anemias

9   **Macrocytic Anemias: Megaloblastic and Nonmegaloblastic Anemias**   59
Peter W. Marks

Part C Hemoglobinopathies

10   **Sickle Cell Syndromes**   66
Maureen Achebe

11   **Structural Hemoglobinopathies**   76
Edward J. Benz, Jr.

Part D Hemolytic Anemias

12   **Autoimmune Hemolytic Anemia**   84
Mark A. Murakami, Edward J. Benz, Jr., and Nancy Berliner

13   **Drug-Induced Hemolytic Anemia**   95
Oreofe O. Odejide

14   **Red Cell Membrane Defects**   100
Patrick G. Gallagher

15   **Malaria**   108
Michael A. McDevitt and Richard Bucala

16   **Microangiopathic Hemolytic Anemia**   113
Elaine M. Majerus and J. Evan Sadler

17   **Extrinsic Nonimmune Hemolytic Anemias**   122
Pavan K. Bendapudi and Ronald P. McCaffrey

Part E Hypoplastic Anemias

18   **Acquired Aplastic Anemia and Pure Red Cell Aplasia**   128
Daria Babushok and Monica Bessler

19   **Paroxysmal Nocturnal Hemoglobinuria**   137
Robert A. Brodsky

20   **Congenital Marrow Failure Syndromes**   143
Anupama Narla and Benjamin L. Ebert

21 **Anemia of Chronic Inflammation** 150
Satish P. Shanbhag and Cindy N. Roy

22 **Myelodysplasia** 156
Ida Wong-Sefidan and Rafael Bejar

Section 4 Secondary Anemias

23 **HIV and Anemia** 167
Owen Seddon, Andrew Freedman,
and David T. Scadden

24 **Anemia in the Patient with Cancer** 172
Murat O. Arcasoy

25 **Secondary Anemias Associated with Hematopoietic
Stem Cell Transplantation** 179
Joseph H. Antin

26 **The Anemia of Aging** 185
Amanda J. Redig and Nancy Berliner

27 **Anemia in Pregnancy** 190
Ariela Marshall and Jean M. Connors

28 **Anemias Due to Systemic Diseases** 194
Giada Bianchi and Ronald P. McCaffrey

29 **Transfusion Therapy for Anemia** 201
Joseph D. Sweeney

30 **Transfusion Reactions** 207
Alex Ryder, Edward Snyder, and David Unold

Section 5 Management of Anemia

31 **Pharmacologic Therapy of Anemia** 217
Nicholas Short and Elisabeth M. Battinelli

32 **Splenectomy: Indications and Consequences** 223
Sophia Fircanis Rizk, Andrew Brunner, and Fred
J. Schiffman

Section 6 Summary

33 **Anemias: Summary, Conclusions, and Future
Prospects** 229
Edward J. Benz, Jr.

Index 234

Contributors

Maureen Achebe, MD, MPH
Assistant Professor, Harvard Medical School, Clinical Director, Dana-Farber Cancer Institute Hematology Services, Division of Hematology, Brigham and Women's Hospital, Boston, MA, USA

Joseph H. Antin, MD
Professor of Medicine, Harvard Medical School, Chief, Stem Cell Transplantation, Dana-Farber Cancer Institute, Boston, MA, USA

Murat O. Arcasoy, MD, FACP
Professor of Medicine, Divisions of Hematology and Hematologic Malignancies / Cellular Therapy, Vice Chief for Clinical Affairs, Division of Hematology, Department of Medicine and Duke Cancer Institute, Duke University School of Medicine, Durham, NC, USA

Daria Babushok, MD, PhD
Instructor in Hematology-Oncology, Comprehensive Bone Marrow Failure Center, Division of Hematology, Department of Pediatrics, Children's Hospital of Philadelphia, and Division of Hematology, Department of Medicine, Hospital of the University of Pennsylvania, Philadelphia, PA, USA

Elisabeth M. Battinelli, MD, PhD
Assistant Professor of Medicine, Department of Medicine, Division of Hematology, Brigham and Women's Hospital, Boston, MA, USA

Rafael Befar, MD, PhD
Assistant Professor, Division of Hematology and Oncology, UCSD Moores Cancer Center, La Jolla, CA, USA

Pavan K. Bendapudi, MD
Instructor in Medicine, Division of Hematology and Blood Transfusion Service, Massachusetts General Hospital, Boston, MA, USA

Edward J. Benz Jr., MD
Richard and Susan Smith Distinguished Professor of Medicine, Professor of Pediatrics, Professor of Genetics, Harvard Medical School, President and CEO Emeritus, Dana-Farber Cancer Institute, Director and Principal Investigator Emeritus, Dana-Farber / Harvard Cancer Center, Boston, MA, USA

Nancy Berliner, MD
H. Franklin Bunn Professor of Medicine, Chief, Division of Hematology, Department of Medicine, Brigham and Women's Hospital, Harvard Medical School, Boston, MA, USA

Monica Bessler, MD, PhD
Adjunct Professor of Pediatrics, Comprehensive Bone Marrow Failure Center, Division of Hematology, Department of Pediatrics, Children's Hospital of Philadelphia, and Division of Hematology, Department of Medicine, Hospital of the University of Pennsylvania, Philadelphia, PA, USA

Giada Bianchi, MD
Instructor in Medicine, Dana-Farber Cancer Institute, Department of Medical Oncology, Boston, MA, USA

Robert A. Brodsky, MD
Professor of Medicine and Oncology, Director, Division of Hematology, Johns Hopkins University School of Medicine, Baltimore, MD, USA

Andrew Brunner, MD
Instructor in Medicine, Harvard Medical School, Assistant in Medicine, Center for Leukemia, Massachusetts General Hospital, Boston, MA, USA

Richard Bucala, MD, PhD
Professor of Medicine, Pathology, and Epidemiology and Public Health, Yale Schools of Medicine and Public Health, New Haven, CT, USA

David H. K. Chui, MD, FRCPC
Professor of Medicine, Pathology, and Laboratory Medicine, Boston University School of Medicine, Boston, MA, USA

Nathan T. Connell, MD, MPH
Assistant Professor of Medicine, Harvard Medical School, Division of Hematology, Brigham and Women's Hospital, Boston, MA, USA

Jean M. Connors, MD
Associate Professor of Medicine, Harvard Medical School, Hematology Division, Brigham and Women's Hospital, Boston, MA, USA

Benjamin L. Ebert, MD, PhD
Professor of Medicine, Harvard Medical School, Chair, Medical Oncology, Dana-Farber Cancer Institute, Boston, MA, USA

Sophia Fircanis Rizk, MD
Medical Oncologist, Department of Hematology and Medical Oncology, SouthCoast Centers for Cancer Care, Fairhaven, MA, USA

Paula Fraenkel, MD
Assistant Professor, Department of Medicine, Harvard Medical School, Division of Hematology/Oncology, Beth Israel Deaconess Medical Center, Boston, MA, USA

Andrew Freedman, MD
Reader in Infectious Diseases / Honorary Consultant Physician, Cardiff University School of Medicine, Cardiff, UK

Patrick G. Gallagher, MD
Professor of Pediatrics, Pathology, and Genetics, Yale University School of Medicine, New Haven, CT, USA

Bertil Glader, MD, PhD
Professor of Pediatrics and Pathology, Stanford University School of Medicine, Stanford, CA, USA

Alina Huang, MD
Hematologist and Medical Oncologist, Virginia Cancer Specialists, Alexandra, VA, USA

Richard Kaufman, MD
Associate Professor of Pathology, Harvard Medical School, Division of Transfusion Medicine, Brigham and Women's Hospital, Boston, MA, USA

Elaine M. Majerus, MD, PhD
Professor of Medicine, Division of Hematology, Department of Medicine, Washington University School of Medicine, St. Louis, MO, USA

Peter W. Marks, MD, PhD
Director, Center for Biologics Evaluation and Research / FDA, Silver Springs, MD, USA

Ariela Marshall, MD
Assistant Professor of Medicine, Division of Hematology, Assistant Professor of Laboratory Medicine and Pathology, Mayo Clinic, Rochester, MN, USA

Ronald P. McCaffrey, MD
Professor of Medicine, Harvard Medical School, Hematology Division, Brigham and Women's Hospital, Boston, MA, USA

Michael A. McDevitt, MD, PhD
Assistant Professor, Department of Internal Medicine and Hematology, Johns Hopkins University School of Medicine, Baltimore, MD, USA

Mark A. Murakami, MD
Instructor in Medicine, Harvard Medical School, Department of Medical Oncology, Dana-Farber Cancer Institute, Boston, MA, USA

Anupama Narla, MD
Assistant Professor of Pediatrics, Stanford University, Stanford, CA, USA

Oreofe O. Odejide, MD, MPH
Instructor in Medicine, Harvard Medical School, Division of Hematologic Malignancies, Dana-Farber Cancer Institute, Boston, MA, USA

Matthew Quesenberry, MD
Assistant Professor of Medicine, Brown University Division of Hematology/Oncology, Rhode Island Hospital, Providence, RI, USA

Amanda J. Redig, MD
Instructor in Medicine, Dana-Farber Cancer Institute/ Partners Cancer Care, Boston, MA, USA

Cindy N. Roy, MD, PhD
Assistant Professor of Medicine, Geriatric Medicine and Gerontology, Department of Medicine, Johns Hopkins University School of Medicine, Baltimore, MD, USA

Alex Ryder, MD, PhD
Assistant Professor Pediatrics and Pathology, University of Tennessee Health Science Center, Medical Director, Transfusion Services, Le Bonheur Children's Memphis, TN, USA

J. Evan Sadler, MD, PhD
Professor of Medicine, Director, Division of Hematology, Department of Medicine, Washington University School of Medicine, St. Louis, MO, USA

David T. Scadden, MD
Gerald and Darlene Jordan Professor of Medicine, Harvard Stem Cell Institute, Massachusetts General Hospital, Harvard University, Cambridge, MA, USA

Fred J. Schiffman, MD, MACP
Sigal Family Professor of Humanistic Medicine, Vice Chair, Department of Medicine, Warren Alpert Medical School of Brown University, Providence, RI, USA

Owen Seddon, MB, BCh
Senior Registrar in Infectious Diseases, Department of Infectious Diseases, University Hospital of Wales, Cardiff, UK

Satish P. Shanbhag, MD
Assistant Professor of Medicine, Division of Hematology, Johns Hopkins University School of Medicine, Baltimore, MD, USA

Nicholas Short, MD
Assistant Professor, Department of Leukemia, Division of Cancer Medicine, The University of Texas MD Anderson Cancer Center, Houston, TX, USA

Edward Snyder, MD
Professor, Laboratory Medicine, Yale School of Medicine, New Haven, CT, USA

Joseph D. Sweeney, MD, FACP, FRCPath
Professor of Pathology and Laboratory Medicine, Brown University, Director, Coagulation and Transfusion Medicine, Providence, RI, USA

David Unold, MD
Health Sciences Assistant Clinical Professor, Department of Pathology and Laboratory Medicine, UC Davis School of Medicine, Sacramento, CA, USA

Madeleine M. Verhovsek, MD, FRCPC
Associate Professor of Medicine, Department of Medicine, McMaster University School of Medicine, Hamilton, ON, Canada

Wendy Wong, MD
Adjunct Clinical Associate Professor, Stanford University, Stanford, CA, USA

Ida Wong-Sefidan, MD
Assistant Professor, Division of Hematology and Oncology, University of California, San Diego, La Jolla, CA, USA

Preface

The erythrocyte (red cell) is the nearly universal means by which aerobic animals larger than insects deliver oxygen to the tissues. Red cells are able to achieve oxygen acquisition and delivery by accommodating high cytoplasmic concentrations of dissolved hemoglobin. Hemoglobin is a pigmented protein that enfolds an iron-containing heme moiety in a manner that permits the reversible binding and unbinding of oxygen over the physiologic range of oxygen pressures present in our environment. Sufficient numbers of adequately hemoglobinized erythrocytes in the circulation are essential for the sustenance of life. Until recently, the red cell was regarded as having relatively little in the way of functions or impacts save for its vital role in oxygen transport. As discussed in this volume, recent insights show that red cells, partly because of their sheer numbers and bulk, can also have physiologic effects on other vital functions including hemostasis, vascular tone, and energy metabolism. Any understanding of physiology or of the pathobiology of human diseases requires a grasp of the production, survival, and destruction of red cells and the structures and functions of their major components, including hemoglobin.

Anemias are conditions in which the number of red cells or their hemoglobin content is insufficient to sustain the normal cardiovascular, neurologic, and metabolic needs of the body. Anemias as a group are among the most common abnormalities encountered in medicine. Since the introduction of red cell transfusions and readily available hematinics such as iron, folic acid, and vitamin B12, anemia *per se* is infrequently the primary cause of death when treatment is available. Yet anemia represents a significant complicating comorbidity in a variety of human diseases, one that is often associated with reduced survival. Indeed, support of the red cell mass has led to the creation of an entire specialty: transfusion medicine. While there are many causes of anemia that result from primary abnormalities in the production, survival, or destruction of red cells, anemias are every bit as important as indicators of physiologic distress in other organs and tissues. For example, blood loss anemia can provide a clue to gastrointestinal bleeding from ulcers or intestinal neoplasms. Anemias often accompany or can even be the presenting finding in patients with hematologic malignancies or autoimmune disorders. Anemias may also accompany conditions such as multiple myeloma or leukemia, where other lineages are affected. Mastery of the causes, diagnostic approaches, and clinical management of anemias is essential to any high-quality medical practice in almost every specialty area.

This textbook is intended to provide both an introduction to the general features of anemia and concise but thorough descriptions of the major causes of anemias. Also discussed are the pathophysiologic mechanisms involved, the best diagnostic strategies to pursue, and the state-of-the-art approaches to management. Finally, we consider some of the prospects for progress toward better understanding and management of anemias in the future. Each of the editors and authors is a hematologist with expertise in the field of red cell pathobiology. Each is an experienced clinician who has managed anemias in numerous patients. Each has also taught various aspects of this field to students, practitioners, investigators, and allied health professionals.

We have attempted to provide coverage of anemias that is comprehensive yet accessible in a relatively small and readable volume, enriched by abundant illustrations, graphs, and tables. It is our hope that this text will be useful to those entering the field of health care sciences but also as a refresher and reference source for more experienced clinicians. Because the study of the red cell has, for many decades, served as an entry point for the cutting edge of life sciences into the investigation of human diseases, we have also taken pains to provide, in a readable way, some sense of the scientific and biological basis for the abnormalities that lead to particular forms of anemia.

There is a strong scientific foundation upon which our understanding of red cell structure, function, production, and survival is based. Familiarity with new developments in this field is therefore relevant to a wide variety of medical disciplines and specialties. We have had the good fortune to prepare this volume in a dynamic time in the history of red cell research, one that is yielding promising new approaches to the management of red cell disorders that could be prototypical for other applications. Gene therapy clinical trials are in progress and providing promising early results. Engineered stem cells are being used to generate large quantities of red cells, which can provide a means for red cell transfusion support that is free of the immunological and infectious consequences of donor-based transfusion. Multiple start-up companies share this goal.

The recognition of the importance of the red cell interactions with the vascular wall and with other components of the hemostatic, immune, and inflammatory networks has altered the approach to understanding many diseases for which the red cell was not previously thought to be relevant. We have attempted to preview some of these impending developments for the reader.

The completion of this volume clearly required the efforts of many more people than the editors. We are indebted to the authors who prepared excellent chapters about specific topics in this textbook and to their staff who assisted in the preparation of their contributions. We are also extraordinarily grateful to Addy Donnelly, Bernadette Sessa, and Jacqueline Gifford, without whose expert support and persistent organizational efforts this book would not have been possible. We are equally appreciative of our colleagues at Cambridge University Press for their guidance and their patience with the long process of manuscript submission. We thank the many thousands of patients whose willingness to be studied and to participate in clinical trials has made all of the advances noted on this book possible. Finally, and perhaps most importantly, we are each grateful to our spouses, Margaret Ann Vettese, Alan Plattus, and Gerri Schiffman, and to our families for their ongoing support throughout our careers. We sincerely hope that our readers will find this volume enjoyable as well as edifying and, most especially, useful in enhancing their care of anemic patients.

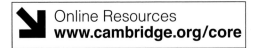

Online Resources
www.cambridge.org/core

Chapter

Anemias, Red Cells, and the Essential Elements of Red Cell Homeostasis

Edward J. Benz, Jr., MD

This monograph is focused on anemias. Among the most common disorders in the world, anemias are conditions that cause the number of red blood cells (erythrocytes) in the circulation to fall. In humans, red cells provide the sole means for efficient oxygen acquisition (in the lungs), transport (in the circulation), and delivery (via capillaries perfusing vital tissues). They are thus essential for survival. In the most severe cases, anemias can lead to major organ dysfunction or non-function due to oxygen deprivation, producing heart failure, coma, or even death. In more moderate situations, anemia can produce protean symptoms and physical signs of inadequate oxygen transport, such as pallor, exercise intolerance, malaise, cognitive changes, congestive heart failure, and weakness. In many cases, however, anemias tend to be milder and can be entirely asymptomatic, detectable only as deviations from the patient's normal red cell values in laboratory tests.

As discussed in detail in many chapters of this book, literally hundreds of factors govern the production, destruction, or loss, via bleeding, of red cells. Reductions in the red cell mass can thus have many hundreds of possible causes. While a number of these arise from intrinsic abnormalities in the production (erythropoiesis), structure, or function of erythrocytes themselves, in most patients with anemia, the fall in red cell mass is due to extrinsic factors that impair erythropoiesis, cause hemorrhage, or lead to accelerated destruction of red cells. Thus, a very mild anemia can be a sign of a potentially fatal condition, such as colon cancer or a myelodysplastic syndrome, while some of the most severe anemias, though requiring emergent lifesaving interventions, can be due to relatively readily managed conditions such as severe folate or vitamin B12 deficiency. Discerning the reason for an individual's anemia, however mild, is thus an imperative of good clinical practice.

The body's need for large quantities of red cells is intimately related to the need for large quantities of hemoglobin, the body's major oxygen transport protein. Since oxygen is minimally soluble in plasma, a higher-efficiency means of transport from the lungs to the tissues is required. In most metazoan species, this bulk transport depends on "heme" or "heme-like" pigments. These consist of a transition metal (e.g., iron or cobalt) coordinately bound to a planar porphyrin molecule. In mammals, this compound is invariably heme, consisting of reduced iron (Fe^{++}) encased in protoporphyrin IX. Unfortunately, heme is minimally soluble in plasma. It would, in any event, be rapidly catabolized and excreted by the liver and kidneys. In order to achieve a sufficient capacity for oxygen transport, heme is packaged in a highly soluble, tetrameric group of proteins called hemoglobins. In addition to allowing enough heme to be soluble, hemoglobins also modulate the interaction between heme and oxygen so as to ensure reversible binding and release of oxygen over the physiologic range of oxygen tensions encountered in the lungs and the vascular beds perfusing the interior tissues of the body.

Enormous quantities of hemoglobin are needed to ensure life-sustaining oxygen transport. Unfortunately, hemoglobins themselves cannot persist for more than a few minutes in the circulation, where they dissociate into dimers and are rapidly cleared by the kidneys. The amount of energy and nutrients needed to replenish literally pounds of hemoglobin lost every day would overwhelm the entire resources of the body. Nature has addressed this problem by packaging hemoglobin into erythrocytes. These highly durable cells are capable of lasting 4 months in the blood. All of the vital cells, tissues, organs, and physiologic functions of the body thus depend on the continued production and prolonged survival of red cells to provide them with life-sustaining amounts of oxygen.

The abundance of red cells in the circulation is assessed clinically by a series of laboratory tests. They measure the "concentration" of red cells or hemoglobin in whole blood, or the volume of red cells as a percentage of the volume of whole blood. These are summarized in Table 1.1, along with a number of other basic laboratory tests useful for characterizing anemias and assessing possible underlying causes. The *red cell count* (RBC) is measured by automated particulate counters and tabulated as the number of cells per cubic millimeter of whole blood; normal values range from 4 to 5.5 cells/cu.mm. The *hemoglobin value (Hb or Hgb)* measures the concentration of hemoglobin, calculated as grams of hemoglobin per 100 cubic centimeters of whole blood. Normal values range from 12.5 to 15.5 mg/100 cc. Finally, the *hematocrit* measures the total volume of red cells as a percentage of the volume of whole blood; normal values range from 38 to 45%. As noted in the table, "normal" values vary somewhat by age and gender.

Table 1.1 Clinical Laboratory Assessments of Red Cell Homeostasis

TEST	NORMAL VALUES	RED CELL PROPERTY MEASURED
Hematocrit (HCT)	38–48%	% of WB volume occupied by RBC
Hemoglobin (Hb)	12.5–15.5 gm%	Grams Hb per 100 ml WB
RBC (millions/cmm)	4.5–5.5 × 10⁶/cmm	# of red cells per cmm WB
MCV (mean corpuscular volume)	80–95 femtoliters	Average volume of RBC
MCH (mean corpuscular Hb)	27–31 pg/cell	Intracellular concentration of Hb
MCHC (mean corpuscular Hb concentration)	32–36 g/dL	Concentration of Hb per dL of RBC's
RDW (RBC distribution width)	11.5–14.5%	Variation in RBC size/volume
Reticulocyte count	0.5–2.0%	% of "new" RBCs in blood
Bilirubin	0.1–1.2 mg	Hemolysis elevates indirect fraction
LDH (Lactic Dehydrogenase)	122–222	Elevated during hemolysis
Haptoglobin	41–165 gm/dL	Reduced by hemolysis

Abbreviations: WB – whole blood; ml – milliliters; dL – deciliters; cmm – cubic millimeter; pg – picogram; fl – femtoliter; gm – gram; RBC – red blood cell

The table shows the most commonly used tests to assess the adequacy of red cell content in the peripheral blood, the major features of cell size or hemoglobinization and red cell production, for the purpose of evaluating the differential diagnosis of anemias, and a few tests useful for detecting increases in red blood cell destruction. In many laboratories, the values will also be shown in international units (IU) rather than as outlined in the table.

These measurements of the amount of red blood cells are invariably included as part of the routine complete blood count (CBC), which also provides information about the numbers and types of white blood cells and platelets, and some additional information useful for further assessment of anemias. These include the ***mean corpuscular volume (MCV)***, which is expressed as the average volume, in femtoliters, of the red cells in the circulation. Certain forms of anemia in femtoliters, are associated with smaller- or larger-than-normal-sized red cells in the circulation. Recognizing the change in size can be a very useful first step in narrowing down the possible causes of anemia. The ***mean corpuscular hemoglobin*** or ***MCH*** measures the total amount of hemoglobin in picograms per microliter of red cells, while the ***mean corpuscular hemoglobin concentration (MCHC)*** measures the concentration of hemoglobin within red cell cytoplasm and is expressed as picograms of hemoglobin per picoliter of cytoplasm. The ***reticulocyte count*** is a measure of the percentage of total red cells that are newly released into the circulation ("reticulocytes"). These cells retain traces of their bone marrow progenitors that alter their staining properties on peripheral blood smears, as discussed later in this chapter, but only for about one day out of the roughly 100- to 120-day lifespan of normal red cells. The normal value for the reticulocyte count in the setting of a normal hemoglobin and hematocrit is thus about 0.8–1%. Given the relative persistence of reticulocytes and mature erythrocytes in the circulation, this percentage represents the physiological replacement needs. Levels above this indicate increased production of red cells, usually in response to red cell loss or destruction, while levels at or below normal values despite the presence of anemia indicate inadequate marrow response to the need for more red cells. This value is thus very helpful in assessing whether anemias are due to failure to produce sufficient numbers of red cells or to excess red cell loss or destruction, or both.

The definitions and utility of the other tests listed in Table 1.1 are addressed later in this chapter or in the subsequent relevant parts of this textbook. For our present purpose, it is sufficient to note that anemias can be detected and at least partially characterized by a relatively simple set of tests readily obtained from a small peripheral blood sample. When combined with an adequate history and physical examination, the etiology of most anemias can be determined with relatively simple and inexpensive follow-up tests. The clinical approach to the assessment of anemias is discussed in more detail in Chapter 4.

The fairly broad-based normal ranges listed in Table 1.1 are useful as an indicator of the normal ranges of the population. However, an individual's "normal" red cell parameters can vary on the basis of gender, age, environment, and physiologic circumstances. It is thus inadvisable to define anemia by arbitrary numerical standards. For example, an individual living in the high ranges of the Andes requires a higher red cell mass than a similar individual at sea level. Fetuses require higher hematocrits in utero than children and adults at later ages. Women tend to have slightly lower "normal" blood count ranges than men, even when corrections are made for blood loss due to menstruation and pregnancy. Children with cyanotic congenital heart disease require higher hematocrits than those without that malady, while hematocrits tend to decline modestly as we age.

It is important to reiterate the point noted earlier that an operational definition of "anemia" need not necessarily require a reduction in red cell mass sufficient to compromise normal physiologic function, such as cardiovascular status, exercise tolerance, and the like. Indeed, some of the most important reasons for a decline in red cell mass from the patient's "norm" might not cause any symptoms or even cause the blood counts to fall outside of the "normal" range. The underlying reason for an altered red cell mass often is more important than the actual extent of the change in the amounts of red cells.

Chapter 2 describes the process by which red cells are produced in the bone marrow and the mechanisms by which accelerated red cell production is stimulated in response to excessive red cell loss or destruction. Chapter 3 describes the mechanisms by which senescent or infected red cells are removed from the circulation, thereby potentially shortening red cell survival. This chapter outlines the essential components of the red cell that allow for its prolonged survival in the circulation. An understanding of these components is required for understanding anemia, because derangements in the structure, function, or physical status of these components represent major etiologies of anemia.

Essential Components of the Red Cell

The mammalian erythrocyte develops over 2–3 weeks through a highly concerted cellular differentiation program called erythropoiesis. Erythropoiesis begins with the pluripotent hematopoietic stem cell. After a complex series of differentiation events and maturation processes, each red cell circulates as a biconcave disk-shaped cell exquisitely adapted to provide oxygen transport for nearly 120 days. Along the way, it loses its nucleus and all of its cytoplasmic organelles. It enters the blood stream as a reticulocyte, distinguished from its more mature erythrocyte descendants by the retention of a few polyribosomes that support a limited repertoire of protein synthesis, 90% of which is devoted to producing hemoglobin. Within 24 hours, even that capacity is lost. The mature erythrocyte thus has no ability to reproduce or to generate new proteins, lipids, or nucleic acids. It retains only a rudimentary system for generating energy (ATP) from glucose and a modest ability to rebalance redox status in the presence of oxidative stresses.

Despite these limitations, the circulating human erythrocyte is remarkably resilient. In normal individuals, it traverses the circulation nearly 300,000 times during its 4-month lifespan. During this journey, it encounters enormous mechanical, osmotic, and biochemical stresses. The diameters of capillaries in many capillary beds are only 2–3 μm, whereas the erythrocyte has a normal diameter of 7.5 μm. Because of the geometric redundancy of its disk shape and the pliability and tensile strength of its membrane, the red cell is able to withstand the considerable shear stress and distortion of being "squeezed" through these narrow passages. Indeed, it recovers its normal biconcave disk shape as it enters the more capacious venous circulation. Erythrocytes also encounter striking and rapid changes in osmolarity when passing through the collecting system of the kidney, enormous changes

in pH in the renal pelvis, spleen, and other "stagnant" vascular beds, and massive shifts in oxygen tension while traversing the pulmonary arteries, capillaries, and veins. During each passage through the hepatic and splenic circulation, the red cell is brought into proximity with the (RE) system of macrophages, which detect flaws on its surfaces. Cells deemed too damaged are ingested and catabolized. Given these enormous stresses and the limited repertoire it possesses for repair and replacement of essential components, the red cell's endurance is indeed remarkable.

Hemoglobin: The Predominant Component of the Circulating Erythrocyte

Red cells can support the oxygen demands of the organism only because they are able to carry enough hemoglobin for a sufficient period of time to support oxidative metabolism and, therefore, life. Hemoglobin is the overwhelmingly predominant component of the erythrocyte. Red cells do have other important functions, such as contributing to the regulation of blood pH and modulating vascular tone via uptake and release of nitrous oxide. However, these other, "minor" physiologic impacts of erythrocytes are also largely mediated by hemoglobin. It is thus important to review first the structure, function, and regulated biosynthesis of hemoglobin.

Hemoglobin Structure and Function

As shown in Figure 1.1, the predominant hemoglobins produced during fetal and adult life are "heterotetramers" comprised of two "α" globin polypeptide subunits, and two "non-α" or "β-like" subunits. Each of these globin chains is a helical protein that enfolds a single heme moiety. Heme, in turn, consists of protoporphyrin IX coordinately complexed to a single reduced (Fe^{++}) iron ion. In humans, α chains are 141 amino acids long, and non-α chains are 146 amino acids long. The chains are folded into seven (α) or eight (β) helical segments in such a way as to create a highly hydrophobic core. This interior pocket holds the planar heme moiety at an angle appropriate to interact reversibly with oxygen over the physiologic range of partial pressures of oxygen. The helical segments present mostly hydrophilic (charged) amino acid side chains to the aqueous environment of the erythrocyte cytoplasm while maintaining an interlocking set of neutral and hydrophobic amino acids in the interior of the molecule. In addition to promoting the proper tight binding of heme, these surfaces also support a series of hydrogen bonds, electrostatic, weak-force, and hydrophobic interactions that hold the tetramer together.

Two functional parameters are most critical to understanding the derangements of hemoglobin structure or function that can lead to abnormalities of red cell number. The first is the extraordinarily high intracytoplasmic solubility of the hemoglobin tetramer, required because hemoglobin must

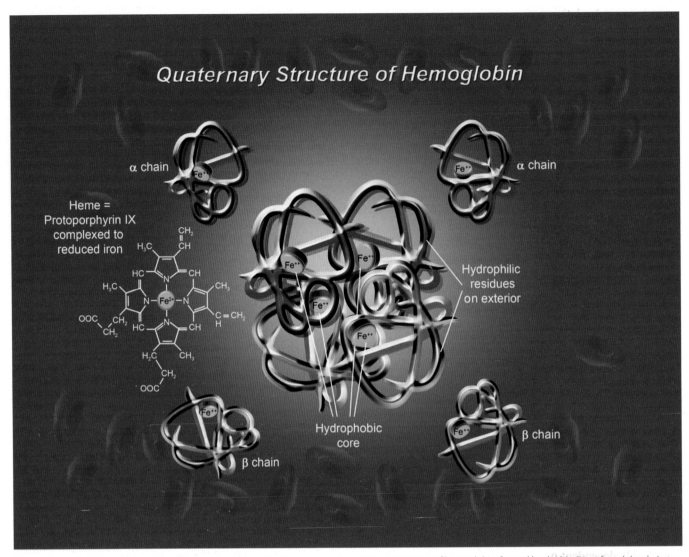

Figure 1.1. The basic structure of the hemoglobin tetramer. The figure shows the tetrameric structure of hemoglobin, formed by the binding of an alpha chain to a beta chain to form alpha-beta dimers, and the pairing of two dimers to form the tetramer. The highly helical chains are illustrated schematically. The fact that hydrophobic residues are clustered around the inner hydrophobic core and toward points of chain–chain contact are indicated, while the hydrophilic residues are shown to be on the outside, facing the aqueous environment. The enfolded heme groups are shown. The structure of heme, a complex of protoporphyrin IX to a reduced iron ion, is illustrated at the left of the tetramer.

accumulate in very high concentrations. Red cells are inherently viscous. If red cells accumulate in excessive numbers (hematocrits greater than 50–55), their viscosity creates significant resistance to blood flow, increasing cardiac afterload. This puts a "cap" on how many red cells can safely circulate. Within that number, there must be sufficient numbers of hemoglobin molecules to carry adequate oxygen to tissues. Thus, if the red cell mass is maintained at the rheological optimal hematocrit level of 35–50, then each red cell must carry roughly 30–35 grams of hemoglobin per 100 cc of red cell cytoplasm. This is a very high level of protein to be maintained in a soluble state. The circulatory system, the regulation of red cell mass, and the cytoplasmic hemoglobin concentration are exquisitely evolved to balance these two parameters.

Hemoglobin tetramers are sufficiently soluble to be present at these concentrations. However, each of the individual components (Fe ions, heme, protophoryins, and individual globin chains) is minimally soluble in physiologic aqueous solutions. It follows that the enormous amount of hemoglobin production needed during the relatively short (5–7 day) period of terminal erythroblast maturation (see below) must be accomplished in such a way that significant excess amounts of free globin, free heme, or Fe are not permitted to accumulate. Conversely, the structural integrity of the intact tetramer and its enfolded heme moieties must be preserved during the circulating life of the erythrocyte. Finally, hemoglobins must be protected from noxious biochemical alterations, most prominently oxidation of either their amino acid residues or their heme moieties. When oxidized, hemoglobins lose the exquisite spatial relationships among their components that maintain the tetramer's state; they then dissociate into their insoluble components and precipitate.

Precipitated hemoglobins, as well as the insoluble inclusions formed by dissociated heme-bearing globin subunits, are rapidly catabolized into highly reactive, toxic aggregates known as hemipyrroles. They oxidize the delicate lipids and proteins of the red cell membrane and cytoskeleton, deranging their structure and function. These in turn render the red cell rigid and create surface abnormalities that are detected by the RE system as a damaged or infected cell destined to be removed from the circulation.

Hemoglobin tetramers can also associate with one another in more ordered ways to form polymers rather than frank precipitated aggregates (Heinz bodies). Hemoglobin tends to polymerize when the hemoglobin molecules carry mutated amino acids that increase the affinity of one intact tetramer for others. These "tactoids" of hemoglobin form fibrous and viscous structures within the cytoplasm, thereby altering the fluid dynamics of the cells in the circulation. Red cells bearing such polymers tend to be viscous and rigid. In addition, polymers often adhere to, and alter, the membrane and its cytoskeleton, causing a variety of surface abnormalities that can produce a hemolytic anemia. The altered membrane exteriors can also make the cells more adherent to the vascular wall itself ("sticky" red cells). The most prominent and clinically important example is HbS, or sickle hemoglobin. As described in Chapter 10, HbS arises from a single amino acid mutation that favors polymer formation, but only when hemoglobin is deoxygenated. These polymers alter the red cell as described earlier, producing hemolytic anemia and impaired blood flow in the microvasculature, causing a protean set of clinical manifestations.

The solubility of hemoglobin in erythrocyte cytoplasm is also highly dependent on a system of metabolic enzymes that generate reducing compounds, notably reduced glutathione. Reduced glutathione reverses oxidative damage to hemoglobin and membrane components. In the circulation, erythrocytes are constantly exposed to oxidant molecules generated by infection, inflammation, and the byproducts of energy metabolism, rendering hemoglobin susceptible to being oxidized and precipitated. Indeed, a significant cause of hemolytic anemia (see Chapters 13 and 17) is impairment of one or more of the enzymes in these reducing pathways, especially when the reduced antioxidant capacity is overly stressed by exposure to oxidative stress, notably by certain drugs, toxins, and dietary components.

The other clinically relevant hemoglobin structure–function relationships are those affecting reversible oxygen binding. The hemoglobin tetramer has evolved to possess an oxygen affinity that actually increases as the concentration of oxygen in its environment increases. This creates the so-called "sigmoidal" oxygen binding curve shown in Figure 1.2. A detailed description of the physical chemistry of this phenomenon is beyond the scope of this discussion. Nonetheless,

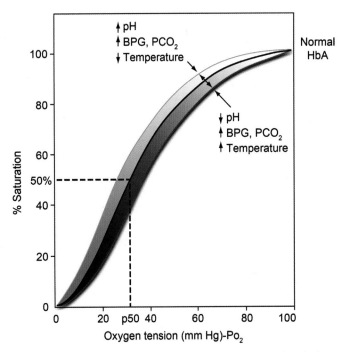

Figure 1.2 Oxygen affinity curve for normal hemoglobin A. As described in the text, the sigmoidal shape of the hemoglobin oxygen affinity curve is shown. The point at which hemoglobins are 50% saturated is called the "p50" value and is about 26–28 mm Hg for normal hemoglobin A. As discussed in the text, normal hemoglobin is nearly fully saturated at p02 of about 60 mm Hg, so that most of the oxygen in normal alveoli provides an excess supply. Normal factors causing hemoglobin affinity to increase ("shift to the left") or decrease ("shift to the right") are indicated by the shaded areas. Fetal hemoglobin (HbF), which fails to bind 2, 3, BPG would thus have a left-shifted oxygen affinity curve relative to HbA.

it is important to note that, at low oxygen tensions, hemoglobin has a low affinity for oxygen until the oxygen concentration is sufficient to break so-called salt bridges that would otherwise bar access of oxygen to the iron moiety within heme. This binding shifts the configuration of heme molecules within the remaining chains of the tetramer to make the breakage of those salt bridges easier. Thus, as oxygen tension rises, the hemoglobin becomes more avid for oxygen, and the amount of binding increases steeply over a relatively narrow range of oxygen tension. In other words, "oxygen binding begets more oxygen binding." At about 60–65 mm Hg PaO$_2$, all four of the heme groups become fully oxygen saturated. Further increases in oxygen concentration have little effect on the oxygen-carrying capacity of the blood because the additional amount of nonhemoglobin oxygen that can be dissolved in the blood is virtually negligible.

Figure 1.2 reveals one very important aspect of the oxygen-binding properties of hemoglobin, namely that it is virtually completely saturated with oxygen at an arterial PaO$_2$ of 60–65 mm Hg. This is far below the PaO$_2$ (90–100 mm Hg) in the normal pulmonary capillary circulation. Thus, the ability of red cells to acquire their maximum payload of oxygen in the lungs is protected by the oxygen binding properties of normal human hemoglobins. Figure 1.2 also reveals that, at the normal PaO_2 of mixed capillary blood (roughly 40 mm Hg), hemoglobin rapidly loses much of its oxygen over a relatively narrow range of PaO_2. Changes in the inherent oxygen affinity of hemoglobin thus tend to have a much greater impact on the *delivery* of oxygen to the tissues than they do on the ability to *acquire* oxygen in normal lungs. Increased oxygen affinity offers virtually no advantage in terms of acquiring oxygen unless the ambient oxygen is extremely low or pulmonary function is seriously compromised. However, "high-affinity" hemoglobins are disadvantageous at the capillary level, where much less oxygen is released (see Figure 1.2). Tissue hypoxia triggers erythropoietin release because the kidney perceives the . reduced oxygen delivery as reflecting reduced red cell mass. This leads to erythrocytosis; when the red cell mass increases beyond hematocrits of 50–55, blood viscosity increases and hemodynamics are compromised.

Conversely, the oxygen affinity of hemoglobin can be reduced significantly without substantially reducing the amount of oxygen acquired in the lung. As shown once again by Figure 1.2, the wide range of PaO_2s over which hemoglobins will be fully saturated allows for this change. However, at the PaO_2 of capillary beds, low-affinity hemoglobins deliver far more oxygen to the tissues than "normal" hemoglobins. These individuals thus have little or no erythropoietin drive and can function physiologically quite well at lower red cell masses, which, when measured in routine blood labs, appear to be "anemias."

The clinical aspects of inheriting high-affinity and low-affinity hemoglobins are discussed in Chapter 11. Even though these are not major causes of anemia, they are instructive because they demonstrate *in vivo* the impact of tissue oxygen delivery on the regulation of red cell mass.

Genetics, Ontogeny, and Biosynthesis of Hemoglobin

Humans produce different hemoglobins at different stages of embryonic, fetal, and adult development. The primary sites of erythropoiesis also change at these different stages of development, from the yolk sac in embryonic life to the liver during fetal life, and then, permanently, to the bone marrow in the latter stages of gestation. The production of hemoglobin is tightly coupled to the process of erythropoiesis, which is described in more detail in Chapter 2. Briefly, pluripotent hematopoietic stem cells become committed to erythropoiesis at early stages of development under the influence of a complex array of growth factors. These activate the production or repression of an equally complex network of transcription factors and cofactors. Under their direction, the progenitors progress through a series of differentiation steps until they emerge as the earliest definable fully committed erythroid progenitors, the so-called burst forming units – erythroid (BFU-E). BFU-E give rise to so-called colony forming units – erythroid (CFU-E) that then differentiate to the earliest morphologic state of erythropoiesis, the proerythroblast. This cellular progression is accompanied by an increasing sensitivity to erythropoietin, which serves to promote both survival and proliferation. BFU-E appear to be more flexible than CFU-E as to which globin genes they will ultimately express.

Although completely committed to produce only erythrocytes, progenitors at the early proerythroblast stage express globin at minimal levels. As the proerythroblast matures, the globin genes, which have been poised for high levels of expression via their chromatin configuration, unleash a remarkably high level of transcriptional activity. During the next 5–7 days, this burst gives rise to the abundant amounts of hemoglobin needed for oxygen transport.

At about the same time, iron uptake increases. The increased intracellular levels of iron then trigger a complex series of gene expression events, largely at the posttranscriptional level, which greatly increase the amount and activities of the heme biosynthetic enzymes. In this manner, rapid increases in the amounts of iron, heme, and globin are coordinated. Maturation beyond the proerythroblast stage also marks the beginning of a progressive decline in the expression of most other genes except those required for producing the red cell membrane cytoskeleton and the few metabolic enzymes that will persist in the circulation. The production of hemoglobin thus ultimately constitutes nearly 95% of the total gene expression activity of late erythroblasts and reticulocytes. This progression is evident by observing the progressive morphologic stages of erythroblast maturation. As these cells mature from proerythroblasts to metachromatophilic erythroblasts to orthochromatic erythroblasts, there is progressive hemoglobinization ("pinking") of the cytoplasm, reduced basophilia (due to declining amounts of ribosomes and nucleic acids), and condensation of active nuclear chromatin (euchromatin) into heterochromatin-producing nuclear pyknosis. In the very terminal stages of maturation, the nucleus is ejected, mitochondria and other organelles disappear, and the enucleate reticulocyte is released into the circulation. Hemoglobin synthesis persists for about 24 hours in the circulation before the reticulocyte matures into fully developed erythrocytes.

A highly coordinated production of α globin, non-α globins, the protoporphyrin IX component of heme, and the incorporation of iron cause each to accumulate in roughly equal amounts. Since each component is rapidly incorporated with the others to form hemoglobin, excesses of none of them occur. This ensures that only highly soluble hemoglobin tetramers and none of their insoluble components accumulate in the cytoplasm.

The Globin Genes

The globin genes map to two compact clusters on chromosome 16 (the ζ globin and α globin genes) and chromosome 11 (the β-like globin genes, β, γ, δ, and ε). As shown in Figure 1.3, the embryonic, fetal, and adult hemoglobins are defined by their globin chain composition. Embryonic hemoglobins are

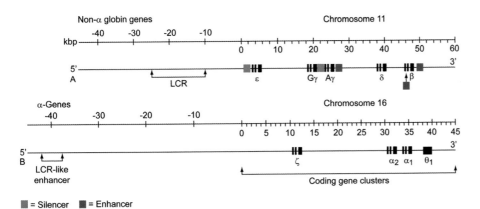

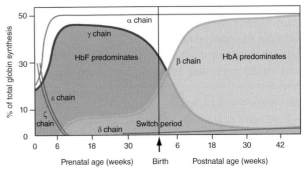

Figure 1.3A. Organization of the globin gene clusters. The organization of the linked clusters alpha and alpha-like globin genes (chromosome 16) and the beta and beta-like globin genes (chromosome 11) are shown. The LCRs (locus control regions) serve as "super-enhancers" or "master switches," which open the chromatin of the entire cluster, making the globin gene complexes available for expression. Expression of the individual genes is strongly influenced by the silencer (S) and enhancer (E) sequences shown. Note that the alpha genes are duplicated, as are the gamma genes, but the beta gene exists in a single copy. (See text for additional details).

Figure 1.3B. Ontogeny of globin gene expression. As discussed in the text, the expression of individual globin genes varies during prenatal and postnatal life. As shown by the shading in the figure, fetal hemoglobin (HbF) predominates during fetal life and persists for several months after birth even though the switch from expression of gamma globin to beta globin occurs just prior to birth. Adult Hemoglobin (Hb A) predominates throughout postnatal life. Fetal hemoglobin is a very minor component from about 18 months of age onward. Embryonic globins are expressed in the yolk sac during the first few weeks of gestation but are not clinically relevant for the purposes of this text.

produced in the yolk sack during embryonic life, beginning at about 5–6 weeks of gestation: Hb Portland I ($\zeta_2\gamma_2$), Hb Portland II ($\zeta_2\beta_2$), Hb Gower-1 ($\zeta_2\epsilon_2$), and Hb Gower-2 ($\alpha_2\epsilon_2$). For our purposes, no further discussion of these hemoglobins is necessary. By the gestational age of 10–11 weeks, red cell production has largely switched to the fetal liver, where the predominant hemoglobin is HbF ($\alpha_2\gamma_2$), i.e., fetal hemoglobin. β globin genes are expressed, but at very low levels, throughout gestation. Production of hemoglobin F predominates until approximately 34–37 weeks' gestation, when a largely irreversible switch to the production of adult hemoglobins (Hb A: $\alpha_2\beta_2$ and Hb A$_2$: $\alpha_2\delta_2$) begins (the Hb F > Hb A switch). At birth, virtually all new hemoglobins being produced are adult hemoglobins. Hb A is the most abundant adult hemoglobin, comprising more than 95% of total adult red cell hemoglobin. Hb A$_2$ accounts for 2–3.5% and residual HbF about 1%, in the normal adult array of red cells. HbF is confined after birth to a small subpopulation of red cells ("F cells"), within which the HbF content is very high.

Even though the switch to *biosynthesis* of adult hemoglobin is virtually complete at the time of birth, the composition of hemoglobins in the peripheral blood changes more slowly. This reflects the long life span of the erythrocytes. HbF persists for a long time after the switch in biosynthesis in circulating red cells that were launched into the circulation before the switch occurred. The transition to the adult pattern of hemoglobin content in the peripheral blood is usually not complete until the latter half of the first year of life.

As discussed in Chapter 8, "hemoglobin switching" has clinical relevance for the understanding and potential therapy of anemias due to certain hemoglobinopathies. Reference to Figure 1.3B shows that individuals inheriting anemia due to α or γ globin gene defects will be affected *in utero* as well as in adult life, provided that the severity of the anemia is compatible with survival through gestation. However, individuals inheriting abnormalities of the β chain will be asymptomatic in utero, since dependence on β globin becomes physiologically important only several months after birth. Sickle cell anemia, a β chain hemoglobinopathy, and β thalassemia comprise major causes of morbidity and mortality among hemoglobinopathies. These patients generally do not present with symptoms until infancy, childhood, or even, in milder situations, adult life. It follows that prevention or reversal of the fetal to adult hemoglobin switch could potentially eliminate the clinical consequences of β globin chain hemoglobinopathies.

Reference to Figure 1.3A also shows that the α globin loci are duplicated, whereas the β globin locus exists as a single copy. Thus, individuals inheriting a mutation in one of the α globin alleles will tend to have a smaller percentage of their total hemoglobin affected by that mutation than individuals inheriting a comparably "severe" abnormality of the single β globin locus. The latter will impair half of all the hemoglobin produced, the former only about 25%. This feature may account for the fact that fetuses are often able to survive gestation despite the phenotypic impact of abnormal α globin production during fetal life.

A great deal of research has been devoted to understanding how the globin genes first become poised to express themselves and then execute their programs of abundant yet tightly regulated fetal and adult globin gene expression. Globin genes are completely silent in all other tissues, and in other hematopoietic progenitors, except for the 5- to 7-day period between the early erythroblast and reticulocyte stages of terminal maturation. It has become clear that the two tightly clustered arrays of globin genes are under the control of a series of promoters and enhancers that regulate their individual function but are also subservient to "super enhancers" or "master switches" called the LCR, for locus control region (Figure 1.3). Evidence suggests that the LCRs, when bound to the transcription factors and cofactors mentioned earlier, form "loops" of chromatin that connect with the promoters and enhancers flanking a particular globin gene. These looped-out regions provide access for additional factors and cofactors that form the transcriptional complex needed to produce globin mRNA. Many of these key proteins have been identified and characterized. Manipulation of LCR interactions is being attempted experimentally to modulate hemoglobin switching as a potential therapeutic modality.

Although the process of hemoglobin biosynthesis is exquisitely and tightly regulated, there is little or no direct "cross talk" between the α-like and β-like gene clusters. The fact that equal amounts of α and β globin are produced is the result of intrinsic structural features of the genes and their mRNA products. The production of globin mRNA is regulated exclusively at the transcriptional level. Globin pre-mRNAs do not undergo alternative pre-mRNA splicing. The rate of production of α globin mRNA exceeds that of β globin mRNA by about 50%, particularly in the earlier stages of erythroblast maturation. However, β globin mRNA is translated into β protein more efficiently than α globin mRNA by nearly the same relative percentages. These differences in translational efficiency are due to differences in the structure of the 5' untranslated regions of the mRNAs. β globin mRNA has a 5' untranslated conformation more amenable to formation of the initiation complex for binding to polyribosomes. β globin mRNA is also slightly more stable than α globin mRNA, having a cytoplasmic survival time of about 54 hours, in contrast to about 38 hours for α globin mRNA. These differences produce a net result that α and β chain production is very nearly equal. Only a very slight excess of α globin is produced, much of it in the earlier stages of maturation. The small pools of excess α globin chains are catabolized by an ubiquitin-mediated pathway, thereby preempting the formation of precipitated inclusions. However, as discussed in Chapter 8, this catabolizing capacity can be easily overcome if the α globin burden increases as the result of impairments in β globin production.

Assembly of hemoglobin from newly synthesized globin chains requires the presence of chaperone proteins. To date, there are no well-described forms of anemia due to the failure of these assembly mechanisms. However, some mutations in the globin chains themselves appear to alter globin structure sufficiently that posttranslational formation of tetramers is impaired, producing a thalassemia-like syndrome.

Hemoglobins are susceptible to many posttranslational modifications. Of note is the affinity of HbA for (2,3-BPG, bisphosphoglycerate, 2,3-BPG), a metabolite of the glycolytic pathway present in the circulating red cell. 2,3-BPG decreases the oxygen affinity of hemoglobin (Figure 1.2). HbF has very low affinity for 2,3-BPG. Even though fully purified ("stripped") preparations of HbF and HbA have nearly identical oxygen affinity, HbF-rich red cells tend to have a higher oxygen affinity *in vivo* and thus can "steal" oxygen from HbA. It also delivers oxygen less efficiently, which accounts at least partially for the high hematocrits of fetuses and neonates.

By virtue of its prolonged exposure to a variety of substances in the circulation, hemoglobin can also be non–enzymatically modified. These modified hemoglobins accumulate as the red cell ages. The most important modifications include the binding of hemoglobin to carbon monoxide in the environment, which can produce carbon monoxide poisoning, the creation of sulfated hemoglobins from exposure to sulfurous compounds, and the glycosylation of the hemoglobin by exposure to glucose. Indeed, "HbA$_{1C}$", the best known of the glycosylated hemoglobins, tends to increase or decrease as a percentage of the total hemoglobin as a reflection of the red cell's exposure to the amounts of glucose in the blood. HbA$_{1C}$ has thus become an important and useful biomarker for the chronic control of blood sugar in diabetic patients.

While interesting physiologically and in other clinical contexts, most posttranslational modifications of hemoglobin are not especially relevant for the purposes of assessing the causes of anemia or developing strategies for their management. A few exceptions are discussed in Chapter 11. However, it is worth noting that anemia can modify the utility of HbA$_{1C}$ measurements in diabetic patients who also have shortened red cell survivals. Since HbA$_{1C}$ tends to accumulate in red cells over time, HbA$_{1C}$ levels can be artefactually low in patients with severe hemolytic anemia.

The Red Cell Membrane and Its Cytoskeleton

The circulating erythrocyte faces daunting challenges in the circulation. These include the physical stresses of circulating under high hydrostatic pressures through sometimes turbulent vascular beds. In the microcirculation, many of the capillaries are 2–3-fold narrower than the normal red cell diameter. To return to the venous circulation in the spleen, RBCs must also slither through interendothelial cell slits only a few microns in width. The high concentration of hemoglobin exerts a tremendous internal oncotic pressure, which causes swelling and contraction of the red cell as it passes through environments that are either hypotonic or extraordinarily hypertonic, for example, in the collecting system of the kidney. Moreover, circulating erythrocytes are subjected to enormous biochemical challenges including redox fluxes in sluggish vascular beds and wide swings in oxygen tension as the red cell passes from the venous circulation into the lungs, through the arteries, and back into the capillary beds. Erythrocytes must therefore possess not only the high tensile strength but also the pliability and flexibility needed to tolerate extraordinary changes in cell

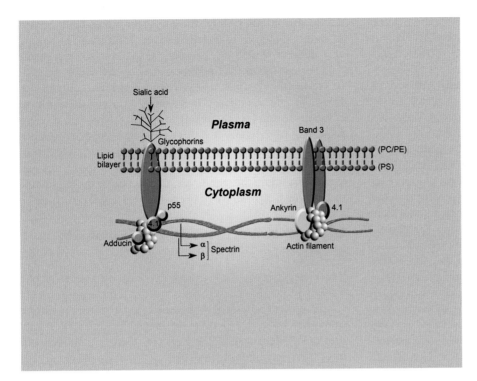

Figure 1.4 The red cell membrane and its cytoskeleton. As discussed in the text, the red cell membrane consists of an asymmetrical lipid bilayer. Phosphatidyl choline (PC) and phosphatidyl ethanolamine (PE) predominate on the outer leaflet, while phosphatidyl serine (PS) is largely confined to the inner leaflet of the lipid bilayer. Transmembrane proteins "poke through" to the outer surface of the membrane. Exteriorly exposed portions of these proteins and lipids are heavily modified by glycolytic groups such as sialic acid (the only one illustrated in this figure). The fragile lipid bilayer is strengthened by attachment of a hexagonal cytoskeletal protein lattice to the cytoplasmic domains of the transmembrane proteins. The basic latticework of the cytoskeleton is formed by highly helical spectrin dimers, which attach head to tail to form the array. These attachments, as well as the attachments to the cytoplasmic domains transmembrane proteins, are strengthened and stabilized by a variety of proteins. Adducin, ankyrin, protein 4.1, and p55 protein are shown here for illustrative purposes.

volume, shape, and biochemistry. Finally, red cells must be able to resist adherence to the walls of the vascular tree and to one another despite their exposure to adherence molecules when passing in intimate contact with small capillaries and venules. If red cells adhered to one another, they would form aggregates that would tend to block small vessels as well. An essential adaptation for these challenges is the unique structure and function of the erythrocyte membrane and its underlying cortical cytoskeleton. Derangements of these elements that can lead to anemia are considered in considerable detail in Chapter 14. For our present purposes, it is sufficient to note the special features of this integrated membrane/cytoskeleton structure and the ways in which they provide for the longevity of the circulating red cell.

The red cell membrane consists of a phospholipid and cholesterol bilayer punctuated with transmembrane proteins (Figure 1.4). These support ion and nutrient transport. The vast majority of these molecules are glycoproteins or lipoproteins whose attached residues tend to be negatively charged, thus creating a repellent electrostatic "cloud" around the outer surface of the cell. Most abundant among these is glycophorin, which is heavily modified by sialic acid on its outer surface. In addition to their functional role, these exterior-facing moieties are polymorphic both at the amino acid sequence level and in the composition of their carbohydrate and lipid modifications. These polymorphisms are recognized clinically as the major and minor blood group antigens. As discussed in Chapters 12, 29, and 30, the blood group antigens are important in the characterization and management of immune hemolytic anemias, in bone marrow transplantation, and in transfusion medicine.

The lipid components that make up the phospholipid bilayer of the membrane are also critical both structurally and functionally. The major lipid component of the erythrocyte membrane is cholesterol, but a wide variety of lipids and phospholipids, including sphingomyelin, also contribute to the stability of the red cell membrane and its interaction with its external environment. It is important to note that three major phospholipid classes – phosphotidylserine, phosphatidylcholine, and phosphatidylethanolamine – are particularly germane to the pathophysiology of a number of the anemias discussed in this text. Phosphatidylserine can act as a cofactor in the activation of prothrombin; thus, its presence on the outer leaflet, facing into plasma, could cause the red cell to have procoagulant activity. Given the mass of red cells in the circulation, this could create a thrombophilic state. In normal erythrocytes, phosphotidylserine is maintained almost exclusively on the *inner* leaflet of the lipid bilayer. Phosphatidylcholine and phosphatidylethanolamine predominate on the *outer* surfaces of the lipid bilayer.

Lipid asymmetry is maintained by a system of enzymes called "flippases," "floppases," and "scramblases." As suggested by their names, these enzyme systems have the effect of "flipping" the polar heads of specific phospholipids in one direction (inward), in the other direction (outward), or in both directions, respectively. In erythrocytes, as in other cells, influx of calcium into the cytoplasm causes eversion of phosphotidylserine to the outer leaflet. As discussed in other chapters, this is relevant in hemolytic anemias such as sickle cell anemia, in which oxidation of membrane structures by precipitation or polymerization leads to altered ion transport, calcium influx, and alterations of the phospholipid translocating systems, resulting in eversion of phosphotidylserine. While the pathophysiologic importance of this phenomenon is unknown, it is clear that sickle red cells are more adherent to the vascular wall, and appear to be somewhat prothrombotic. Failure of an impaired RE system to remove red cells with everted phosphotidylserine in patients who have been splenectomized might also contribute to the hypercoagulable state seen postsplenectomy.

The cytoplasmic domains of the key transmembrane proteins are important for the physical strength and flexibility of the red cell, because these are sites at which the phospholipid bilayer becomes attached to the underlying protein cytoskeleton (Figure 1.4). Indeed, without anchorage to an underlying protein meshwork, the red cell membrane has the physical properties of a soap bubble. In the circulation, red cells would quickly be emulsified into small vesicles as they are pushed through small capillaries under high hydrostatic pressure. Fortunately, the erythrocyte membrane cytoskeleton is uniquely adapted to circulate in that vasculature. The underlying protein scaffold consists primarily of spectrin. Spectrins are large (ca250 kD) helical proteins. In erythrocytes, the functional unit of spectrin is a dimer of α spectrin and β spectrin. These chains bind to one another in a head-to-tail fashion in such a way as to become entwined along a series of more than 20 helices. This structure allows the protein to be highly extensible and compressible, roughly like a spring.

Spectrins form a hexagonal latticework underneath the lipid bilayer and are attached at the junctions of one dimer with another to the cytoplasmic domains of several transmembrane proteins, the most critical of which quantitatively and functionally are the glycophorins and the anion exchange transporter ("Band 3"). These two proteins are the most abundant in the red cell membrane. They provide multiple attachment points for the spectrin cytoskeleton. Additional flexibility is provided by binding to actin at these critical junctions.

Binding of the spectrin lattice to the cytoplasmic domains of the transmembrane proteins is mediated primarily by two multifunctional proteins, protein 4.1R and Ankyrin (Figure 1.4). Each of these molecules has separate binding regions for the cytoplasmic domains of transmembrane proteins and for the spectrin–actin cytoskeleton. They thus provide strong yet flexible attachment, much like "molecular swivels" or "molecular hinges," conferring the freedom of motion needed for the twisting or sliding of the cytoskeleton across the inner surfaces of the phospholipid bilayer when the cells are distorted by shear stress and stretched or shriveled by osmotic changes. An added effect of these two proteins is to stabilize spectrin–spectrin and spectrin–actin interactions, thus stabilizing the entire complex. A number of other molecules, mentioned in more detail in Chapter 14, participate in this complex set of linkages and contribute to stability. Figure 1.4 illustrates these structural and functional features.

In summary, the red cell membrane and its cytoskeleton are adapted to the cellular transport and communication needs of the circulating erythrocyte and also provide the critical tensile strength, flexibility, and metabolic adaptability needed to endure 4 months in the circulation. Unfortunately, they are also delicate structures. They are susceptible to irreversible damage because of the limited capacity of circulating red cells to regenerate or repair damaged and destroyed components. Inherited defects in or acquired damage to any of these protein components can lead to hemolytic anemias. However, it is also important to recognize that other conditions, such as enzymopathies, immune damage to red cells, polymerization of hemoglobin in sickle cell anemia, or exposure to drugs or ingested agents that injure the membrane, can also cause the membrane to be a key intermediary of premature red cell destruction.

Enzymes of Red Blood Cell Intermediary Metabolism

The systems supporting energy homeostasis and metabolic stability of the red cell were once thought to be extraordinarily simple. Recent studies have revealed that red cells possess a somewhat broader repertoire of metabolic capabilities than previously appreciated. For example, there are limited but important signal transduction pathways that persist in red cells and appear to help control interactions between the red cell, other blood cell types, and the vascular wall. Similarly, enzymes involved in nitric oxide metabolism remain in the circulation for quite a long time. However, compared to most cells or even cell remnants like the platelet, the red cell is rather simple metabolically. For the purposes of understanding anemias, it is sufficient for us to review its three major metabolic capabilities, one for generating energy (ATP) and two for maintaining the balance of oxidized and reduced molecules (redox state).

As shown in Figure 1.5, the anaerobic pathway for glycolysis in red cells is rather primitive in comparison to other cell types. Lacking mitochondria, erythrocytes are unable to sustain oxidative metabolism of the metabolites of glucose. Oxidative metabolism of glucose generates 38 ATPs per glucose molecule and nets 36, but the fermentative pathway available to erythrocytes generates only 3 ATPs. In fact, there is a net of only 2 ATPs/glucose because of the ATP requirement for one of the steps in this Embden-Meyerhof pathway (Figure 1.5). Red cells are thus significant consumers of glucose and must have an efficient system for glucose uptake. This is facilitated by the glucose transporter, GLUT-1, which catalyzes facilitated transmembrane uptake of glucose from the plasma into the red cell cytoplasm.

In red cells, a shunt also exists within the Embden-Meyerhof pathway. Known as the Rapoport-Luebering shunt, this bypass mechanism (Figure 1.5) generates 2,3 biphosphoglyceric acid (2,3-BPG). 2,3-BPG is an important cofactor of hemoglobin. Its binding to hemoglobin reduces the affinity of the hemoglobin molecule for oxygen. As discussed in other chapters, this can affect red cell homeostasis by modulating the ability of hemoglobin to acquire or deliver oxygen under physiologic conditions.

Intermediary Metabolism in the Red Cell

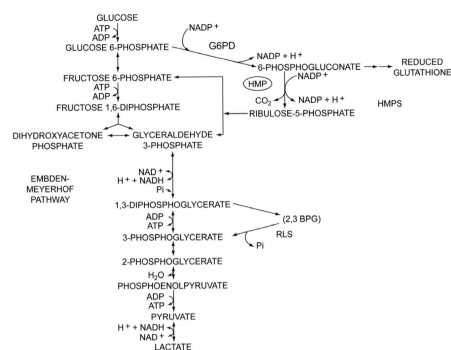

Figure 1.5 Intermediary metabolism of the red cell. The vertically organized set of metabolic reactions shows the Embden Meyerhof pathway of anaerobic glycolysis, generating a net gain of two ATP molecules and generating lactic acid as a byproduct. However, two major shunts exist. The first, hexose monophosphate shunt (HMPS), for which glucose-6-phosphate-dehydrogenase is the rate-limiting first enzyme, generates reduced nucleotides and, ultimately reduced glutathione to combat oxidative stresses in the red cell. The Rappaport Luebering Shunt (RLS) is also shown. This generates 2,3 biphosphoglycerate (2,3 BPG), which can modulate oxygen affinity in accordance with metabolic needs.

ATP within red cells is required for membrane homeostasis and to fuel the other two metabolic pathways needed to generate intracellular reducing power. ATP is needed to maintain red cell phospholipid levels, to fuel membrane pumps, and to support kinase reactions that modulate the behavior of membrane cytoskeletal proteins and signaling components. For example, reversible phosphorylation of protein 4.1R alters its tightness of binding to the spectrin actin cytoskeleton and thus modulates membrane fluidity and, thereby, red cell hemodynamics.

The hexose monophosphate shunt (HMPS) begins with the rate-limiting enzyme glucose-6-phosphate-dehydrogenase (G6PD). Its connection to glycolytic metabolism is shown in Figure 1.5. Through a series of enzyme reactions, the HMPS generates reduced glutathione molecules critical for correcting oxidative damage to hemoglobin and red cell membrane proteins. Deficiencies of these enzymes due to inherited mutations are associated with diminished reducing power and consequent oxidation and precipitation of hemoglobin. By far the most common of these conditions is G6PD deficiency. It is discussed in more detail in Chapter 13. Exposure to toxic levels of oxidizing compounds (e.g., phenylhydrazine) can also overwhelm even the normal complement of glutathione and produce very similar types of hemolysis.

The cytochrome B5 reductase ("methemoglobin reductase system") system is a complex of several enzymes that are expressed in multiple isoforms during red cell development and remain intact for much of the red cell lifespan. As noted elsewhere, the iron moiety within hemoglobin is susceptible to oxidation from its reduced ferrous Fe^{++} to oxidized ferric state

Fe^{+++}, generating methemoglobin, which is a useless respiratory pigment and can also be unstable in the red cell. The cytochrome B5 reductase system generates reduced nicotinamide adenine dinucleotide (NADH), which can reduce ferric Fe^{+++} iron to ferrous Fe^{++} iron. Deficiency of this system by virtue of inherited defects or by exposure to toxins such as nitrite or nitrate compounds results in methemoglobinemia.

Even though the red cell is limited in its arsenal of metabolic capabilities, it manages, at the price of high levels of glucose consumption, to generate sufficient ATP and reducing power to preserve the normal lifespan of the red cell. The consequences, direct or indirect, of impairments in this system can cause multiple forms of anemia that are discussed in other chapters.

Red Cell Synthesis and Destruction

While discussed in much more detail in Chapter 3, it is worth mentioning here a few of the basic mechanisms of normal red cell synthesis and destruction. Anemias resulting from excessive red cell destruction invariably result from alterations within or on the red cell that signal systems intended normally for the removal of senescent red cells. These alterations cause the RE system to catabolize these altered red cells before their intended time. Three basic mechanisms are postulated to result in the eventual loss of red cells from the circulation.

The metabolic hypothesis derives from the inability of red cells to replace their proteins. Although launched with a completely normal array of proteins, key enzymes "wear out," and oxidative damage to membrane components and to hemoglobin accumulates. It is believed that these changes eventually create sufficient damage to the red cell membrane that abnormalities are sensed on the exterior of the cell (e.g., exteriorization of phosphotidylserine), creating signals that activate macrophages in the RE system to engulf the red cell and catabolize it.

The second hypothesis, the "immunological" hypothesis, is based on the observation that at least one abundant membrane protein, the anion exchange transporter (Band 3), forms, over time, tetramers that are antigenic and are recognized by iso-antibodies present in nearly every normal human. It is possible these are only examples of other preformed antibodies that recognize exteriorized antigens that accumulate over time. What is clear is that red cells contain, in their early phases of circulating life, abundant supplies of the membrane protein CD47. CD47 is known to be a "don't eat me" signal by virtue of its interaction with a macrophage protein SHPS-1. CD47 levels decline on the surface of the red cell as it ages, making macrophages more likely to recognize and ingest red cells bearing any of these antigen–antibody complexes.

The third mechanism, the geometric hypothesis, may simply be a final common pathway of the aforementioned aging phenomena. In order to traverse the tortuous and sluggish microcirculation of the RE system in the spleen and liver, red cells must maintain their "slipperiness," pliability, and elasticity. Even normal red cells have "bits" of their membrane removed as they come in intimate contact with RE system macrophages. These lost membrane "bits" are likely surface abnormalities that are "polished" away by the RE system to facilitate the red cell's ability to circulate efficiently. As the red cell ages and loses more and more membrane to this polishing process, it begins to be unable to maintain its biconcave disk shape and becomes rounder (a spherocyte), because the smallest surface that can enclose the interior volume of hemoglobin and cytoplasm is a sphere. The sphere, however, is a rigid structure. It is thus less able to navigate the microcirculation of the RE system and has a higher probability of being catabolized.

It is likely that all three of these mechanisms contribute to the eventual demise of senescence of red cells. It is well documented that most metabolic enzymes decline as the red cells age, albeit at different rates, reducing both energy-generating and reducing capability. It is clear that the immunological factors considered above cause erythrocytes to be more recognizable as targets for immune clearance as cells age. In addition, either of these mechanisms will result in gradual loss of membrane function, causing the cells to become more rigid spherocytes.

Regardless of how red cells get destroyed, the process of red cell death generates molecules that serve as important markers of the rate of red cell destruction and are thus critical tools for assessing whether anemia is due to premature red cell destruction (i.e., a hemolytic anemia). Once an erythrocyte is engulfed by the macrophage, its membrane, hemoglobin, and enzyme systems are efficiently catabolized to their component parts. Notably, the iron moieties of hemoglobin are recycled by being transferred to circulating transferrin, which carries the iron either to the bone marrow for use in producing hemoglobin from newly developing red cells or, if present in excess supply, to the liver and the marrow macrophages for storage in the form of ferritin and hemosiderin. The heme moiety is catabolized to biliverdin and then to bilirubin (See Chapter 6). Bilirubin is released into the circulation and is conjugated in the liver. When red cell destruction levels are increased, the bilirubin level rises. When hemolysis is brisk, the newly released "unconjugated" or "indirect" bilirubin fraction rises disproportionately high compared to bilirubin that is hepatically conjugated. Thus, hemolytic anemia is accompanied by higher serum bilirubin levels with a preponderance of increase in the indirect bilirubin fraction.

Some enzymes that are abundant in the red cell, such as lactic dehydrogenase (LDH), also "leak" out of the macrophage, resulting in increased LDH levels in the circulation. The leakage of free heme and hemoglobin subunits, while a small percentage of the total in red cells, is sufficient to saturate the available supplies of circulating proteins, such as haptoglobin and hemopexin, designed to bind and sequester them. The levels of free haptoglobin and hemopexin thus tend to decline during periods of hemolysis. Finally, when hemolysis is brisk, there is hypertrophy of the spleen and liver due to an increase in the proliferation of macrophages attempting to destroy the abnormal red cells. In particularly prolonged or severe states of hemolysis, this can also occur in the liver so that hepatosplenomegaly is a cardinal sign of a brisk hemolytic anemia.

The normal pathway for destruction of red cells at the end of their lifespan is almost exclusively "extravascular," meaning that it occurs in the sinusoids of the RE system, which, technically, are not part of the normal vascular tree (because they are not lined by endothelial cells). However, in some circumstances, such as extreme oxidative stress, overt mechanical destruction (e.g., due to heart valves or arteriovenous malformation), certain autoimmune conditions in which the classical pathway of complement is fully activated, acute fresh water drowning, severe thermal burns, and so forth, direct fragmentation of red cells can occur within the circulation. Under these conditions, large quantities of hemoglobin are released directly into the blood, where it disassociates into its subunits and is filtered through the kidneys. This results in the generation of red urine that looks like hematuria but is in fact hemoglobinuria. Plasma hemoglobin levels also rise; serum LDH levels can rise to extremely high levels because the enzyme is released directly into the blood. Hemoglobin was once thought to be damaging to the renal tubules. However, the primary damage to the kidneys in states of extreme intravascular hemolysis appears to be due to the trapping of other components of the destroyed red cells such as the red cell membrane and its cytoskeleton in the interstices of the renal tubules.

Conclusion

Red cells are critical to human survival. Without them, little or no oxygen can reach our vital organs. To serve their function, each red cell must support the substantial metabolic and osmotic burdens placed on it by the high intracellular concentration of the hemoglobin molecules needed to transport adequate amounts of oxygen. These demands are met because each red cell is the product of a remarkable set of maturation and differentiation events that provide for the physical and biochemical strength and flexibility needed to traverse the circulation with its payload of hemoglobin and oxygen nearly 300,000 times during its lifespan. Many intrinsic and extrinsic factors can damage the highly evolved and adaptive yet fragile membrane and metabolic components that ensure this durability and/or impair the high rates of erythropoiesis needed to replace worn-out or lost red cells. These comprise the basic causes of anemia. They determine the clinical management challenges that are reviewed in the remainder of this text.

Further Reading

Bain B. Diagnosis from the blood smear. *N Engl J Med.* 2005; 353:498.

Semenza GL. Involvement of oxygen-sensing pathways in physiologic and pathophysiologic erythropoiesis. *Blood.* 2015; 2009:114.

Stamatoyannopoulos G. Control of globin gene expression during development and erythroid differentiation. *Exp Hematol.* 2005; 33:259.

Steinberg MH, Benz EJ, Jr., Adeboye HA, Ebert BL. Pathobiology of the human erythrocyte and its hemoglobins. In: Hoffman R, Benz EJ, Jr., Silberstein LE, Heslop HE, Weitz JI, Anastasi J., *Hematology Basic Principles and Practice*, ed 6, Elsevier; 2013, Chapter 31.

Steinberg MH, Forget BG, Higgs DR, et al. *Disorders of Hemoglobin: Genetics, Pathophysiology, and Clinical Management.* Cambridge, MA: Cambridge University Press; 2001.

Weatherall DJ, Clegg JB. *The Thalassaemia Syndromes*, 4th edn. Oxford: Blackwell Science Limited; 2001.

Chapter

Red Cell Production

Anupama Narla, MD, and Benjamin L. Ebert, MD, PhD

Introduction

"[F]irst consider the evolutionary beauty of our bi-concave discocytic RBC."
– *Stanley L. Schrier[1]* and Figure 2.1

The production of mature red blood cells (RBCs) from hematopoietic stem cells is a tightly regulated process that is dependent on growth factors, specific niches, and physiologic needs. Erythropoiesis normally proceeds at a basal rate, allowing for the replacement of senescent red blood cells, which constitute 1% of red cell mass, with young reticulocytes produced within the bone marrow. However, red cell production can be enhanced by as much as 10- to 20-fold in a variety of clinical settings where there is decreased arterial blood oxygenation and/or oxygen delivery to the tissues. This chapter will review the highly regulated process of erythropoiesis with a focus on definitive erythropoiesis in the adult bone marrow rather than embryonic and fetal erythropoiesis in the yolk sac and fetal liver. For the purposes of this discussion, we will divide the process into three stages: early erythropoiesis, terminal erythroid differentiation, and reticulocyte maturation.

Early Erythropoiesis

Erythropoiesis is derived from the lineage commitment and differentiation of a small pool of pluripotent hematopoietic stem cells (HSCs) to committed erythroid progenitors. The most primitive single-lineage committed erythroid precursor that can be defined functionally is the erythroid burst-forming unit (BFU-E), followed by erythroid colony-forming unit (CFU-E) that ultimately differentiate into proerythroblasts,

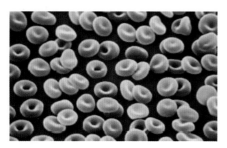

Figure 2.1 Transmission electron micrograph image of normal red blood cells. Image courtesy of Narla Mohandas.

the first morphologically recognizable erythroid precursor in the bone marrow.

HSCs are first committed to either the lymphoid or myeloid lineage. The common myeloid progenitor (CMP) differentiates into all of the progenitors of blood cells other than lymphoid cells. Early-acting hematopoietic growth factors such as IL-3, GM-CSF, Flt3 ligand, IL-11, IL-6, and thrombopoietin (tPO) help determine whether the CMP becomes a more committed progenitor of the granulocyte, monocyte (GMP), eosinophil lineage, basophil lineage, or the megakaryocyte/erythroid (MEP) lineages.[Rev in 2] There is also evidence suggesting a direct pathway from the HSC to the MEP.[3] A simplified schema of the proposed pathways involved in adult blood cell lineage commitment is shown in Figure 2.2.

A precise balance of several different classes of factors regulates the specification and differentiation of MEPs into erythroid cells or megakaryocytes. These include the GATA binding transcription factors GATA-1 and GATA-2, ETS factors (FLI-1 and GABPα), Krüppel-containing factors (KLF1, also known as EKLF, and Leukemia/lymphoma Related Factor [LRF]), basic helix-loop-helix factors (SCL also known as TAL-1), and multiple adaptors (Friend of GATA-1 [FOG-1] and LDB1).[4] In recent years, microRNAs have also been linked to the regulation of different stages of erythropoiesis including miR-144, 451, 221, 222, 24, 15a, 16–1, 16–2, and 191.[5] The role of some of these factors is highlighted in Figure 2.2.

GATA-1 is the best-studied hematopoietic transcription factor and is critical for erythropoiesis. This is evidenced by mutations in GATA-1 leading to diseases including dyserythropoietic anemia[6] and Diamond Blackfan anemia.[7] The major binding partner of GATA-1, FOG-1, is also one of its primary target genes, and they function in a feed-forward regulatory circuit to activate β-globin gene expression.[8] The interaction between FOG-1 and NuRD (nucleosome remodeling and histone deacetylase) components is critical for GATA-1-mediated repression of GATA-2 and c-Kit, which is critical for the maintenance of lineage fidelity.[9]

Once committed to the erythroid lineage, cells are regulated by lineage-specific hematopoietic growth factors, specifically erythropoietin (EPO). Erythropoietin was purified from the urine of anemic patients in 1977, and the gene was isolated and cloned in 1985.[10,11] EPO is the principal stimulator of

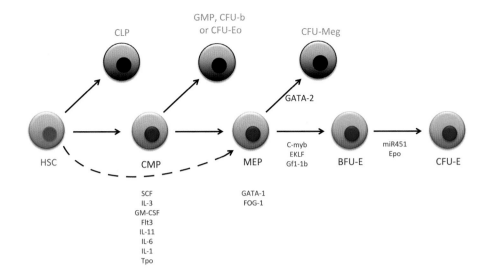

Figure 2.2 A simplified overview of the progenitor cells and transcription factors involved in erythropoiesis
HSC = hematopoietic stem cell, CMP = common myeloid progenitor, MEP = megakaryocyte erythroid progenitor, BFU-E = burst-forming unit-erythroid, CFU-E = colony-forming unit-erythroid. Progenitors not involved in red cell production are shown in gray, and further details are not included; CLP = common lymphoid progenitor, GMP = granulocyte monocyte progenitor, CFU-b = colony-forming unit-basophil, CFU-Eo = colony-forming unit-eosinophil, CFU-Meg = colony-forming unit-megakaryocyte.

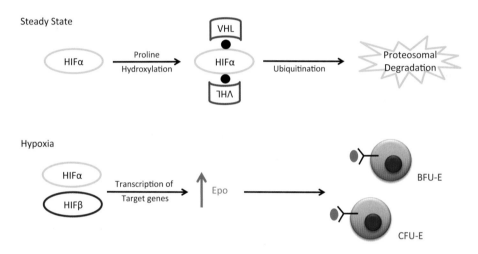

Figure 2.3 A simplified schematic of the oxygen sensor mechanism in erythropoiesis. Under steady-state conditions (top panel), the α unit of HIF is regulated by the HIF prolyl-hydroxylase domain enzymes (PHDs). The PHDs hydroxylate HIF, allowing for poly-ubiquitination by the von Hippel-Lindau (VHL) tumor suppressor complex. This process ultimately leads to proteolytic degradation and prevents the subsequent transcription of EPO. Under conditions of hypoxia (bottom panel), the two HIF subunits are stabilized, allowing for increased transcription of target genes, including EPO. The increased levels of EPO bind to EPO receptors on committed erythroid progenitor cells, promoting erythropoiesis.

erythropoiesis, and the kidney is the primary EPO-producing organ in adult mammals. Hypoxia induces an increase in EPO hormone production in the kidney, which then circulates in the plasma and binds to receptors expressed on erythroid progenitor cells. The hypoxic induction of EPO depends in large part on the transcription factor hypoxia inducible factor (HIF-1).[Rev in 12]

If oxygen demand is adequate, the α subunit (HIF1α, which is ubiquitously expressed) is hydroxylated by HIF prolyl-hydroxylase domain enzymes (PHDs) and subsequently degraded after ubiquitination by the von Hippel-Lindau tumor suppressor complex. Low oxygen tension abrogates this process, allowing accumulation of the HIF1α subunit; it translocates to the nucleus, binds to its heterodimerization partner HIFβ, and leads to transcriptional activation of target genes that harbor hypoxia-responsive elements (HRE) which includes the 3′ enhancer region of the EPO gene.[Rev in 13] and Figure 2.3.

The major effects of EPO appear to be at the level of the CFU-E, and these progenitors do not survive *in vitro* in the absence of EPO. BFU-E are so named because of the burstlike morphology of the colonies in semisolid (methylcellulose) *in vitro* cultures. Less-mature BFU-Es can survive in culture without the presence of EPO as long as either SCF, IL-3, or granulocyte-macrophage colony stimulating factor (GM-CSF) is present, and mice lacking the EPO receptor can still form BFU-E. A second subset of presumably more mature BFU-E will respond to the combination of EPO and either IL-3, SCF, or GM-CSF by forming subpopulations of CFU-E.[14 and Rev in 15] Each of the CFU-E go on to form a large colony of proerythroblasts, which ultimately culminates in an increase in red blood cell mass, increased tissue oxygen tension, and a feedback loop that suppresses further expression of EPO.

The EPO receptor (EPOR) is present in very low levels until the CFU-E stage. The receptor is present as a homodimer and, upon binding to EPO, undergoes a conformational change that brings its intracellular domains into close apposition. This enables cross-phosphorylation via binding of Jak2 kinase, which activates multiple pathways including Stat5, phosphoinositide-3 kinase/Akt, and p42/44 mitogen-activated protein kinase.[Rev in 16] The initiation of this signal transduction cascade reduces apoptosis and promotes expansion and differentiation of erythroid progenitors.

Progression of progenitor cells to terminal differentiation is marked not only by the acquisition of specific responses to growth factors but also by the acquisition of phenotypic markers. BFU-E tend to have a similar antigenic profile to progenitor cells of other lineages, whereas CFU-E begin to express more of the markers specific to mature erythroid cells such as glycophorin A and blood group antigens. Recent work has systematically examined the changes of red cell membrane proteins during human terminal erythroid differentiation and will be summarized in the next section.

Terminal Erythroid Differentiation

During this process, proerythroblasts undergo sequential divisions to become basophilic, polychromatic, and orthochromatic erythroblasts that enucleate to become reticulocytes. One remarkable feature of this stage of erythropoiesis is that each cell division is simultaneously coupled with differentiation so that the daughter cells are structurally and functionally different from the mother cell. The average transit time from proerythroblast to emergence of the reticulocyte into the circulation is 5–7 days. During this time, several important changes occur including a series of sequential mitoses with increased chromatin condensation, accumulation of erythroid-specific proteins, assembly of these proteins into functional complexes (such as hemoglobin and cell membrane proteins), and enucleation. Additionally, the expression of major red cell membrane proteins increases, while the expression of most adhesion molecules decreases.[17]

While the early phases of erythroid maturation are exclusively regulated by EPO, the later phases are EPO independent and appear to be more transferrin receptor dependent. These changes in growth factor sensitivity are reflected by the progressive reduction in EPO-R number.[Rev in 18] The signaling pathways activated by both EPO and transferrin receptors affect erythroid-specific proteins, which are responsible for cell surface remodeling and several of the cytoplasmic and nuclear changes during the process of terminal maturation.

Iron and heme play a critical role in erythroid cell differentiation as well as in hemoglobin synthesis. Heme iron accounts for the majority of the iron in the human body, and hemoglobin contains as much as 70% of the total iron content of a healthy adult. Iron homeostasis is regulated systematically by the hormone hepcidin, which is mainly produced in hepatocytes. The expression of hepcidin is decreased by iron deficiency, anemia, increased erythropoietic activity, and hypoxia; conversely, hepcidin expression is increased by iron loading and inflammatory signals. Hepcidin inhibits iron absorption and recycling by binding to the iron exporter ferroportin, located on the basal side of enterocytes, triggering its internalization and lysosomal degradation.[Rev in 19] Recently, a role for HIF-2 in the expression of key genes involved in iron transport has been identified, further cementing the role of the HIF transcription factors as central mediators of cellular adaptation to hypoxia.[20]

There is a unique association between heme and globin synthesis. Heme regulates hemoglobin synthesis by affecting both the transcription and translation of β-globin mRNA through a heme-regulated eIF2α kinase (HRI). The binding of heme to HRI inhibits the phosphorylation of eIF2α, resulting in the promotion of the translation of globin and other proteins in erythroid cells. The orderly assembly of heme and globin is essential for the formation of a functional heme protein. In the reticulocyte, the proportions of α subunits, non-α subunits, and heme are almost always equal, which suggests that there is a close regulation in the cytoplasm for these components. After the association of heme with globin chains, an α subunit and a β subunit interact to form an αβ-dimer.[Rev in 21] Two of the dimers then bind to each other to form the $\alpha_2\beta_2$ tetramer, hemoglobin A.

Key players throughout terminal erythroid differentiation are the erythroblastic islands, unique stromal environments within the bone marrow cavity. In steady-state erythropoiesis, cells from proerythroblasts through multilobulated, young reticulocytes surround central macrophages. These central macrophages not only anchor erythroblasts within island niches, they also affect erythroid proliferation and/or differentiation. In addition, they transfer iron directly to the attached erythroid progenitors and phagocytose the extruded erythroblast nuclei.[22] These findings support the idea that disruptions of macrophage function can result in decreased red blood cell production and anemia.

Reticulocyte Maturation

At the end of erythroid differentiation, orthochromatic erythroblasts expel their nuclei to produce reticulocytes. The enucleation process involves membrane remodeling, chromatin condensation (mediated in part by histone deacetylase [HDAC] 2), and formation of a spindle-independent motor that drives the separation of the pyknotic nuclei from the early reticulocyte.

Enucleation generates the nascent reticulocyte (with abundant cytoplasm and hemoglobin) and a pyrenocyte (membrane-bound nucleus). Enucleation is also accompanied by a sorting process in which cytoskeletal and membrane proteins important for red cell function are directed to the nascent reticulocyte, whereas other proteins, such as those which mediate intercellular attachment, are directed to the pyrenocyte. Aberrant protein sorting is one mechanistic basis for the protein deficiencies seen in hereditary eliptocytosis and hereditary spherocytosis.

The final step in erythropoiesis involves the enucleate multilobular reticulocytes maturing into the classic discoid red blood cells. This brief period of erythropoiesis (2–3 days) is a time of rapid change. After a short period of time in the bone marrow, reticulocytes are released into circulation, where they eliminate their residual RNA and mature into erythrocytes. The dramatic shape transformation involves the loss of mitochondria and ribosomes as well as extensive remodeling of the plasma membrane. This remodeling includes loss of surface area, decrease in cell volume, increase in mechanical stability, and acquisition of the classic biconcave shape.[Rev in 23] The red blood cell is unique in that its principal physical structure is its membrane, which encloses a concentrated hemoglobin solution; there are no cytoplasmic structures or organelles.

The plasma membrane of the mature red blood cell is ultimately composed of a lipid bilayer anchored to a filamentous network of proteins underlying the cytoplasmic surface of the membrane as shown in Figure 2.4. The membrane proteins are divided into integral proteins that are tightly embedded through hydrophobic interactions and peripheral proteins located on the cytoplasmic side that can be readily released from the membrane. Examples of the former include Band 3, aquaporin-1, and Glut1, while the latter group includes constituents of the membrane skeleton such as spectrin, actin, protein 4.1, band 4.2, ankyrin, adducin, tropomodulin, and tropomyosin.[24] The ability of the red cell to undergo extensive deformation is essential for both its function and its survival.

Our understanding of the specific molecular changes that accompany terminal erythroid differentiation and reticulocyte maturation has increased over the past several years. In mice, during reticulocyte maturation, tubulin and cytosolic actin are lost, in part mediated by the ubiquitin-proteasome pathway, and the membrane content of myosin, tropomyosin, ICAM-4, GLUT4, Na-K-ATPase, NHE1, GPA, CD47, Duffy, and Kell is reduced (www.ncbi.nlm.nih.gov/pmc/articles/PMC2837329). By examining the dynamic changes of expression of membrane proteins during in vitro human terminal erythroid differentiation, An and colleagues used band3 and α4 integrin to isolate erythroblasts at successive developmental stages.[17] This work, along with the findings of several other groups, should facilitate a more comprehensive characterization of each specific developmental stage of human erythroblasts in the future.

Conclusion

The production of the red blood cell is a unique and fascinating process in human biology. The red blood cell needs to coordinate the production of all of the proteins that will be required for its 120-day lifespan in circulation during erythroid differentiation, followed by enucleation and elimination of ribosomes and mitochondria, leaving the cell fixed in its content of cellular proteins. The goal of this process is to produce a cell optimally designed to be packed with hemoglobin at extraordinarily high concentrations to maximize oxygen transport.

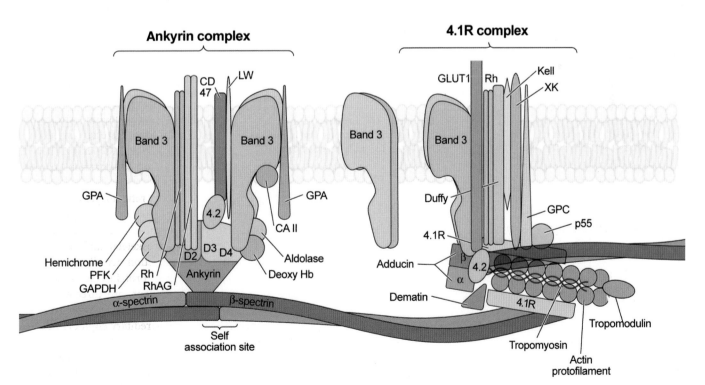

Figure 2.4 Schematic representation of the red cell membrane. Image courtesy of N. Mohandas. Reprinted from *PNAS* 2008 Jun 10; 105(23); Protein 4.1R-dependent multiprotein complex: new insights into the structural organization of the red blood cell membrane; Salamoa M, Zhang X, Yang Y, Lee S, Hartwig JH, Chassis JA, Mohandas N, and An X.[24]

References

1 Schrier SL. What does the spleen see? *Blood.* 2012 Jul 12; 120(2):242–243.

2 Sieff CA, Zon LI. Anatomy and physiology of hematopoiesis. In: Orkin SH, Nathan DG, et al., eds. *Nathan and Oski's Hematology of Infancy and Childhood Edition 7.* Philadelphia, Saunders Elsevier Press; 2009: 195–273.

3 Adolfsson J, Mansson R, Buza-Vidas N, et al. Identification of Flt3+ lympho-myeloid stem cells lacking erythro-megakaryocytic potential a revised road map for adult blood lineage commitment. *Cell.* 2005 Apr 22; 121(2):295–606.

4 Dore LC and Crispino JD. Transcription factor networks in erythroid cell and megakaryocyte development. *Blood.* 2011 Jul 14; 118(2):231–239.

5 Zhang L, Sankaran VG, Lodish HF. MicroRNAs in erythroid and megakaryocytic differentiation and megakaryocyte-erythroid progenitor lineage commitment. *Leukemia.* 2012 Nov; 26(11):2310–2316.

6 Hollanda LM, Lima CS, Cunha AF, et al. An inherited mutation leading to production of only the short isoform of GATA-1 is associated with impaired erythropoiesis. *Nat Genet.* 2006; 38(7):807–812.

7 Sankaran VG, Ghazvinian R, Do R, et al. Exome sequencing identifies GATA1 mutations resulting in Diamond-Blackfan anemia. *J Clin Invest.* 2012; 122(7):2439–2443.

8 Welch JJ, Watts JA, Vakoc CR, et al. Global regulation of erythroid gene expression by transcription factor GATA-1. *Blood.* 2004 Nov 15; 104(10):3136–3147.

9 Gregory GD, Miccio A, Bersenev A, et al. FOG1 requires NuRD to promote hematopoiesis and maintain lineage fidelity within the megakaryocytic-erythroid compartment. *Blood.* 2010 Mar 18; 115(11):2156–2166.

10 Jacobs K, Shoemaker C, Rudersdorf R, et al. Isolation and characterization of genomic and cDNA clones of human erythropoietin. *Nature.* 1985 Feb 28–Mar 6; 313(6005):806–810.

11 Lin FK, Suggs S, Lin CH, et al. Cloning and expression of the human erythropoietin gene. *Proc Natl Acad Sci USA.* 1985 Nov; 82(22):7580–7584.

12 Bunn HF. Erythropoietin. *Cold Spring Harb Perspect Med.* 2013 Mar 1; 3:a011619.

13 Franke K, Gassman M, Wielockx B. Erythrocytosis: the HIF pathway in control. *Blood.* 2013 Aug 15; 122 (7):1122–1128.

14 Flygare J, Rayon Estrada V, Shin C, et al. HIF1alpha synergizes with glucocorticoids to promote BFU-E progenitor self-renewal. *Blood.* 2011 Mar 24; 117(12):3435–3444.

15 Palis J. Primitive and definitive erythropoiesis in mammals. *Front Physiol.* 2014 Jan 28; 5:3. eCollection 2014.

16 Broxmeyer HE. Erythropoietin: multiple targets, actions, and modifying influences for biological and clinical consideration. *J Exp Med.* 2013 Feb 11; 210(2):205–208.

17 Hu J, Liu J, Xue F, et al. Isolation and functional characterization of human erythroblasts at distinct stages: implications for understanding of normal and disordered erythropoiesis in vivo. *Blood.* 2013 Apr 18; 121(16):3246–3253.

18 Migliaccio AR and Papayannopoulou. Erythropoiesis and the normal red cell. In: Warrel DA, Cox TM, and Firth JD, eds. *Oxford Textbook of Medicine.* Oxford: Oxford University Press; 2012.

19 Ganz T. Hepcidin and iron regulation, 10 years later. *Blood.* 2011 Apr 28; 117(17):4425–4433.

20 Wilkinson N, Pantapoulos K. IRP1 regulates erythropoiesis and systemic iron homeostasis by controlling HIF2α mRNA translation. *Blood.* 2013 Aug 29; 122(9):1658–1668.

21 Chen JJ. Regulation of protein synthesis by the heme-regulated eIF2alpha kinase: relevance to anemias. *Blood.* 2007 Apr 1; 109(7):2693–2699.

22 Chasis JA, Mohandas N. Erythroblastic islands: niches for erythropoiesis. *Blood.* 2008 Aug 1; 112(3):470–478.

23 Ney PA. Normal and disordered reticulocyte maturation. *Curr Opin Hematol.* 2011 May; 18(3):152–157.

24 Salomao M, Zhang X, Yang Y, et al. Protein 4.1R-dependent multiprotein complex: new insights into the structural organization of the red blood cell membrane. *Proc Natl Acad Aci USA.* 2008 Jun 10; 105 (23):8026–8031.

Chapter

3

Red Blood Cell Life Span, Senescence, and Destruction

Richard Kaufman, MD

Reticulocyte Maturation

Erythropoiesis in the bone marrow proceeds as described in Chapter 1. Enucleation of the erythroblast produces a nascent reticulocyte, along with the membrane-bound nuclear remnant ("pyrenocyte").[1] In contrast to its parent reticulocyte, the nuclear remnant rapidly externalizes high levels of membrane phosphatidylserine (PS). This appears to signal local macrophages to engulf the nuclear remnant, while the reticulocyte is safely ignored, allowing it to develop further into a mature red blood cell (RBC). The final erythroid maturation process, from reticulocyte to mature erythrocyte, takes about 4 days and involves profound cellular changes. The reticulocyte will spend 3 of these days within the marrow and the fourth day in the peripheral circulation. Early reticulocytes are larger than mature RBCs, with a mean cell volume in the range of 120–150 fL. Reticulocytes are also more spherical and less deformable than mature RBCs. Membrane remodeling, mediated by rapid, extensive vesiculation, causes loss of about 20% of the reticulocyte's surface area.[2] Over 1–2 days, the reticulocyte sheds an area of membrane equal to that lost gradually over the next 4 months as a mature RBC in the circulation.[3] Membrane loss is accompanied by loss of intracellular water, as the reticulocyte contracts down to a final cell volume of approximately 80–99 fL. The net result is a high surface area/volume ratio as the RBC assumes its characteristic biconcave disk shape.

The expression levels of many membrane proteins change during reticulocyte maturation. Proteins such as cytosolic actin and tubulin are lost. Expression of surface transferrin receptor 1 (CD71) is downregulated; this prevents potentially toxic iron uptake by the nascent RBC. Expression of membrane proteins such as myosin, CD47, Duffy, Kell, and others decreases but remains detectable, while proteins of the band 3 complex, including Rh, RhAG, GPC, and XK appear to increase after maturation.[4,5] Mitochondria are degraded and cleared from reticulocytes. The teleological view is that the primary mission of the RBC is to transport oxygen; mitochondria consume oxygen and are therefore undesirable. Other organelles of no use to an anucleate cell are discarded as well: endoplasmic reticulum, ribosomes, and Golgi bodies are all rapidly degraded via as-yet poorly characterized mechanisms.

The final product of this intense development process is a mature RBC, uniquely durable and built to travel. The absence of a nucleus, a strong and flexible membrane, and a biconcave disk morphology all combine to produce a cell capable of tolerating extreme passive deformations. RBCs are typically 8 μm wide but are regularly required to squeeze through capillaries and splenic fenestrations only 2–3 μm wide.[6] RBCs must survive harsh osmotic environments as they traverse the renal and pulmonary capillary systems. And RBCs must be able to withstand oxidative damage accumulated over months, even as their lack of a nucleus and translational apparatus renders them incapable of generating new proteins.

RBC Life Span

Normal RBCs have a life span in the circulation of approximately 120 days. Some variability exists among individuals, but within a given individual, RBC survival is highly consistent. A few different experimental approaches have been used to measure RBC life span. The first accurate observations of the RBC life span were published in 1919 by Winifred Ashby, who transfused type O RBCs to type A or B recipients and detected the transfused cells using serologic methods.[7] Beginning in the 1940s, it became possible to radiolabel samples of RBCs with ^{51}Cr. In the form of $Na_2{}^{51}CrO_4$, this agent is taken up by RBCs, and it binds noncovalently to hemoglobin. It is an imperfect label – about 1% of ^{51}Cr is eluted from labeled RBCs per day – but standardized methods to measure RBC survival using ^{51}Cr have been well established. More recently, biotin labeling has been used for studies of RBC life span determination. This method offers several advantages over earlier techniques: it is nonradioactive, there is less elution of the label, and it is possible to quantify RBCs precisely using flow cytometry. However, biotin labeling shares the main limitation of radiolabeling: a random cohort of RBCs of mixed ages is typically labeled.[8] Labeling a synchronized cohort of new reticulocytes would be desirable from an experimental standpoint, but this approach has not traditionally been used due to technical hurdles.

The RBC life span of ~120 days gives rise to the normal reticulocyte count of 0.5–1.5%. If each consecutive day approximately 1 out of 120 RBCs (0.8%) is removed from the circulation, then that is the fraction that must be replaced by reticulocytes daily to maintain a constant RBC mass. (The absolute numbers are fairly daunting: assuming a normal 120-day life span, approximately 2 million RBCs must be cleared from the circulation each second.[9]) Higher reticulocyte counts reflect the marrow's response to an increased rate of RBC clearance, as detailed in other chapters. A small fraction of RBCs, perhaps 0.1% per day, are destroyed randomly, in an RBC age-independent fashion. The vast majority of normal RBC loss occurs due to the still poorly understood age-dependent process known as RBC senescence.

RBC Senescence

Several mechanisms have been hypothesized to serve as the "clock" that signals the end of RBC life after 120 days in the circulation. To date, no single mechanism has been definitively established to control RBC life span. The proposed mechanisms summarized in what follows are not mutually exclusive, and they may actually play interrelated roles in determining how long RBCs circulate.

Gradual loss of membrane surface area occurs during the mature RBC's ~120 days in the circulation. Over the same time period, approximately 20% of the RBC's hemoglobin is lost.[10] Together, these observations strongly suggest the existence of an RBC vesiculation mechanism, and indeed, RBC-derived vesicles (more commonly known as "microparticles") containing RBC membrane and cytoplasmic constituents are well described. How RBC microparticles form continues to be investigated. It has been hypothesized that microparticles may serve as a means for RBCs to shed patches of membrane that have sustained damage over time, allowing the healthy remaining cell to continue circulating.[10] As a consequence of losing membrane (and therefore surface area), RBCs gradually become more spherical and less deformable. These geometric and mechanical changes eventually progress to a point that senescent RBCs are cleared from the circulation by phagocytes of the reticuloendothelial system, as discussed in the next section.

Circulating RBCs accumulate various traumatic lesions over time. They are thought to endure a kind of "death by a thousand cuts." Lacking a nucleus and translational machinery, RBCs start their 4-month journey through the circulation with all of the enzymes that they will ever have, and these stores gradually become depleted. RBCs may suffer mechanical damage due to shear forces in the circulation. Perhaps most importantly, RBCs constantly encounter reactive oxygen species (ROS), both in the circulation and generated internally, as approximately 3% of hemoglobin undergoes auto-oxidation daily. Hemoglobin oxidation yields both methemoglobin and superoxide radicals. To prevent oxidative damage by ROS, RBCs have evolved multiple antioxidant pathways. Normally, about 90% of the glucose present in an RBC is metabolized by glycolysis, while the other 10% is routed to the hexose monophosphate shunt (pentose shunt). Under conditions of oxidant stress, the metabolic contribution of the pentose shunt may be greatly increased, boosting production of the major RBC antioxidant, reduced glutathione (GSH). GSH serves as the electron donor in several critical biochemical reactions that result

in ROS neutralization, such as the reduction of H_2O_2 to water catalyzed by glutathione peroxidase.

But when ROS manage to escape the RBC's antioxidant defenses, they can cause irreversible cellular damage. Hemoglobin is the primary target. Oxidation of hemoglobin to methemoglobin, unchecked, can progress to form denatured methemoglobin derivatives called hemichromes. Further oxidative damage can cause the hemoglobin tetramer to break apart and heme groups to dissociate from their globin chains. Denatured globin precipitates out of solution, becoming detectable microscopically as Heinz bodies. Hemichromes may form covalent cross-links with spectrin and other RBC membrane proteins such as the anion exchanger band 3, damaging the membrane and impairing cellular deformability.[11] Experiments conducted during the 1970s and 1980s led to the development of a model proposing that cross-linking of band 3 by denatured/oxidized hemoglobin causes band 3 clustering and/or conformational changes, leading to the formation of neoantigens (originally termed "senescent cell antigens") on the RBC surface. In turn, binding of universally present, naturally occurring IgG autoantibodies directed against senescent cell antigens triggers RBC phagocytosis and destruction.[12–15] Exactly how band 3 becomes altered and immunogenic remains poorly understood, and the degree to which this mechanism contributes to normal RBC homeostasis remains unclear. It is clear, for example, that both antibody-dependent and antibody-independent mechanisms of phagocytosis exist.

A second proposed RBC senescence signal is the display of PS on the external surface of the RBC membrane.[16,17] Due to the activity of membrane phospholipid translocases ("flipases," "flopases," and "scramblases"), phospholipids are asymmetrically distributed in eukaryotic cell membranes, with amino-containing phospholipids (PS and phosphatidylethanolamine) localized to the inner leaflet and choline-containing phospholipids (phosphatidylcholine and sphingomyelin) localized to the outer leaflet. Surface exposure of PS is characteristically observed in nucleated cells undergoing apoptotic death, and PS externalization has also been observed in various RBC pathologic states (e.g., sickle cell disease), so it was natural to hypothesize that PS expression on the RBC surface might mark RBCs undergoing terminal senescence. In support of this concept, liver-specific knockdown of the PS receptors stabilin-1 and stabilin-2 was recently shown to inhibit hepatic elimination of RBCs in a mouse model system.[18] However, PS externalization during RBC aging has been variably observed in different experimental systems, and the role of PS as a signal for RBC senescence remains controversial.[19]

Still another potential RBC senescence signal involves the membrane surface protein CD47. A 50 kDa cell glycoprotein belonging to the immunoglobulin superfamily, CD47 is expressed on all human cells. On many types of cells, CD47 is associated with integrins (hence its original name, integrin-associated protein, IAP). RBCs do not express integrins, yet CD47 is expressed on the RBC surface at a high level. Some erythroid CD47 appears to be associated with the Rh and band 3 membrane complexes. There additionally appears to be a more mobile CD47 membrane pool that is unassociated with the RBC cytoskeleton. In addition to integrins, CD47 interacts with thrombospondin 1 (TSP-1).[20] Most intriguingly, CD47 can bind to SIRPα (signal regulatory protein α), a cell-surface glycoprotein expressed by macrophages and other cells. Like CD47, SIRPα belongs to the immunoglobulin superfamily. The cytoplasmic tail of SIRPα contains two immunoreceptor tyrosine-based inhibitory motifs (ITIMs), which allow signaling through downstream molecules such as the tyrosine phosphatase SHP-1. Considerable experimental evidence supports the idea that CD47 serves as a marker of "self." The engagement of RBC CD47 with macrophage SIRPα delivers an inhibitory ("don't eat me") signal to the macrophage, preventing phagocytosis. As an example, in murine models, CD47-deficient RBCs are cleared far more rapidly than control RBCs by splenic macrophages.[21] But CD47's functional role in RBCs appears to be more complicated than simply inhibiting phagocytosis. In studies of many types of cells undergoing apoptosis, the CD47-SIRPα interaction has been shown to serve as an important signal promoting phagocytosis. Recent data suggest that CD47 molecules may undergo conformational changes as RBCs age, perhaps as a result of accumulated oxidative damage. After adopting its alternate conformation, RBC CD47 may provide an activating ("eat me") signal to the macrophage via SIRPα ligation rather than the usual inhibitory/"don't eat me" signal.[22,23]

RBC Destruction

The final common pathway for senescent RBC destruction is extravascular clearance by the reticuloendothelial system. Ordinarily, the primary site for RBC clearance is the spleen, although other sites within the reticuloendothelial system such as the liver support a normal rate of RBC clearance (and therefore a normal RBC life span) in individuals who have undergone splenectomy. The red pulp of the spleen has been proposed to provide an RBC "quality control" function.[24] The splenic cords of Billroth have an architectural structure not found elsewhere in the circulatory system: they form dead ends. In order to keep circulating, RBCs in the splenic cords are required to squeeze through approximately 2-μm-wide slits in the walls that form the splenic sinuses. Those RBCs unable to make it through are ingested rapidly by local macrophages surveying the area. Recent experiments examined the ability of RBC cohorts subjected to varying degrees of lysophosphatidylcholine (LPC)-induced membrane loss to successfully transit through an ex vivo spleen. The data from this model strongly suggest that the normal RBC's high surface area/volume ratio is the dominant factor allowing it to deform sufficiently to escape from the splenic cords, as opposed to the RBC's cytoplasmic viscosity or the specific protein and lipid content of the RBC membrane.[25] RBCs with a lower surface area/volume ratio (i.e., spherocytes – or aged RBCs that have lost membrane) have a much higher probability of physical entrapment, followed by phagocytic engulfment.

References

1. Ney PA. Normal and disordered reticulocyte maturation. *Curr Opin Hematol.* 2011; 18(3):152–157.

2. Bosman GJCGM, Werre JM, Willekens FLA, Novotný VMJ. Erythrocyte ageing in vivo and in vitro: structural aspects and implications for transfusion. *Transfus Med.* 2008; 18 (6):335–347.

3. Gifford SC, Derganc J, Shevkoplyas SS, Yoshida T, Bitensky MW. A detailed study of time-dependent changes in human red blood cells: from reticulocyte maturation to erythrocyte senescence. *Br J Haematol.* 2006; 135 (3):395–404.

4. Liu J, Guo X, Mohandas N, Chasis JA, An X. Membrane remodeling during reticulocyte maturation. *Blood.* 2010; 115(10):2021–2027.

5. Liu J, Mohandas N, An X. Membrane assembly during erythropoiesis.

6. *Curr Opin Hematol.* 2011; 18(3):133–138.

7. Schrier SL. What does the spleen see? *Blood.* 2012; 120(2):242–243.

7. Ashby W. The determination of the length of life of transfused blood corpuscles in man. *J Exp Med.* 1919; 29 (3):267–281.

8. Franco RS. Measurement of red cell life span and aging. *Transfus Med Hemother.* 2012; 39(5):302–307.

9. Bratosin D, Mazurier J, Tissier JP, et al. Cellular and molecular mechanisms of senescent erythrocyte phagocytosis by macrophages. A review. *Biochimie.* 1998; 80(2):173–195.

10. Willekens FLA, Werre JM, Groenen-Döpp YAM, Roerdinkholder-Stoelwinder B, de Pauw B, Bosman GJCGM. Erythrocyte vesiculation: a self-protective mechanism? *Br J Haematol.* 2008; 141(4):549–556.

11. Low PS, Waugh SM, Zinke K, Drenckhahn D. The role of hemoglobin

denaturation and band 3 clustering in red blood cell aging. *Science.* 1985; 227 (4686):531–533.

12. Lutz HU. Naturally occurring anti-band 3 antibodies in clearance of senescent and oxidatively stressed human red blood cells. *Transfus Med Hemother.* 2012; 39(5):321–327.

13. Kay M. Immunoregulation of cellular life span. *Ann N Y Acad Sci.* 2005; 1057(1):85–111.

14. Kay MM. Isolation of the phagocytosis-inducing IgG-binding antigen on senescent somatic cells. *Nature.* 1981; 289(5797):491–494.

15. Christian JA, Rebar AH, Boon GD, Low PS. Senescence of canine biotinylated erythrocytes: increased autologous immunoglobulin binding occurs on erythrocytes aged in vivo for 104 to 110 days. *Blood.* 1993; 82(11):3469–3473.

16. Freikman I, Fibach E. Distribution and shedding of the membrane

phosphatidylserine during maturation and aging of erythroid cells. *BBA – Biomembranes.* 2011; 1808 (12):2773–2780.

17. Schroit AJ, Madsen JW, Tanaka Y. In vivo recognition and clearance of red blood cells containing phosphatidylserine in their plasma membranes. *J Biol Chem.* 1985; 260 (8):5131–5138.

18. Lee SJ, Park SY, Jung MY, Bae SM, Kim IS. Mechanism for phosphatidylserine-dependent erythrophagocytosis in mouse liver. *Blood.* 2011; 117 (19):5215–5223.

19. Boas FE, Forman L, Beutler E. Phosphatidylserine exposure and red cell viability in red cell aging and in hemolytic anemia. *Proc Natl Acad Sci USA.* 1998; 95(6):3077–3081.

20. Oldenborg PA. CD47: a cell surface glycoprotein which regulates multiple functions of hematopoietic cells in health and disease. *ISRN Hematol.* 2013; 2013(5):1–19.

21. Olsson M, Oldenborg PA. CD47 on experimentally senescent murine RBCs inhibits phagocytosis following Fc receptor-mediated but not scavenger receptor-mediated recognition by macrophages. *Blood.* 2008; 112 (10):4259–4267.

22. Burger P, Hilarius-Stokman P, de Korte D, van den Berg TK, van Bruggen R. CD47 functions as a molecular switch for erythrocyte phagocytosis. *Blood.* 2012; 119(23):5512–5521.

23. Burger P, De Korte D, van den Berg TK, van Bruggen R. CD47 in erythrocyte ageing and clearance – the Dutch point of view. *Transfus Med Hemother.* 2012; 39(5):348–352.

24. Mebius RE, Kraal G. Structure and function of the spleen. *Nat Rev Immunol.* 2005; 5(8):606–616.

25. Safeukui I, Buffet PA, Deplaine G, et al. Quantitative assessment of sensing and sequestration of spherocytic erythrocytes by the human spleen. *Blood.* 2012; 120(2):424–430.

The Clinical Approach to the Patient with Anemia

Matthew Quesenberry, MD, Alina Huang, MD, and Fred J. Schiffman, MD, MACP

Introduction

Anemia is a commonly identified clinical condition and has a broad differential diagnosis. The etiology can be related to hereditary or acquired abnormalities of the red blood cell or can be a manifestation of an underlying disorder. It is important to develop a systematic and thorough approach in identifying the cause of a patient's anemia.

Definition

Anemia is defined as a deficiency of red blood cells or hemoglobin in the blood. The initial definition of anemia was based on a report from a World Health Organization (WHO) expert committee in 1968 that defined sex-specific hemoglobin targets of 12 g/dL in females and 13 g/dL in males.[1] However, these cutoffs were based on small samples of patients. Since that time, numerous sources have provided other definitions of the lower limit of normal of hemoglobin concentration in adult men and women.[2]

The availability of two large databases, the Scripps-Kaiser and NHANES-III (the third US National Health and Nutrition Examination Survey) databases, have provided the means to define age- and sex-specific definitions of anemia by systematically excluding individuals who did not have anemia. Based on these data, anemia has been defined as a hemoglobin level less than 13.7 g/dL in males 20–59 years of age and 13.2 g/dL in men older than 60 years of age. The corresponding values in females are 12.2 g/dL and 12.2 g/dL, respectively, (i.e., no differences with increasing age).

Values defining the range of normal are generally lower in blacks, possibly due in part to the higher prevalence of hemoglobin variants in this group compared to whites.[2] Also, the standard definitions for anemia may not apply to certain populations, notably patients living at higher altitudes, smokers, pregnant patients, and athletes.[3,4]

Because the clinical definition of anemia is based on a Gaussian distribution, 2.5% of normal adults will have hemoglobin values 2 standard deviations below the defined mean. Therefore, in certain situations, the patient should serve as their own reference range, as a change in hemoglobin over time may suggest a change in health status.

Erythropoiesis

Erythropoiesis occurs in the bone marrow, where stem cells are stimulated by the hormone erythropoietin (EPO) to proliferate and differentiate into mature red blood cells (RBCs). EPO is primarily produced by periglomerular cells in the kidney in response to decreased oxygen tension. Proerythroblasts move through several stages in the bone marrow and finally become reticulocytes, cells that have recently extruded their nuclei. These cells still retain RNA and a ribosomal network, allowing them to continue to synthesize proteins, including hemoglobin.[5]

Reticulocytes spend approximately 3 days in the bone marrow and 1 day in the peripheral circulation before they become mature RBCs. However, in circumstances of worsening anemia, reticulocytes spend a shorter time in the marrow and a longer time in the peripheral circulation. RBCs typically circulate for approximately 120 days, after which they are removed by the reticuloendothelial system. Under steady-state conditions and a marrow replete with iron, vitamin B12, and folate, the rate of RBC production equals the rate of RBC loss.[5]

General Diagnostic Approach

Patients with anemia may visit their caregivers with concerns or manifestations that directly relate to their blood disorder. Alternatively, their complaints may represent the underlying illness that has led to a low blood count. Anemia and most other hematologic problems should always serve as a starting point for the search for the pathophysiologic state associated with the low blood count and the related symptoms and signs. Anemia may have a simple, reversible cause or life-threatening etiology, and these must be discovered and addressed by the clinician. For example, a low hematocrit and abdominal pain may have aspirin-associated gastritis as the etiology or a gastric cancer that has ulcerated. It is the clinician's job to make certain that the simple and accessible etiology is the correct one and the clinical scenario does not have a more menacing origin.[16]

The diagnostic approach to patients with anemia begins with a careful history followed by the physical examination that will guide the choice of subsequent laboratory testing.

After gathering historical and physical examination data, the next step should be the careful review of the peripheral blood smear, which might provide clues that could spur a reconsideration of historical and physical exam information and also assist in the coordination of further laboratory testing or imaging studies.

Examples of common RBC abnormalities seen on peripheral blood smear are shown in Table 4.1.

The 10 guidelines outlined in Table 4.2 may help develop an approach to peripheral blood smear review. Table 4.3 offers a similar approach for the review of bone marrow specimens.

The ordering of other laboratory data will be discussed in individual chapters in this book, but in general, as with other illnesses, the least invasive, least expensive testing that yields results with high specificity and sensitivity should be done early on in the hierarchy of laboratory test requisition. However, other factors come into play as one considers the time course and selection of test ordering. For example, in an acutely ill patient, it may be necessary to order many tests simultaneously in the hope that an answer will be found to speed diagnosis and therapy. A linear, ordered, sequential approach to test ordering may be a fine way to approach a stable outpatient with a mild anemia versus a patient in the intensive care unit whose hematocrit is falling by five points a day, whose caregivers require the timely acquisition of as much data as possible using more of a "shotgun" approach.

Classifying Anemia

Red blood cell morphology (size, shape, inclusions) is assessed by peripheral blood smear review. Further determination of the mean corpuscular volume (MCV) and the splay of the size of red blood cells (red cell distribution width or RDW) as calibrated by automated cell counters, can narrow the differential diagnosis of anemia. A low MCV, corresponding to microcytic red blood cells, will help focus on causes such as iron deficiency, thalassemia, or some forms of anemia of chronic or inflammatory disease. A high MCV associated with macrocytosis or other changes associated with bone marrow megaloblastosis may be seen on the peripheral blood smear and might suggest vitamin B12 or folate deficiency to the clinician. And a normal MCV could represent hemolysis, acute blood loss, or mixed microcytic and macrocytic etiologies. Another method is to classify anemia according to RBC kinetics by examining the mechanisms responsible for the fall in hemoglobin. Unless there are concomitant disease states that would blunt or suppress the expected increase in the reticulocyte count, this test is a good indicator of the erythropoietic capability of the bone marrow.

Reticulocyte Count

The reticulocyte count[6] is reported either as a percentage of the number of RBCs counted or as an absolute number. A normal absolute reticulocyte number is typically between 50,000 and 60,000 μL. However, in the presence of anemia, an absolute reticulocyte count less than 100,000/μL indicates a hypoproliferative process, while an absolute reticulocyte count greater than 100,000/μL indicates an appropriate erythropoietic response to blood loss or a hyperproliferative process.

When interpreting a reticulocyte count reported as a percentage of the RBCs counted, it is important to adjust the percentage based on the degree of anemia and the maturation time of reticulocytes, which, taken together, is calculated as the reticulocyte production index (RPI). An RPI less than 2% indicates a hypoproliferative process, and an RPI greater than 2% indicates appropriate erythropoietic response to blood loss or a hyperproliferative process.

Reticulocytes spend roughly 3 days in the bone marrow and 1 day in the peripheral circulation before they become mature RBCs. However, in circumstances of worsening anemia, reticulocytes spend a shorter time in the marrow and a longer time in the peripheral circulation. When the hematocrit (HCT) is 45%, a reticulocyte will spend 1 day in the periphery. However, when the HCT is 35%, 25%, or 15%, a reticulocyte will spend 1.5, 2.5, and 3.5 days in the periphery, respectively. This number of days is termed the maturation factor (MF).

In summary, taking into account the patient's HCT and maturation factor of reticulocytes, the corrected RI is calculated as follows:

$$\text{Reticulocyte index (RPI)} = \%\text{Reticulocytes}$$
$$\times \text{Patient's HCT/Normal HCT}$$
$$\times 1/\text{MF}$$

Integrating morphology with the kinetic approach can usually direct the clinician to one of several causes for the anemia. They are described in what follows (see Table 4.4).

Blood loss is the most common cause of anemia. Bleeding can be obvious or occult in nature. Common sources of bleeding include gastrointestinal, pulmonary, urologic tracts, and menstrual losses. Hemorrhage not only causes the loss of RBCs but also eventually causes the loss of iron, which leads to iron deficiency and decreased RBC production. An overlooked source of blood loss is increased phlebotomy from frequent blood draws or blood donation.

Hypoproliferative anemias are characterized by an inability to produce adequate numbers of erythrocytes, and the hallmark finding is a low reticulocyte count. The most common cause of anemia worldwide is iron deficiency anemia, and it can be found in up to 4% of women 20–49 years of age in the United States.[7–9]

Hypoproliferative anemias occur when the rate of RBC production is less than that of RBC destruction. Common causes of hypoproliferative anemia include nutrient deficiencies (iron, vitamin B12, and folate) due to lack of availability in diet or malabsorption of these substances. Bone marrow suppression (from drugs, infections, chronic illness, prior chemotherapy or radiation), bone marrow infiltration (myelofibrosis,

Table 4.1 Peripheral blood smear descriptions

Category/name	Microscopic appearance	Description	Associated conditions
Normal RBC		Approximately 7 μm in diameter – about the size of a lymphocyte nucleus. Central pallor is approximately 1/3 of the RBC diameter.	
Red Cell Inclusions			
Howell-Jolly bodies		Basophilic red cell inclusions that are residual nuclear fragments. Howell-Jolly bodies are produced in normal individuals but removed by the spleen.	Post splenectomy, spleen atrophy, sickle cell disease, spleen hypofunction.
Platelet overlying an RBC		A halo is seen around the platelet when the overlying platelet indents the RBC cytoplasm and the light that is refracted reveals a halo. With a Howell-Jolly body, no such halo is seen. With babesia or malaria the, chromophobic area is inside the parasitic ring.	Normal condition seen more frequently with thrombocytosis.
Basophilic stippling		Aggregated inclusions of ribosomes in RBC.	Heavy metal poisoning (e.g., lead and arsenic), hemoglobinopathies, thalassemias, sideroblastic anemias.
Pappenheimer bodies (siderosomes)		Dark-blue or purple granules that contain iron in RBC.	Sideroblastic anemia, sickle cell, and hemolytic anemia.
Red blood cell parasites • babesiosis		Red cell inclusions of various size and shape, e.g., babesiosis (tetrad forms and ring forms) and malaria (ring forms).	Babesiosis and malaria.
• malaria			
Heinz bodies		Inclusions of denatured hemoglobin within red blood cells. NOT seen on Wright's stained RBC. Special Heinz body preparation is needed.	Chronic liver disease, G6PD-sp. deficiency, thalassemia, post splenectomy, inherited red cell enzyme deficiencies.

Table 4.1 (*cont.*)

Category/name	Microscopic appearance	Description	Associated conditions
Blister cells		A mature red cell that contains one or more submembranous vacuoles.	Characteristic of glucose-6-phosphate dehydrogenase (G-6-PD) deficiency or autoimmune hemolytic anemia.
Cabot rings		String-like strands in the shape of a loop in RBC. They are likely microtubule or nuclear membrane remnants. Finding these rings often indicates an abnormality in red cell production.	Pernicious anemia, lead poisoning, hemolytic anemia. May be seen in patients with severe anemia of various causes.
Hemoglobin C crystals		Intracellular crystals that are rhomboid or hexagonal in shape. May also be curved and blunt. Lighter area between crystals seen in hemoglobin SC disease.	Hemoglobin C and hemoglobin SC disease.

Abnormal Red Cell Shapes

Schistocytes		Fragmented red blood cells that are typically jagged and irregularly shaped because of direct trauma to the red cell. A true schistocyte does not have central pallor.	Mechanical heart valve prostheses, hemolytic anemia, microangiopathic hemolytic anemia (DIC, TTP), intraaortic balloon pumps, left ventricular assist devices, hypertensive emergency, scleroderma renal crisis.
Teardrop cells (dacryocytes)		RBCs that are shaped like a teardrop, likely formed after having to squeeze through bone marrow packed with normal elements (erythroid hyperplasia) or abnormal ones (malignant cells).	Myelophthisic anemia (particularly myelofibrosis with myeloid metaplasia), but can be found in moderate numbers in beta thalassemia, megaloblastic anemia, infections like tuberculosis, acquired hemolytic anemia, renal failure, hypersplenism, and other hematologic diseases.
Rouleaux formation ("pseudoagglutination")		A stack-of-coins appearance of red blood cells often caused by increased blood concentration of globulin, paraproteins, or fibrinogen.	Acute and chronic inflammatory disorders, Waldenstrom's macroglobulinemia, and multiple myeloma.
Poikilocytes		RBCs appear in bizarre shapes. Fragments are seen.	Burns, hereditary pyropoikilocytosis, myelofibrosis, thalassemia, iron deficiency.

Table 4.1 (*cont.*)

Category/name	Microscopic appearance	Description	Associated conditions
Bite cells (degmacytes)		RBCs appear as if a bite has been taken out of them. Formed when Heinz bodies are removed by the reticuloendothelial system with a portion of cell membrane and hemoglobin.	G6PD deficiency and with unstable hemoglobins.
Sickle cells (drepanocytes)		Irregular curved red blood cells with pointed ends. The abnormal hemoglobin is prone to crystallization when oxygen tension is low, and the red cells change shape into long, thin, curved forms.	Characteristic of the "sickle" hemoglobinopathies. Diseases with Hb S (sickle cell anemia, hemoglobin SC disease, hemoglobin S-beta-thalassemia), but can be seen in other hemoglobinopathies.
Elliptocytes (ovalocytes)		Elliptical-shaped red cells rather than the normal typical biconcave red cell.	Characteristic of hereditary elliptocytosis, but can be prominent in thalassemia, sickle cell trait, and Hb C trait, iron deficiency anemia, megaloblastic anemia, myelophthisic anemia, and mechanical trauma. Elliptocytes (<1%) occur in normal peripheral blood smears.
Spur cells (acanthocytes)		Red blood cell with irregularly arrayed thorny, spiked projections protruding from its cell membrane.	Postsplenectomy, in patients with alcoholic cirrhosis, liver disease, and in hemolytic anemias, sideroblastic anemia, thalassemia, severe burns, and hypothyroidism.
Burr cells (echinocytes)		RBCs demonstrate projections from membrane, but they are smaller and uniform in shape in distribution, unlike the acanthocyte.	Postsplenectomy, after the administration of heparin, in the hemolytic-uremic syndrome, renal failure, uremia, and malabsorption states. Also seen with hypophosphatemia and hypomagnesemia.
Crenated RBC	See above	Very similar to burr cells (echinocytes). Most cells on peripheral blood smear slide will exhibit this artifact. True burr cells may be less numerous.	An underfilled collection tube with a relative excess of EDTA/blood, slow drying of slide, a humid environment, or an alkaline pH.
Abnormal Red Cell Size			
Macrocytes		Red cells that are typically larger than the size of the nucleus of a lymphocyte (7–8 μm). They are more round in liver disease and more oval shaped in B12 or folate deficiency.	Liver disease (obstructive jaundice, alcoholism), impaired DNA synthesis from chemotherapy or inherited diseases, myeloproliferative disorders, myelodysplastic syndromes, B12 or folate deficiency.

Table 4.1 (*cont.*)

Category/name	Microscopic appearance	Description	Associated conditions
Microcytes		An abnormally small red cell that is often less than 5 μm in diameter.	Iron deficiency anemia, thalassemia, anemia of chronic disease, lead poisoning, and sideroblastic anemias.
Nucleated red cell (NRBCs)		Large, immature red blood cells with a nucleus.	Can denote markedly accelerated erythropoiesis, severe bone marrow stress, and/or bone marrow infiltrative disease. Clinical scenarios in which it is seen includes acute bleeding, severe hemolysis, myelofibrosis, leukemia, myelophthisis, and asplenia. The presence of NRBCs in the peripheral blood of an adult almost always indicates a significant disease process.
Spherocytes		Spheroidal red cells with absent central pallor. May be small or large. Cells are dense and hyperchronic. MCHC is high.	Hereditary spherocytosis, hemolytic anemia, can also be seen in smaller amounts in microangiopathic hemolytic anemia, hypersplenism, and postsplenectomy, myelofibrosis with myeloid metaplasia, hemoglobinopathies, malaria, liver disease, recent transfusions, and severe burns.

Abnormal Red Cell Color/Appearance

Category/name	Microscopic appearance	Description	Associated conditions
Hypochromia		Abnormal decrease in the hemoglobin in the red cell that makes the cell appear pale.	Thalassemia, iron deficiency, and the sideroblastic anemias.
Polychromasia		Larger RBCs that lack central pallor and appear bluish gray. The blue-gray appearance is due to the residual RNA in the cell.	Numerous disorders that can cause release of immature red cells (bleeding, hemolytic anemia, infiltrative bone marrow process, etc.).
Target cells (codocytes)		A red cell with a bull's-eye appearance: central hyperchromia surrounded by a ring of hypochromia, which is surrounded by an outer hyperchromic ring.	Postsplenectomy, thalassemia, hemoglobinopathies (hemoglobin SS, SC, CC, EE, AE, sickle cell-thalassemia), iron deficiency anemia, and liver disease.
Stomatocytes		Mature RBCs with a slit-like central pallor. A mouth-like appearance when seen from the side.	Characteristic of hereditary stomatocytosis. They can be seen in small numbers in patients with acute alcoholism, cirrhosis, obstructive liver disease, advanced malignancy, severe infections.

Table 4.2 Guidelines for the review of peripheral blood smear[16]

Guidelines for review of the <u>peripheral blood smear</u> for all clinicians include the following:
1. Develop an approach.
2. Know how a blood smear is made.
3. Know what the stains stain (methylene blue stains acidic structures blue; eosin stains alkaline structures red).
4. Find the sweet spot (the area where there is little or no artifact).
5. Begin at low power (looking for overall pattern, frequency, and distribution of blood cell abnormalities; for example, clumping of red blood cells [as seen in cold agglutinin disease]; frequency of smudge cells [a chronic lymphocyte leukemia marker]).
6. Look at all three cell lines (red blood cells, white blood cells, platelets) one at a time. Be disciplined; don't get distracted.
7. Be a detective.
8. Don't try to identify every cell.
9. Look at many fields.
10. Pay attention to overall configuration, color, consistency/internal structure, shape, size.

Table 4.3 Guidelines for the review of bone marrow aspirate specimens[16]

Guidelines for review of <u>bone marrow aspirate specimens</u> for the advanced clinician include the following:
1. Develop an approach.
2. Know how a bone marrow smear is made.
3. Know what the stains stain (methylene blue stains acidic structures blue; eosin stains alkaline structures red).
4. Find the sweet spot (the area where there is little or no artifact).
5. Begin at low power (looking for overall architecture, tumor, cellularity, fat, heterogeneity, granuloma, fibrosis, lymphoma, infiltrates, megakaryocyte, myeloid-to-erythroid ratio).
6. Examine many fields.
7. Look at all three cell lines (erythroid, myeloid, megakaryocyte) one at a time. Be disciplined; don't get distracted.
8. Be a detective.
9. Don't try to identify every cell.
10. Examine many fields on many different slides.
11. Pay attention to dysmyelopoiesis, megaloblastic changes, lymphocytes and plasma cells, abnormal cells (e.g., Gaucher cells).

acute leukemia, or metastatic disease), other bone marrow disorders (aplastic anemia, RBC aplasia, myelodysplasia), or decreased levels of hormones that stimulate RBC production (low erythropoietin from chronic kidney disease, hypothyroidism, hypoandrogenism) are other causes of hypoproliferative anemias.

Hyperproliferative anemias are those associated with hemolysis or acute blood loss. In these conditions, the reticulocyte count is typically high, as there is a physiologic attempt to compensate for the reduced oxygen-carrying capacity of the blood. Several days may pass before an appropriate increase in the reticulocyte count is noted. However, if nutritional or infiltrative states are also present, the expected reticulocytosis may not be seen.

Causes of hemolytic anemia (where red blood cells are prematurely destroyed) may be categorized by *congenital* versus *acquired* etiologies. Common *congenital* causes of hemolytic anemia include membranopathies (hereditary spherocytosis), enzymopathies (glucose-6-phosphate dehydrogenase deficiency), or hemoglobinopathies (sickle cell disease, thalassemia), all of which are intrinsic states leading to RBC hemolysis. Etiologies outside of the cell membrane, within it, or in the interior or the red blood cell can also be used to guide categorizing hemolytic anemias. (See Part D, Hemolytic Anemias (Chapters 12–17)

Common *acquired* causes of hemolytic anemia include autoimmune hemolytic anemia, microangiopathic hemolytic anemia (thrombotic thrombocytopenic purpura, disseminated

Table 4.4 Classification of anemia using the mean corpuscular volume (MCV) and the reticulocyte count. There are many ways to classify anemia, and one might start to differentiate between various causes by starting with the MCV or the reticulocyte count. This table summarizes the most common causes of anemia based on these two indices.

	Low MCV (<80 fL)	Normal MCV (80–100 fL)	High MCV (>100 fL)
Low reticulocyte count <100,000/μL (Hypoproliferative)	Iron deficiency anemia Anemia of chronic disease Sideroblastic anemia (congenital, lead)	Early iron, vitamin B12, folate deficiency Anemia of chronic disease Anemia of renal disease Bone marrow replacement (metastatic disease, myelofibrosis) Bone marrow disorders (myelodysplasia, aplastic anemia, pure red cell aplasia) Endocrine dysfunction (hypothyroidism)	Folate deficiency Vitamin B12 deficiency Bone marrow suppression (chemotherapy, radiation, ethanol) Drug-induced (anticonvulsants, hydroxyrea, methotrexate, zidovudine) Bone marrow disorders (myelodysplasia, aplastic anemia) Multiple myeloma Chronic liver disease Hemolytic anemia
High reticulocyte count >100,000/μL (Hyperproliferative)	Thalassemias	Acute blood loss Hemolytic anemia (immune, enzymopathies, hemoglobinopathies, microangiopathic) Sickle cell anemia	

intravascular coagulation, hemolytic uremic syndrome, malignant hypertension, HELLP syndrome), infection-related anemia (direct RBC lysis from parasitic infections such as *Babesia microti* or *Plasmodium* species or toxin-mediated RBC lysis from *E. coli* O157:H7 or *Clostridium perfringens*), vascular trauma (from prosthetic cardiac valves or repetitive trauma of vascular beds such as in march hemogloubinuria), or acquired membrane defect (PNH). (See Chapter19)

Specifics of the Approach to the Patient

Following a traditional History and Physical Examination format, we outline an approach and suggestions regarding the search for common symptoms and signs of anemia and selected etiologies.

History

History of Present Illness

Symptoms of anemia are related to the etiology, degree, and rapidity of onset of hemoglobin decrease. Most commonly, anemia leads to weakness, fatigue, pallor, malaise, or sometimes dyspnea or cognitive impairment. Severe or persistent anemia can result in cardiovascular morbidity, causing tachycardia, angina, and eventually heart failure. It is important to identify the cause of anemia before more severe symptoms and potential irreversible organ damage occurs.

In addition to inquiring about specific symptoms of anemia, it is important to know the duration of symptoms. This can potentially differentiate between acute and chronic causes of anemia. Obtaining a history of possible blood loss is essential, taking care to ask specifically about gastrointestinal, urinary, respiratory, and gynecologic sources. It is crucial to inquire about use of medications that can cause bleeding such as anticoagulants, aspirin, and nonsteroidal anti-inflammatory agents and all medications including complementary or alternative ones.

Concomitant symptoms suggesting low white count or low platelet count, such as recurrent infections, fevers, easy bruising, or petechial rash, can suggest an underlying bone marrow disorder. Changes in skin coloration and onset of jaundice as well as changes in urine color suggest hemolytic anemia.

Review of Systems

HEENT: Scleral icterus may suggest active hemolysis. Angular cheilitis (cracking at the edges of the lips) can be associated with B12 or iron deficiency anemia. A large tongue could indicate amyloidosis or hypothyroidism, and a painful, poorly papilled tongue suggests B12 or iron deficiency (see Figure 4.3). Painful or hypertrophy of gums might suggest acute monocytic leukemia. Discolored gums may indicate lead poisoning.

NECK: Neck swelling might be a sign of thyromegaly or goiter, signs of underlying thyroid disorders that can be associated with anemia. Lymphadenopathy may also cause neck swelling.

CARDIOVASCULAR: Symptoms of anemia include palpitations, chest pain, exertional dyspnea.
PULMONARY: Dyspnea is a common symptom of anemia or can be a symptom of infection or malignancy, both of which can cause anemia.

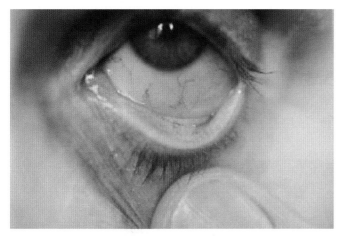

Figure 4.1 Conjunctival pallor. Taken from Sheth TN, Choudhry NK, Bowes M, and Detsky AS. The relation of conjunctival pallor to the presence of anemia. *J Gen Intern Med* 1997; 12:102–106.

GASTROINTESTINAL: Gastroesophageal reflux or epigastric pain may suggest peptic ulcer disease or gastritis, which can cause chronic blood loss anemia. Early satiety can suggest splenomegaly, which can be associated with an underlying lymphoma or chronic hemolytic process. Ascites or history of variceal bleeding suggests underlying liver disease. A history of vomiting blood or passing black or bloody stool suggests the cause for iron deficiency anemia. Benign or malignant lesions in the GI tract are likely reasons. Dysphagia could indicate underlying esophagogastric neoplasm or perhaps be related to esophageal webs seen in Plummer-Vinson syndrome, which is associated with iron deficiency anemia. Biliary colic or right upper-quadrant pain may suggest gallstones, which can be a sign of hyperbilirubinemia resulting from hemolysis.

GENITOURINARY: Pink, red, or dark urine may be a symptom of hematuria, hemoglobinuria suggesting genitourinary blood loss or hemolysis. A history of priapism can be a symptom of sickle cell disease or hyperleukocytosis.

LYMPH NODES: Enlarged lymph nodes may be a sign of underlying malignancy, but the differential diagnosis is quite broad for this problem.

SKIN/INTEGUMENT: Dry skin, fine hair, and brittle nails can be associated with iron deficiency anemia.

BONES: Bony pain, particularly of the vertebral column, can be an indicator of neoplastic disease from primary bone malignancies metastases or multiple myeloma. Patients with chronic sickle cell disease will commonly complain of bony pain. New joint pain can be a clue to an underlying rheumatologic diagnosis, which has associations with anemia of several etiologies.

NEUROLOGIC: Paresthesias, particularly of the lower extremities, can be a sign of vitamin B12 deficiency.

PSYCHIATRIC: Psychiatric symptoms of vitamin B12 deficiency have included depression, acute psychosis, or cognitive slowing.

Past Medical History

It is of value to inquire about chronic inflammatory disorders or chronic infections such as hepatitis, HIV, or tuberculosis to determine the presence of an underlying inflammatory disorder that could cause anemia. A history of renal disease suggests possible inadequate erythropoietin secretion, which can cause anemia. As stated previously, chronic GI inflammation secondary to reflux or gastritis could lead to chronic blood-loss anemia. A history of inflammatory bowel disease, particularly Crohn's disease, can lead to vitamin B12 deficiency. One must inquire about endocrinologic disorders, such as diabetes or hypothyroidism. The cause of anemia from hypothyroidism may be due to decreased stimulation of erythropoietin production.[10] A history of rheumatologic disorders might suggest a predisposition to autoimmune causes of anemia, such as autoimmune hemolytic anemia or pernicious anemia.

Past Gynecologic History

In women, taking a thorough gynecologic history is important to evaluate for blood loss anemia secondary to menorrhagia or pregnancy. Ask details about frequency, duration, and volume of menses.

Past Surgical History

A history of prior gastric bypass surgery or small bowel resection suggests that the patient is at risk for vitamin B12 and/or iron deficiency.

Medications

One should inquire about new medications, complementary herbal supplements, and over-the-counter medications. Common medications implicated in drug-induced autoimmune hemolytic anemia include penicillins, cephalosporins, and α-methyldopa.[11] Antiandrogens are thought to cause anemia by causing decreased testosterone levels, which in turn may cause decreased erythropoiesis.[12] Angiotensin-converting enzyme inhibitors have been associated with anemia presumably by suppressing erythropoietin.[13] Antifolate medications such as methotrexate, hydroxyurea, and anticonvulsants can cause a megaloblastic anemia. Metformin decreases folate absorption. The new use of sulfa medications may suggest hemolytic anemia secondary to glucose-6-phosphate dehydrogenase deficiency. Proton pump inhibitors have recently been found to be associated with malabsorption of iron and B12.

Family History

The physician should ask about ethnicity, particularly in patients in whom there is suspicion of thalassemia, sickle cell disease, or G6PD deficiency. Other causes of hereditary anemia include hereditary spherocytosis.

Social History

One must determine risk factors related to HIV or hepatitis transmission. Occupational exposures regarding lead, benzene, or radiation are potential environmental risk factors. It is critical to obtain a thorough travel history to inquire about risk for contracting babesia or malaria, which can both cause hemolytic anemia. An accurate history of alcohol intake is important because of its bone marrow toxicity and its relation to liver disease, which is associated with many types of anemia. One should ask if the patient donates blood on a regular basis. Questions about diet can elucidate whether a patient is vegetarian, who may be at risk for several forms of anemia. Pica is a common symptom seen in iron deficiency anemia. A history of lead exposure can suggest sideroblastic anemia.

Physical Examination

Vital Signs

Clues about volume status and possible blood loss will manifest initially as tachycardia and, later, as relative hypotension. In a patient with normal blood pressure at rest, orthostatic changes in pulse rate and blood pressure may be evidence of volume loss.

Skin

Commonly, patients will exhibit pallor if the degree of anemia is significant. One must pay attention to the color of conjunctiva, oral mucous membranes, and palm creases (see Figure 4.1). Jaundice can be a sign of underlying liver disease but also of indirect hyperbilirubinemia caused by hemolysis. Other skin findings of chronic liver disease include caput medusa and spider angiomas. Dry skin, fine hair, brittle nails, and koilonychia (spooning of the nails) are all signs of iron deficiency anemia (see Figure 4.2). A variety of skin rashes may alert the observer to systemic lupus, vascullities, or other rheumatologic diseases that have associations with anemia. The presence of petechiae suggests a process that is causing both anemia and thrombocytopenia, such as microangiopathic hemolytic anemia or Evan's syndrome.

HEENT

Signs of frontal bossing in which the frontal bones are prominent are seen with sickle cell disease and thalassemia. Scleral icterus is a sign of hyperbilirubinemia. Proptosis suggests underlying thyroid disorder. An abnormality in the size or texture of the tongue suggests vitamin B12 deficiency, iron deficiency (Figure 4.3), amyloidosis, or hypothyroidism.

Neck

Thyromegaly might suggest anemia caused by thyroid disease. Lymphadenopathy may suggest a whole host of malignancy-associated anemias and other conditions. Kussmaul's sign may suggest constructive pericarditis, which could be associated with anemias from malignancy, inflammation, or infection.

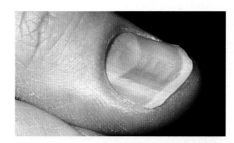

Figure 4.2 Koilonychia. In iron deficiency anemia, nails can be brittle and spoon shaped. (Copyright © 2013, reused with the permission of the Health and Social Care Information Centre. All rights reserved.)

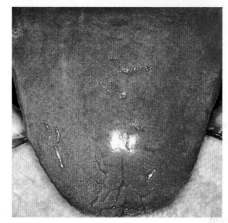

Figure 4.3 Glossitis. The texture of the tongue appears smooth due to the loss of papillae and results in a smooth, beefy, red, painful tongue. This may indicate a deficiency in vitamin B12, iron, riboflavin, niacin, or folic acid. (Reprinted from Cawson RA Oral Pathology 1st ed. London, UK, Gower Medical Publishing, 1987.)

Cardiovascular

One should listen carefully for murmurs, which might originate from a high flow state in the setting of anemia or from new or worsening valvular disease causing valve-related hemolysis. An S3 might indicate congestive heart failure (CHF). Patients with CHF may appear anemic due to increased plasma volume and resultant dilutional anemia. Anemia in CHF has been shown to be an independent predictor of hospital readmission for CHF.[14]

Pulmonary

Dullness to percussion, decreased tactile fremitus, and decreased breath sounds are signs of a pleural effusion, which can be present in the setting of congestive heart failure, infection, inflammation, or malignancy, all of which can cause anemia. One must also auscultate for rales or rhonchi, which may indicate pulmonary parenchymal abnormalities.

Abdomen

Inspection of the abdomen may reveal blood vessel abnormalities such as caput medusa. Abdominal distention may indicate ascites secondary to liver disease or peritoneal involvement by malignancy, both of which can cause anemia. Palpation of the abdomen is important to assess for hepatomegaly or splenomegaly. Presence of splenomegaly can be due to a myriad of causes, but in the setting of anemia, it can suggest underlying malignancy, RBC sequestration, or chronic hemolytic disease. A rectal exam should be performed to look for occult gastrointestinal bleeding, masses, or prostate abnormalities.

Genitourinary

Testicular atrophy in males may be a sign of low androgen state. Studies have shown that sex differences in hemoglobin level do not manifest until after puberty, when it is thought that testosterone independently increases hemoglobin levels in men compared to women.[12] Illnesses such as liver disease or medications that reduce androgen levels are associated with anemia. In women, ovarian or uterine carcinoma can be associated with anemia, and submucosal fibroids might bleed and be associated with blood loss anemia. Genital examinations in men and pelvic examinations in women are essential components of the physical examination.

Extremities

Inspect and palpate joints for signs of synovitis or joint effusions. Arthritis can be caused by underlying infectious or inflammatory states, which can cause or be related to anemia. Patients with sickle cell disease may have swelling of the hands and fingers (dactylitis).

Neurologic

A thorough cranial nerve exam and assessment for peripheral neuropathy is important. Causes of peripheral neuropathy and anemia include vitamin B12 deficiency, paraneoplastic syndromes, and amyloidosis.

Summary

Anemia remains one of the most common hematologic clinical conditions. The definition of anemia varies with sex and race. A thorough understanding of erythropoiesis and the mechanisms of hemoglobin reduction can help the clinician approach and evaluate a patient systematically in determining the cause of anemia. A focused and thorough history and physical exam can provide significant clues for determining the etiology of a patient's anemia. They should be used in an integrated fashion with information obtained from review of the peripheral blood smear and other laboratory and imaging data to both expand and then focus on diagnostic possibilities.

References

1. WHO scientific group. Nutritional Anaemias. World Health Organization Technical Report Series 1968; no. 405:1–37.

2. Beutler E, Waalen J. The definition of anemia: what is the lower limit of normal of the blood hemoglobin concentration? *Blood*. 2006; 107:1747–1750.

3. Ruíz-Argüelles GJ, Sanchez-Medal L, et al. Red cell indices in normal adults residing at altitude from sea level to 2670 meters. *Am J Hematol*. 1980; 8:265–271.

4. Nordenberg D, Yip R, and Binkin NJ. The effect of cigarette smoking on hemoglobin levels and anemia screening. *JAMA*. 1990; 264:1556–1559.

5. Papayannopoulou T, Migliacccio AR. Biology of erythropoiesis, erythroid differentiation, and maturation. In: Hoffman R, et al., eds. *Hematology: Basic Principles and Practice*. 6th ed. Philadelphia, PA: Elsevier; 2013:261–265.

6. Rose MG, Berliner N. Red blood cells. In: Schiffman FJ, ed. *Hematologic Pathophysiology*. Philadelphia, New York: Lippincott – Raven;1998:54–55.

7. Massey AC, et al. Microcytic anemia. Differential diagnosis and management of iron deficiency anemia. *Med Clin North Am*. 1992 May;76 (3):549–566.

8. Looker AC, Dallman PR, Carrol MD, et al. Prevalence of iron deficiency in the United States. *JAMA*. 1997; 277:973–976.

9. Centers for Disease Control and Prevention: Iron Deficiency—United States 1999–2000. *MMWR Morb Mortal Wkly Rep*. 2002; 51:897.

10. Das KC, et al. Erythropoiesis and erythropoietin in hypo- and hyperthyroidism. *J Clin Endocrinol Metab*. 1975; 40:211–220.

11. Garretty G. Drug-induced immune hemolytic anemia. *Hematology*. 2009:73–79.

12. Shahidi NT. Androgens and erythropoiesis. *N Engl J Med*. 1973; 289:72–80.

13. Pratt MC, et. al. Effect of angiotensin converting enzyme inhibitors on erythropoietin concentrations in healthy volunteers. *Br J Clin Pharm*. 1992; 34:363–365.

14. Kosiborod M, et al. Anemia and outcomes in patients with heart failure. A study from the national heart care project. *Arch Intern Med*. 2005; 165:2237–2244.

15. Rees DC, Williams TN, Gladwin MT. Sickle-cell disease. *Lancet*. 2010; 376:2018–2031.

16. Schiffman, Fred J. Clinical approach to the patient with hematologic problems. In: Schiffman FJ, ed. *Hematologic Pathophysiology*. Philadelphia, New York: Lippincott–Raven; 1998:27–28.

5

Anemia in Children

Wendy Wong, MD, and Bertil Glader, MD, PhD

Anemia is a common problem in children. Many of the same types of anemia in adults also occur in children. However, the clinical and diagnostic issues related to these conditions can differ. The types of anemia occurring in newborn infants are particularly unique. To appreciate how anemia is recognized in children, it is important to understand that the normal hemoglobin values and RBC characteristics of childhood change as a function of age.

General Considerations

Hemoglobin F is the major hemoglobin found in fetuses after the first trimester. Its replacement by adult hemoglobin A begins before birth, such that 60 percent to 90 percent of the hemoglobin found in the normal-term infant is hemoglobin F. After birth, gamma chain synthesis declines as beta chain synthesis increases (Figure 5.1). Hemoglobin F declines to a level of approximately 5 percent by 6 months, achieving adult levels of less than 1 percent after 1 year of age. Only trace amounts of hemoglobin A_2 ($\alpha_2\delta_2$) and hemoglobin Barts (γ_4) normally are present in cord blood. Hemoglobin Barts quickly disappears, whereas the hemoglobin A_2 level increases gradually to the adult level of 2.0–3.5 percent by 1 year of age. Beta globin disorders such as sickle cell anemia or beta thalassemia major are not clinical problems until several months of age, after the switch from hemoglobin F to hemoglobin A synthesis. Gamma globin chain abnormalities are most evident in fetal and neonatal life and then disappear by approximately 3 months of age. Alpha globin disorders are evident at all stages of fetal, childhood, and adult life. Homozygous alpha thalassemia (4 alpha globin gene deletions) is usually lethal *in utero* or, if the fetus survives, death usually occurs shortly after birth. Hemoglobin H disease due to deletions of 3 alpha globin genes is not a neonatal problem although it can be detected by finding an increased concentration of Hb Barts (tetramers of gamma globin chains, γ_4) in cord blood.

The normal hemoglobin concentration of neonates is increased (14–20 g/dL), a reflection of the intense erythropoietic activity of the fetus developing in a relatively hypoxic environment. At birth, following the first breath, hemoglobin oxygen saturation increases, erythropoiesis is turned off, and over a few days, reticulocytes decrease and nucleated RBC

disappear. The Hb concentration gradually begins to decrease over 8–12 weeks of life, with the hemoglobin nadir reaching 10–11 g/dL. This process is known as the *physiologic anemia of infancy*. It is a normal neonatal adjustment to extrauterine life. A similar phenomenon occurs in small premature infants (less than 32 weeks' gestation) but it is usually more severe (Hb 7–9 g/dL) and occurs earlier (3–6 weeks). In large part the *anemia of prematurity* is an exaggeration of the normal physiologic anemia of infancy, but other factors (shorter RBC lifespan, decreased erythropoietin production for the degree of anemia) also are involved.[1] Significant anemia can develop in premature neonates, frequently requiring packed RBC transfusion. Controversies exist regarding the appropriate transfusion threshold for premature infants and also on whether recombinant erythropoietin (EPO) supplementation is helpful in treatment of this anemia.[2]

At 1 year of age, the normal Hb concentration is 11–13 g/dL, and it is the same for boys and girls. Subsequently, throughout childhood, Hb concentration gradually increases to reach normal adult levels during puberty. Since children undergo puberty at different ages, it is important to consider Tanner stage in addition to age when determining if an adolescent is

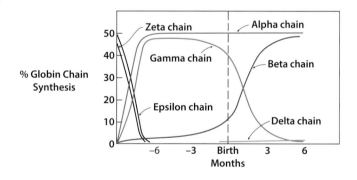

Hemoglobin	Birth	1 year ──▶ adult
F ($\alpha_2\gamma_2$)	60–90%	<1%
A ($\alpha_2\beta_2$)	15–40%	96–98%
A_2 ($\alpha_2\delta_2$)	1%	2–3%

Figure 5.1 Top: Globin chain synthesis in fetus and infants. Bottom: Hemoglobin composition at birth (cord blood) and beyond 1 year of age.

Table 5.1 Red blood cell characteristics in children

Age	Normal Hemoglobin (g/dL)	Normal MCV (fL)
Birth	14–20	100–130
0.5–1 year	11–13	70–85
1–4 years	11–13	70–85
4 years–puberty	11–13	75–90
Pubertal female	12–16	80–100
Pubertal male	14–18	80–100

anemic. The reason for the lower normal hemoglobin levels in children compared to adults is thought to be related to the relative hyperphosphatemia of childhood, resulting in altered RBC organic phosphates and enhanced oxygen release to tissues, the so-called *physiologic anemia of childhood*.[3]

In addition to the age-dependent changes in normal hemoglobin levels, there also are marked variations in RBC size. At birth, the cell volume (MCV) is larger than in adults, ranging from 100 to 130 fL (Table 5.1). This large MCV at birth is a residual of fetal erythropoiesis, since earlier in gestation RBCs are even larger. Following birth, the MCV decreases to 70–85 fL at 1 year of age, then gradually increases to adult values at adolescence. The reason why RBCs of normal healthy children are smaller than in adults is not entirely understood. However, the changing "normal" MCV values in infants and children have diagnostic importance. For example, neonates with an MCV of 85 fL (normal for an adult) actually have neonatal microcytosis. The differential diagnosis of neonatal microcytosis includes the alpha thalassemia syndromes, and if there is significant anemia, it may represent iron deficiency due to chronic fetal–maternal hemorrhage during pregnancy. Another example of how knowledge of normal childhood MCVs is important is the 2-year-old child with an MCV of 74 fL who is referred for microcytosis, only because adult normal values are on the CBC report, and the practitioner doesn't recognize this a normal value for this age child.

There are several causes of anemia that are unique to the newborn infant. These include hemorrhagic anemia related to the pregnancy or delivery and hemolytic anemia due to maternal alloimmunization. Other types of anemia can occur in both infants and older children. These include anemias due to nutritional deficiencies, hemolytic anemias, and red cell hypoplastic anemias. These will be discussed briefly in the following sections.

Neonatal Hemorrhagic Anemia

Newborns are at risk for developing anemia from hemorrhage due to pregnancy or delivery complications such as placental abruption, umbilical cord laceration, or cephalohematoma from vacuum extraction. In addition, they can have occult blood loss due to fetal–maternal hemorrhage. For obvious reasons, the perinatal medical history is very important in assessing an infant with anemia.

Fetal–maternal hemorrhage can be acute or chronic.[4] At delivery, infants who are placed much higher above the placenta are at risk of significant blood loss into the placenta. Also, small amounts of fetal blood loss into the maternal circulation are common during pregnancy, but in 1 in 400 pregnancies, the fetal blood loss is 30 ml or more. These infants with acute blood loss usually are born with a normocytic anemia. On the other hand, chronic fetal–maternal hemorrhage may result in a microcytic anemia due to iron deficiency. If one suspects a fetal–maternal hemorrhage has occurred, the Kleihauer Betke test can detect fetal RBC (containing Hb F) in the maternal circulation, and the volume of fetal hemorrhage can be calculated.

Twin–twin transfusion is a serious pregnancy complication seen in monochorionic twin pregnancies.[5] This is a result of an imbalance of the types of vascular anastomoses between the twins. In these cases, a shift of blood from the donor twin to the recipient twin results in hypervolemia, polyuria, and polyhydraminos in the recipient twin, while the donor twin develops hypovolemia, oligouria, and oligohydraminos.

Neonatal Hemolytic Anemia Due to Maternal Alloimmunization

The most common cause of hemolysis in newborn infants is due to alloimmunization. Prior to 1970, the majority of cases of *hemolytic disease of the newborn (HDN)* were due to maternal alloimmunization to Rhesus (Rh) D antigen. This condition was a result of an Rh-negative mother developing an Rh D antibody from exposure to D antigen in a previous pregnancy or from a prior transfusion with Rh-positive red cells. In the previously sensitized pregnant mother, anti-D antibodies cross the placenta, bind to Rh-positive RBC in the fetus, and lead to a hemolytic anemia in utero. The anemia in these fetuses can be very severe, often resulting in hydrops fetalis. The mortality rates from HDN were as high as 50 percent, and there also was a high rate of perinatal morbidity. In utero, bilirubin from hemolyzed RBC is cleared through the mother's circulation, but following delivery, it is processed by the immature neonatal liver. In healthy-term infants, this normally results in hyperbilirubiemia, reaching a maximum level of 12 mg/dL by day 4 of life. However, in babies with any kind of hemolytic anemia, the bilirubin concentration can become markedly elevated, leading to bilirubin staining of the brain and the development of kernicterus. The morbidity with HDN following birth mainly is due to the increased bilirubin load. In 1970, postnatal administration of anti-D immunoglobulin given to Rh-negative mothers was started, and since then, the incidence of HDN has decreased drastically. Maternal RhD sensitization and HDN still occur, however, usually seen in individuals from areas of the world where medical resources are limited and the anti-D antibody prophylaxis is not available.

With the decreasing incidence of anti-D hemolytic anemia, *ABO incompatibility* has become the leading cause of hemolysis due to maternal alloimmunization. ABO incompatibility hemolytic anemia is seen almost exclusively in mothers with type O blood and neonates with type A or B blood. Maternal IgG anti-A or anti-B antibodies cross the placenta and cause hemolytic anemia. The severity of ABO incompatibility anemia is much milder than that seen with Rh D incompatibility. In part this is due to a lower density of A and B antigens on neonatal red cells. Also, A and B antigens are present on other nonerythroid tissues which can absorb the antibodies and thereby minimize the hit on fetal RBC. Hyperbilirubinemia is the most prominent clinical feature of ABO incompatibility. The peripheral blood smear contains many spherocytes, and the direct antiglobulin test (DAT) is usually positive. However, in up to 40 percent of infants with ABO incompatibility, the DAT is negative. Consequently, in DAT-negative cases with peripheral blood spherocytosis, the diagnosis sometimes is confused with hereditary spherocytosis, since the peripheral blood smears can look identical.

Other common pathologic allo-antibodies include anti-c, anti-E and anti-Kell. Anti-Kell is known to cause very severe anemia without significant hyperbilirubinemia. The reason why the bilirubin levels are not that elevated is that there is also impaired erythropoiesis, a reflection of the fact that anti-Kell antibody targets erythroid precursors.[6]

Anemia Due to Nutritional Deficiencies

Iron deficiency anemia is one of the most common causes of anemia in children. The typical age of presentation is between 1 and 3 years. Due to their rapid growth, children require increased amounts of iron for red cell production. Premature infants are particularly at risk of early iron deficiency because fetuses receive most of their maternal iron during the third trimester of pregnancy. Full–term infants who are exclusively breastfed need iron supplementation at around 4 months of age as recommended by the American Academy of Pediatrics.[7] Children who are exclusively breastfed during first year of life and then take excessive amounts of cow's milk after age 1 are at highest risk of iron deficiency anemia, usually presenting between 1 and 2 years of age. Cow's milk contains no iron but has high calorie content such that iron-deficient children gain weight normally. Children with iron deficiency present have a microcytic anemia, usually with a low MCV (50–60 fL) and decreased hemoglobin, sometimes as low as 2–3 g/dL. In children older than 3 years of age, iron deficiency due to inadequate dietary intake can occur, but this is a diagnosis of exclusion. Just as in adults, older children with iron-deficiency anemia need to be scrutinized for other causes such as bleeding or gastrointestinal disease that impairs iron absorption.

Vitamin B12 deficiency is an uncommon cause of anemia in children. Dietary causes are extremely rare but sometimes are seen in children who are true vegans. In some cases there are congenital disorders that impair vitamin B12 absorption. More commonly it is found in children who have had ileal surgery and thereby impaired B12 absorption. Premature infants with necrotizing enterocolitis (NEC) requiring significant bowel resection but who are not provided with vitamin B12 supplementation can present later with vitamin B12 deficiency. The peripheral blood findings are the same as in adults: macroovalocytosis with hypersegmented neutrophils.

Hemolytic Anemia in Children: General Considerations

Hemolytic anemia in children most commonly reflects an inherited disorder. However, acquired causes also occur, such as autoimmune hemolysis or microangiopathic hemolytic anemia, as seen in the hemolytic-uremic syndrome. Congenital causes of hemolytic anemia often lead to severe problems in infancy or early childhood or may remain silent until a stressor is encountered later in life, provoking a crisis (e.g., G6PD deficiency). These disorders are discussed in detail throughout this book. The comments here reflect some of the pediatric issues related to a few of the common causes of hemolytic anemia in children.

Children with hemolysis usually have indirect hyperbilirubinemia, reticulocytosis, and low serum haptoglobin levels as indicators of hemolysis. However, using these markers to identify hemolytic anemia in neonates is challenging. Indirect hyperbilirubinemia presenting earlier and in excess of the expected physiologic levels is the most common and, occasionally, the only sign of hemolytic anemia in neonates. The physiologic anemia of infancy can limit reticulocytosis even in the presence of hemolysis if it is mild. However, reticulocytosis and persistence of nucleated RBC beyond third day of life are reasons to consider the possibility of hemolytic anemia. Decreased serum haptoglobin concentration as a marker of hemolysis in neonates is problematic, since infant levels of this protein are reduced and don't reach normal adult levels until 3–6 months of age.

Children with chronic hemolytic disorders occasionally have a sudden worsening of their anemia. Commonly this is due to accelerated hemolysis in association with some nonspecific infection, and usually these episodes are associated with increased scleral icterus and the passing of dark urine. In some cases, however, this acute exacerbation of anemia is due to an "aplastic crisis," and it is not unusual for this to be the reason a child with hemolytic disease first comes to medical attention. Aplastic crises are observed in all types of chronic hemolytic anemia, and they usually happen only once, with a majority of cases occurring in children. The etiologic agent responsible for almost all of these hypoplastic episodes is parvovirus B19, which is known to be cytotoxic for human erythroid progenitor cells. Characteristically, there is a sudden change in the usual degree of pallor, and the magnitude of anemia can be quite severe because hemolysis of abnormal RBC continues during the period of aplasia. In patients with chronic hemolytic anemia, it generally is easy to recognize RBC aplastic crises because the steady-state hemoglobin and reticulocyte counts are markedly reduced, whereas the bilirubin concentration may be normal or minimally elevated due to ongoing hemolysis of defective RBC. Usually only one RBC transfusion is required, since reticulocytosis occurs within 2–14 days of presentation. In families where more than one member has the congenital hemolytic disorder, it is not uncommon for other siblings to experience the same problem within a few days.

Hemolysis–RBC Membrane Disorders

Hereditary spherocytosis (HS) is the most common congenital hemolytic anemia resulting from a red cell membrane defect (Chapter 14).[8] In the neonatal period, jaundice is likely to be the most prominent feature of HS. Thirty to fifty percent of adult HS patients report a history of neonatal jaundice. The magnitude of hyperbilirubinemia may be severe, requiring phototherapy or exchange transfusion. Despite the jaundice, most newborns with HS are not anemic. Spherocytosis on the peripheral blood smear and reticulocytosis are frequently minimal or absent. As noted before, spherocytes also are found in infants with ABO incompatibility, sometimes confusing the diagnosis. Over the first few weeks of life, significant anemia develops in many HS infants. This increased rate of hemolysis after birth is thought to be due to maturation of splenic filtering and the development of the splenic circulation. Since the erythropoietic response to anemia is blunted in neonates, the anemia can be severe, often requiring red cell transfusions. Within a few months, erythropoiesis increases, anemia improves, and the need for red cell transfusions disappears in almost all affected infants. Chronic hemolysis persists throughout childhood until splenectomy. Splenectomy is the definitive treatment for HS. However, the indications for this surgery depend on severity of disease (Chapter 32). Even in the most severe cases, splenectomy is delayed until a at least 5 years of age given the increased risk of life-threatening sepsis with encapsulated organisms in young children. There is evidence that partial splenectomy can mitigate hemolysis and also protect against sepsis. (See Chapter 32 for further discussion.)

Hemolysis–RBC Enzyme Disorders

Glucose-6-Phosphate Dehydrogenase (G6PD) deficiency is the most common red blood cell enzymopathy in the world (Chapter 13). In older children and adults, episodic hemolysis occurs in association with infections and certain drugs. In neonates with G6PD deficiency, there is more jaundice than anemia; and there is an increased risk of very severe jaundice with kernicterus. It is of interest that data from the USA Kernicterus Registry from 1992 to 2004 indicate that more than 30 percent of kernicterus cases are associated with G6PD deficiency.[9] Neonatal hyperbilirubinemia is seen with G6PD Mediterranean (Class II) variants and also is seen in neonates from Southeast Asia and China. It has been suggested that hyperbilirubinemia may be due to impaired liver clearance of bilirubin. Also, it is now thought that the variable degree of hyperbilirubinemia in G6PD-deficient neonates reflects the presence or absence of the variant form of uridine-diphosphoglucoronylsyl-transferase responsible for Gilbert's syndrome.[10]

Favism refers to the acute hemolytic anemia in some people with G6PD deficiency following exposure to the fava bean (*Vicia fava*, broad bean). Symptoms of acute intravascular hemolysis occur within 5–24 hours of ingestion of the bean. Headache, nausea, back pain, chills, and fever are followed by hemoglobinuria, anemia, and jaundice. The drop in hemoglobin concentration is precipitous, often severe, and may require a red cell transfusion. Favism occurs most commonly in children between the ages of 1 and 5 years. The G6PD variant most frequently implicated is G6PD Mediterranean and, as a result, favism is encountered commonly in people from Italy, Greece, and the Middle East, areas where fava beans are a dietary staple; but it also occurs in the Asian G6PD variants. Favism usually results from ingestion of fresh beans. However, hemolysis of comparable severity can follow consumption of fried fava beans, a popular Chinese snack. Favism also has been observed in nursing infants of mothers who have eaten the beans.

Pyruvate kinase (PK) deficiency is the second most common cause of congenital anemia secondary to RBC enzyme deficiency (Chapter 17).[11] Neonates with PK deficiency can develop hydrops fetalis in utero. Often there is pronounced neonatal jaundice and usually anemia and reticulocytosis. Most PK-deficient children require regular transfusions starting in the first year of life. Patients with more severe forms of PK deficiency often are transfusion dependent until they undergo splenectomy, usually after 5 years of age. Postsplenectomy, transfusion needs will decrease or resolve, but the hemolytic anemia persists with a more exaggerated reticulocytosis due to improved survival of reticulocytes postsplenectomy. Since hemolysis persists after splenectomy, gallstones invariably occur over time.

Hemolysis–Hemoglobin Disorders

In the past, it was not uncommon for a child with sickle cell anemia to present in the first few months of life with overwhelming sepsis due to pneumococcus, and often this occurred before the diagnosis of sickle cell disease had been established. Several years ago in a landmark study, it was demonstrated that serious morbidity and mortality could be prevented by giving prophylactic penicillin to infants diagnosed with sickle cell anemia at birth.[12] This observation became the basis of newborn screening for hemoglobinopathies that now occurs throughout the USA. In addition to identifying neonates with sickle cell syndromes, the newborn screen also detects other hemoglobin disorders such as beta thalassemia, hemoglobin E-beta thalassemia, and Hemoglobin H Disease. General practice is to refer these identified infants and parents to a hematology center for counseling and early institution of therapy if indicated. The childhood course of sickle cell disorders involves mainly infectious problems, vaso-occlussive crises, acute chest disorders, and, in a small fraction, stroke (Chapter 10). For most children with beta thalassemia major and hemoglobin E-thalassemia, the clinical course during childhood includes regular RBC transfusions, iron chelation therapy, and consideration for stem cell transplantation (Chapter 8).

Red Cell Hypoplastic Disorders

Anemia due to RBC aplasia is a common problem in pediatric hematology seen with a variety of disorders including leukemia and aplastic anemia. However, in many instances, RBC aplasia in children presents as a "relatively pure erythroid abnormality" without an associated disease. Two major causes of pure red cell aplasia in children are Diamond Blackfan anemia (DBA) and transient erythroblastopenia of childhood (TEC). The characteristic feature of RBC aplasia is anemia with reticulocytopenia.

Diamond Blackfan anemia (DBA) is a lifelong disorder most commonly presenting in the first year of life, usually with persistent macrocytosis lasting beyond infancy and also associated with a variety of congenital abnormalities (Chapter 20).[13]

With the discovery of multiple ribosomal gene mutations in DBA patients, it is now firmly established that DBA is a ribosomopathy. The mechanism of erythroid failure is thought to be due to accelerated apoptosis, but how this relates to abnormalities in ribosome biogenesis is not known. More than 80 percent of DBA patients have elevated erythrocyte adenosine deaminase (eADA), and this is a useful marker to recognize DBA, particularly in neonates, because of the normally high neonatal MCV.

Transient erythroblastopenia of childhood (TEC) is an acquired immunologic red blood cell aplasia lasting a few weeks, occurring in otherwise normal children between 1 and 3 years of age. MCV in children with TEC is normal for age, thus distinguishing them from children with iron deficiency (low MCV) or Diamond Blackfan anemia (high MCV).[14] TEC occurs in previously healthy children who usually have had a viral infection several weeks prior, although no specific viral etiology has been identified. These children present with a moderate normocytic anemia (hemoglobin of 5–8 g/dL range) with reticulocytopenia. In contrast to Diamond Blackfan anemia, red blood cells usually lack markers of fetal erythropoiesis like elevated hemoglobin F, and eADA levels usually are normal. The anemia in TEC typically self-resolves within 1 to 2 months. Children with symptomatic anemia often require an RBC cell transfusion.

References

1. Strauss RG. *Anaemia of prematurity: pathophysiology and treatment. Blood Rev.* 2010; **24**(6):221–225.

2. Bishara N, Ohls RK. *Current controversies in the management of the anemia of prematurity. Semin Perinatol.* 2009; **33**(1):29–34.

3. Card RT, Brain MC. *The "anemia" of childhood: evidence for a physiologic response to hyperphosphatemia. N Engl J Med.* 1973; **288**(8):388–392.

4. Sebring ES, Polesky HF. *Fetomaternal hemorrhage: incidence, risk factors, time of occurrence, and clinical effects. Transfusion.* 1990; **30**(4):344–357.

5. Chalouhi, GE, et al. *Specific complications of monochorionic twin pregnancies: twin-twin transfusion syndrome and twin reversed arterial perfusion sequence. Semin Fetal Neonatal Med.* 2010; **15**(6):349–356.

6. Vaughan JI, et al. *Inhibition of erythroid progenitor cells by anti-Kell antibodies in fetal alloimmune anemia. N Engl J Med.* 1998; **338**(12):798–803.

7. Baker RD, Greer FR. *Diagnosis and prevention of iron deficiency and iron-deficiency anemia in infants and young children (0–3 years of age). Pediatrics.* 2010; **126**(5):1040–1050.

8. Gallagher PG. *Abnormalities of the erythrocyte membrane. Pediatr Clin North Am.* 2013; **60**(6):1349–1362.

9. Johnson L, et al. *Clinical report from the pilot USA Kernicterus Registry (1992 to 2004). J Perinatol.* 2009; **29** Suppl 1: S25–45.

10. Kaplan M, Algur N, Hammerman C. *Onset of jaundice in glucose-6-phosphate dehydrogenase-deficient neonates. Pediatrics.* 2001; **108**(4):956–959.

11. Zanella A, Bianchi P. *Red cell pyruvate kinase deficiency: from genetics to clinical manifestations. Baillieres Best Pract Res Clin Haematol.* 2000; **13**(1): 57–81.

12. Gaston MH, et al. *Prophylaxis with oral penicillin in children with sickle cell anemia. A randomized trial. N Engl J Med.* 1986; **314**(25): 1593–1599.

13. Lipton JM, Ellis SR. *Diamond-Blackfan anemia: diagnosis, treatment, and molecular pathogenesis. Hematol Oncol Clin North Am.* 2009; **23** (2):261–282.

14. Glader BE. *Diagnosis and management of red cell aplasia in children. Hematol Oncol Clin North Am.* 1987; **1**(3): 431–447.

Chapter

Iron Deficiency Anemia

6

Paula Fraenkel, MD

Epidemiology

Anemia is a global problem affecting 47% of preschool-age children and 42% of pregnant women, with rates greater than 65% in preschool-age children in Africa and South-East Asia. Iron deficiency anemia (IDA) causes half of the worldwide burden of anemia. Thus IDA is estimated to affect 810 billion people, or one-eighth of the world's population.[1] IDA is associated with impaired child cognition and increased risk of maternal mortality. The magnitude of the effect is proportional to the severity of the anemia.[2] Improving our understanding of the causes and clinical effects of IDA will facilitate the prevention and treatment of IDA.

Pathophysiology

Iron is a critical element for human survival. It is required for the transport of oxygen throughout the body, for DNA synthesis, and for respiration. Because of its ability to catalyze the production of reactive oxygen species via the Fenton reaction,[3] iron excess causes tissue injury and even organ failure. An adult male has a total body iron store of 4 g: 2.5 g in hemoglobin, 1 g in hepatocytes and reticuloendothelial cells, and 0.5 g in myoglobin, cytochromes and other proteins.[3] Under normal circumstances, the majority of iron is retained within the body, with losses of only 1–2 mg per day in nonmenstruating adults, <0.1% per day of total body iron stores.[4]

Iron absorption from the diet requires an acid environment in the stomach and healthy villous enterocytes in the duodenum. Most dietary iron is in the ferric (Fe^{3+}) form. It is reduced to ferrous (Fe^{2+}) iron by duodenal cytochrome B (DCYTB). Ferrous iron is taken up at the apical surface of the enterocyte by the divalent metal transporter 1 (DMT1) in a process requiring gastric acid as a source for proton cotransport (Figure 6.1). Ferrous iron exits the basolateral surface of the enterocyte via the iron exporter, ferroportin1 (Fpn1).[5] The iron oxidases, hephaestin and ceruloplasmin, oxidize ferrous iron, facilitating its loading onto transferrin.[6] Transferrin transports iron through the bloodstream to the other cells in the body. Transferrin receptor 1 is ubiquitously expressed in human cells and facilitates the uptake of transferrin-bound iron. Transferrin receptor 2 is specifically expressed in the liver and does not take up transferrin-bound iron efficiently, but does participate in sensing body iron stores.[6]

In response to iron overload, human hepatocytes produce hepcidin,[7–9] a peptide hormone that downregulates intestinal iron absorption (Figure 6.2). Inflammatory stimuli that increase interleukin-6 production[10,11] also increase hepcidin expression by increasing Stat3 binding to the *Hepcidin* promoter.[4] Conversely, increased erythropoietic drive, iron deficiency, and hypoxia[12] are each associated with decreased *Hepcidin* expression and increased intestinal iron absorption. Hepcidin appears to be the key regulator of iron homeostasis, because loss of function mutations in genes that regulate hepcidin expression, such as transferrin receptor 2, HFE, hemojuvelin, or in hepcidin itself, have each been associated with hereditary iron overload syndromes.[3]

Maintaining appropriate hepcidin levels depends on a complex interaction of regulatory factors including bone morphogenic proteins (BMPs), the BMP coreceptor, hemojuvelin, proteases such as furin and matriptase-2, and inflammatory cytokines (Figure 6.3). Recent studies in mouse models[13] indicate that hepatic iron overload upregulates bone morphogenic protein 6 (BMP6), which stimulates *Hepcidin* transcription by increasing Smad4 binding at Smad4-binding motifs, termed BMP response elements (BREs), in the *Hepcidin* promoter.[14] Membrane-bound hemojuvelin (Hjv or RGMc),

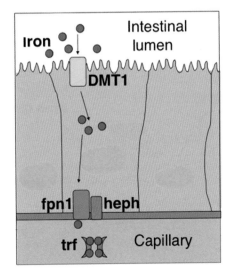

Figure 6.1 Intestinal iron absorption. Iron is absorbed from the diet at the apical surface of the villous enterocyte by the divalent metal transporter, DMT1. Iron is then exported from the enterocyte by ferroportin1, fpn1. The membrane-bound oxidase hephaestin, Heph, oxidizes iron to the ferric form for loading onto transferrin, Trf, which transports iron through the bloodstream.

increases intracellular iron accumulation and enhances BMP-mediated induction of *Hepcidin* expression in vitro. Iron deficiency induces production of soluble Hjv,[15] while iron loading inhibits release of soluble Hjv.[15,16] Soluble Hjv, produced via proteolysis of membrane-bound Hjv by Furin[16,17] or Matriptase-2 (TMPRSS-6),[18] antagonizes the function of membrane-bound Hjv,[19, 20] resulting in low levels of *Hepcidin* expression.[21]

Hepcidin suppresses intestinal iron absorption by binding fpn1 on the surface of the absorptive enterocyte, resulting in the internalization and degradation of the transporter.[4,22] Hepcidin also binds Fpn1 on the surface of macrophages, where it limits the release of iron to developing erythrocytes.[4] In states of severe iron deficiency resulting in anemia, hepcidin levels will be depressed, resulting in increased Fpn1 protein levels on the basolateral surface of the enterocyte. This will facilitate correction of the iron deficiency when oral iron supplementation is provided.

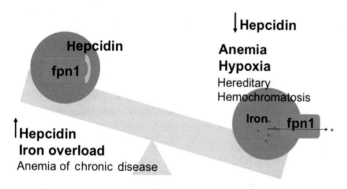

Figure 6.2 The iron regulatory hormone, hepcidin, is produced in the liver in response to iron overload or inflammation, while increased erythropoietic drive secondary to anemia or hypoxia decreases *Hepcidin* expression. Hepcidin binds Fpn1, causing its internalization and degradation and thus terminating iron export.

The majority of iron in the human body is recycled efficiently in a process that depends on Fpn1.[23] As erythroid progenitors mature, they express increasing amounts of transferrin receptor 1[6] to acquire iron for the production of hemoglobin. Macrophages consume senescent erythrocytes, degrade hemoglobin, and store the liberated iron in ferritin for subsequent release of iron to developing erythrocytes via fpn1.[6] Thus iron deficiency anemia requires either dietary iron restriction, deficiency of gastrointestinal iron absorption, or blood loss via menstruation, pregnancy, splenic sequestration, or intravascular hemolysis resulting in hemoglobinuria.

Clinical Presentation and Diagnostic Evaluation

Given the importance of iron for every tissue in the body, it is not surprising that individuals affected by IDA will present with a wide variety of symptoms. They may present with fatigue, poor exercise tolerance, headaches, feeling cold, poor memory, restless leg syndrome, and pica, the desire to eat ice or dirt. On physical examination, iron-deficiency patients may exhibit koilonychias (spooning of the nails).[5]

Review of the peripheral blood smear will often reveal small, pale erythrocytes of varying sizes (anisopoikilocytosis; see Figure 6.4). These findings are consistent with a decrease in mean corpuscular volume (MCV) and an increase in red cell distribution width (RDW).[5] With severe iron deficiency, thrombocytosis may also occur.

The classic chemical findings in IDA include a low serum iron level, high transferrin level or total iron-binding capacity (TIBC), and low serum ferritin. The serum ferritin level is the most strongly correlated with bone marrow iron stores. A serum ferritin level <15 µg/L can also be considered diagnostic for IDA.[5] In states of inflammation, serum transferrin

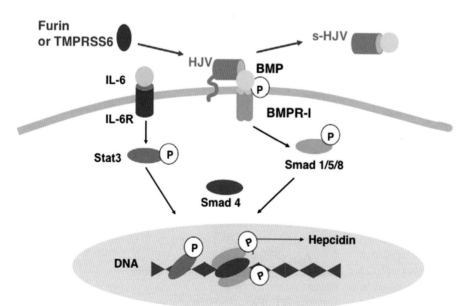

Figure 6.3 A mammalian model of iron homeostasis. In response to high iron states, bone morphogenic proteins, BMPs, bind the BMP receptor, BMPR-I, and the BMP coreceptor, hemojuvelin, HJV, facilitating phosphorylation of Smad proteins that bind the *Hepcidin* promoter and enhance *Hepcidin* transcription. The proteases TMPRSS6 and furin cleave HJV, resulting in decreased *Hepcidin* expression. In inflammatory conditions, interleukin-6, IL-6, binds its receptor, leading to phosphorylation of Stat3 and Stat3-dependent enhancement of *Hepcidin* expression.

A

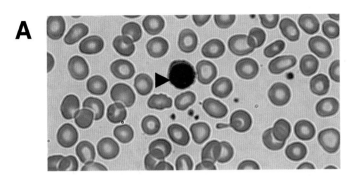

B

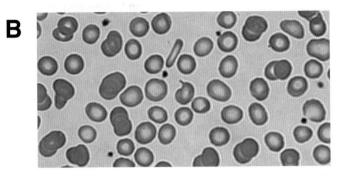

Figure 6.4 Photomicrographs of peripheral blood smears from patients with iron deficiency anemia. The erythrocytes are microcytic relative to the size of a normal lymphocyte nucleus (arrowhead), hypochromic, and exhibit irregularity of size and shape.
A. The patient was a 42-year-old woman 6 years status post–gastric bypass surgery for obesity who has chronic menorrhagia. Although she had taken oral iron supplements for 4 months, her hematocrit was 32, MCV 78 fL, serum iron 32 mg/dL, total iron binding capacity 534 mg/dL, ferritin 11 ng/ml.
B. The patient was a 48-year-old woman with type I diabetes mellitus who had iron deficiency anemia for 5 years. The IDA persisted despite relief of menorrhagia by endometrial ablation and supplementation with oral iron. Hematocrit was 29.7, MCV 70 fL, RDW 17.6%, serum iron 18 mg/dL, total iron binding capacity 373 mg/dL, B12 292 pg/ml, ferritin 2.9 ng/ml. Tissue transglutaminase antibody, IgA was >100 units. Enterogastroduodenoscopy revealed diffuse continuous atrophy of the mucosa, with scalloping folds in the duodenum compatible with celiac disease.

levels may be elevated in the absence of adequate marrow iron stores. The transferrin saturation (TSAT) can be used as an additional test for IDA. The TSAT is calculated by dividing the serum iron by the TIBC. In many cases, the TSAT will be <15%.[5] Specialized testing including the ratio of zinc protoporphyrin to heme or soluble transferrin receptor to ferritin may also be used to confirm the diagnosis.[5] The most rigorous standard for diagnosing IDA, which should be used in ambiguous cases, is a bone marrow biopsy that reveals low macrophage iron stores on Perls' staining for nonheme iron.

Evaluation of Causes

In the developing world, where consumption of beef, poultry, and fish is lower than in the developed world, nutritional deficiency is the most common cause of IDA.[2] Nutritional IDA is particularly common in children and pregnant women whose iron requirements exceed the amount of iron in their diets. In the developed world, strict vegetarians or vegans who do not consume iron supplements are also at increased risk for IDA. In addition, there are rare individuals with genetic impairments in dietary iron absorption caused by mutations in *DMT1, Transferrin, Ceruloplasmin,* or *TMPPRS6.*[6]

After nutritional iron deficiency, chronic blood loss is the most common cause of IDA worldwide. In the developing world, infections with malaria or hookworm are major causes of blood loss,[5] while in the developed world, blood loss in adult men and postmenopausal women is more commonly caused by colon polyps, arterial-venous malformations, hemorrhoids, gastric or duodenal ulcers, gastroesophageal varices, gastritis, inflammatory bowel disease, and malignancies of the stomach, small intestine, colon, or rectum. Gastrointestinal blood loss often occurs very gradually so that the bleeding is unnoticed. In this population, evaluation for occult blood loss may include rectal examination, fecal occult blood testing, colonoscopy, enterogastroduodenoscopy (EGD), and capsule endoscopy to evaluate the small bowel.[5] Chronic gastritis, often caused by *Helicobacter pylori* infection, can impair iron absorption by impairing stomach acidification, which is required for iron absorption.[6] Celiac sprue damages the intestine, impairing iron absorption. One can screen for these conditions serologically by measuring antibody titers against *Helicobacter pylori* and tissue trans-gliadin (tTg). Because iron absorption occurs in the same part of the intestine as cyanocobalamin (B12) absorption, iron malabsorption may also be associated with cyanocobalamin deficiency. Thus it is advisable to evaluate cyanocobalamin levels in patients with evidence of iron malabsorption.

In women, it is important to obtain a reproductive and menstrual history to rule out abnormal vaginal bleeding, pregnancy, breastfeeding, or benign or malignant gynecologic tumors as a potential cause of iron deficiency. Von Willebrand's disease is a common, treatable cause of excessive menstrual bleeding in premenopausal women[24] and can be diagnosed by assessing the partial thromboplastin time (PTT), factor VIII, and von Willebrand's factor activities. Less common bleeding disorders including deficiencies of factors I, II, V, X, XI, or XIII, or platelet disorders are also associated with a high prevalence of menorrhagia.[24]

Prevention and Treatment

To prevent IDA, individuals should ingest the appropriate amount of iron each day. The recommended daily dietary allowance for iron in nonpregnant adults is 8 mg, while the recommended daily dietary allowance for pregnant women is 27 mg. Breastfeeding women require 10 mg of dietary iron per day.[25] Once IDA is established, the options for treatment include oral iron supplementation, intravenous iron infusion, or blood transfusion. Oral iron supplementation, most commonly with ferrous sulfate, is the least expensive approach. However, patients often discontinue the supplement because of gastrointestinal side effects[26] including nausea, diarrhea, and constipation. Some studies indicate that lower doses of oral iron are still effective, but are associated with a lower incidence of side effects.

Even compliant patients with IDA may not respond to oral iron supplementation because of impaired intestinal iron absorption. The potential causes of iron malabsorption include high hepcidin levels secondary to inflammation, hereditary defects in iron-related proteins, intestinal injury secondary to inflammatory bowel disease or celiac sprue, anatomical defects caused by gastric bypass surgery, impaired stomach acid production related to medications, or chelating effects of other medications. A recent study[27] indicates that high serum hepcidin levels predict nonresponsiveness to oral iron supplementation in IDA patients.

Initial usage of parenteral iron salts in the early 20th century was limited by severe toxicity from the rapid delivery of large amounts of iron, causing oxidative damage. To prevent this toxicity, the currently available parenteral iron formulations include an iron-oxyhydroxy gel surrounded by a carbohydrate shell.[28] Following phagocytosis by macrophages, iron releases slowly from the complex and either is stored as ferritin in the macrophage or exported out of the cell by fpn1[28] Administration of iron dextran, the original iron–carbohydrate complex, has declined in favor of ferric gluconate, iron sucrose, and ferumoxytol, which are associated with lower rates of severe allergic reactions and are approved by the Food and Drug Administration for administration at higher dosages and without a test dose.[28]

The development of safer parenteral iron products has broadened usage of parenteral iron to include the treatment of pregnant women and renal failure patients. Several prospective studies in pregnant women with IDA comparing oral iron supplementation with intravenous iron infusion have demonstrated that intravenous iron treatment is associated with greater improvements in hemoglobin levels (reviewed in[25]). Higher hemoglobin and ferritin levels postpartum were, in turn, associated with a longer period of breastfeeding and improvements in maternal health.[29]

Parenteral iron is commonly used in conjunction with erythropoiesis stimulating agents (ESAs) in hemodialysis patients, who often suffer from a multifactorial anemia related to impaired erythropoietin production, impaired iron mobilization secondary to chronic inflammation, and chronic iron deficiency related to blood loss and hemolysis during hemodialysis. Although current guidelines allow administration of parenteral iron in hemodialysis patients with serum ferritins up to 900 ng/ml, recent studies indicate that iron overload can occur in hemodialysis patients receiving chronic parenteral iron therapy.[30] Despite elevations in ferritin related to chronic inflammation, a serum ferritin >350 ng/ml has been associated with increased total-body iron stores in hemodialysis patients,[30]; thus it is important to monitor for signs of iron overload in this population.

Conclusion

Iron deficiency remains a common cause of anemia and an important cause of disability and death, particularly in the developing world. Evaluation for the causes of IDA in individual patients often reveals important underlying diseases, such as gastrointestinal malignancies, bleeding disorders, celiac sprue, or parasitic infections. Studying patients with refractory IDA has also led to the identification of new genes involved in the regulation of iron metabolism. Recent developments in the field of iron biology promise to improve our ability to prevent, evaluate, and treat IDA in safer and more cost-effective ways.

References

1. WHO. World prevalence of anaemia 1993–2005. WHO Global Database on Anaemia 2008.

2. Black RE, Allen LH, Bhutta ZA, Caulfield LE, de Onis M, Ezzati M, Mathers C, et al. Maternal and child undernutrition: global and regional exposures and health consequences. *Lancet.* 2008; 371:243–260.

3. Ganz T, Nemeth E. Iron metabolism: interactions with normal and disordered erythropoiesis. *Cold Spring Harb Perspect Med.* 2012; 2:a011668.

4. Ganz T, Nemeth E. Hepcidin and iron homeostasis. *Biochim Biophys Acta.* 2012; 1823:1434–1443.

5. Miller JL. Iron deficiency anemia: a common and curable disease. *Cold Spring Harb Perspect Med.* 2013; 3.

6. Andrews NC. Forging a field: the golden age of iron biology. *Blood.* 2008; 112:219–230.

7. Hentze MW, Muckenthaler MU, Andrews NC. Balancing acts: molecular control of mammalian iron metabolism. *Cell.* 2004; 117:285–297.

8. Pigeon C, Ilyin G, Courselaud B, Leroyer P, Turlin B, Brissot P, Loreal O. A new mouse liver-specific gene, encoding a protein homologous to human antimicrobial peptide hepcidin, is overexpressed during iron overload. *J Biol Chem.* 2001; 276:7811–7819.

9. Bolondi G, Garuti C, Corradini E, Zoller H, Vogel W, Finkenstedt A, Babitt JL, et al. Altered hepatic BMP signaling pathway in human HFE hemochromatosis. *Blood Cells Mol Dis.* 2010; 45:308–312.

10. Kemna E, Pickkers P, Nemeth E, van der Hoeven H, Swinkels D. Time-course analysis of hepcidin, serum iron, and plasma cytokine levels in humans injected with LPS. *Blood.* 2005; 106:1864–1866.

11. Nemeth E, Rivera S, Gabayan V, Keller C, Taudorf S, Pedersen BK, Ganz T. IL-6 mediates hypoferremia of inflammation by inducing the synthesis of the iron regulatory hormone hepcidin. *J Clin Invest.* 2004; 113:1271–1276.

12. Nicolas G, Chauvet C, Viatte L, Danan JL, Bigard X, Devaux I, Beaumont C, et al. The gene encoding the iron regulatory peptide hepcidin is regulated by anemia, hypoxia, and inflammation. *J Clin Invest.* 2002; 110:1037–1044.

13. Andriopoulos B, Jr., Corradini E, Xia Y, Faasse SA, Chen S, Grgurevic L, Knutson MD, et al. BMP6 is a key endogenous regulator of hepcidin expression and iron metabolism. *Nat Genet.* 2009; 41:482–487.

14. Verga Falzacappa MV, Casanovas G, Hentze MW, Muckenthaler MU. A bone morphogenetic protein (BMP)-responsive element in the hepcidin promoter controls HFE2-mediated

hepatic hepcidin expression and its response to IL-6 in cultured cells. *J Mol Med (Berl)*. 2008; 86:531–540.

15. Zhang AS, Anderson SA, Meyers KR, Hernandez C, Eisenstein RS, Enns CA. Evidence that inhibition of hemojuvelin shedding in response to iron is mediated through neogenin. *J Biol Chem*. 2007; 282:12547–12556.

16. Lin L, Nemeth E, Goodnough JB, Thapa DR, Gabayan V, Ganz T. Soluble hemojuvelin is released by proprotein convertase-mediated cleavage at a conserved polybasic RNRR site. *Blood Cells Mol Dis*. 2008; 40:122–131.

17. Silvestri L, Pagani A, Camaschella C. Furin-mediated release of soluble hemojuvelin: a new link between hypoxia and iron homeostasis. *Blood*. 2008; 111:924–931.

18. Silvestri L, Pagani A, Nai A, De Domenico I, Kaplan J, Camaschella C. The serine protease matriptase-2 (TMPRSS6) inhibits hepcidin activation by cleaving membrane hemojuvelin. *Cell Metab*. 2008; 8:502–511.

19. Lin L, Goldberg YP, Ganz T. Competitive regulation of hepcidin mRNA by soluble and cell-associated hemojuvelin. *Blood*. 2005; 106:2884–2889.

20. Babitt JL, Huang FW, Xia Y, Sidis Y, Andrews NC, Lin HY. Modulation of bone morphogenetic protein signaling in vivo regulates systemic iron balance. *J Clin Invest*. 2007; 117:1933–1939.

21. Du X, She E, Gelbart T, Truksa J, Lee P, Xia Y, Khovananth K, et al. The serine protease TMPRSS6 is required to sense iron deficiency. *Science*. 2008; 320:1088–1092.

22. Nemeth E, Tuttle MS, Powelson J, Vaughn MB, Donovan A, Ward DM, Ganz T, et al. Hepcidin regulates cellular iron efflux by binding to ferroportin and inducing its internalization. *Science*. 2004; 306:2090–2093.

23. Fraenkel PG, Traver D, Donovan A, Zahrieh D, Zon LI. Ferroportin1 is required for normal iron cycling in zebrafish. *J Clin Invest*. 2005; 115:1532–1541.

24. James AH, Kouides PA, Abdul-Kadir R, Dietrich JE, Edlund M, Federici AB, Halimeh S, et al. Evaluation and management of acute menorrhagia in women with and without underlying bleeding disorders: consensus from an international expert panel. *Eur J Obstet Gynecol Reprod Biol*. 2011; 158:124–134.

25. Khalafallah AA, Dennis AE. Iron deficiency anaemia in pregnancy and postpartum: pathophysiology and effect of oral versus intravenous iron therapy. *J Pregnancy*. 2012; 2012:630519.

26. Christensen L, Sguassero Y, Cuesta CB. Anemia and compliance to oral iron supplementation in a sample of children attending the public health network of Rosario, Santa Fe. *Arch Argent Pediatr*. 2013; 111:288–294.

27. Bregman DB, Morris D, Koch TA, He A, Goodnough LT. Hepcidin levels predict nonresponsiveness to oral iron therapy in patients with iron deficiency anemia. *Am J Hematol*. 2013; 88:97–101.

28. Auerbach M, Ballard H. Clinical use of intravenous iron: administration, efficacy, and safety. *Hematology Am Soc Hematol Educ Program*. 2010; 2010:338–347.

29. Khalafallah AA, Dennis AE, Ogden K, Robertson I, Charlton RH, Bellette JM, Shady JL, et al. Three-year follow-up of a randomised clinical trial of intravenous versus oral iron for anaemia in pregnancy. *BMJ Open*. 2012; 2.

30. Vaziri ND. Understanding iron: promoting its safe use in patients with chronic kidney failure treated by hemodialysis. *Am J Kidney Dis*. 2013; 61:992–1000.

Sideroblastic Anemias

Nathan T. Connell, MD, MPH, and Edward J. Benz, Jr., MD

Introduction

The sideroblastic anemias are a diverse group of anemias – characterized as either hereditary or acquired – due to impaired heme synthesis in the bone marrow. The degree of anemia is variable, but all forms show the presence of ring sideroblasts in the bone marrow aspirate when stained with Prussian blue.[1] Ring sideroblasts are erythroblasts with iron-laden granules surrounding the nucleus. In addition, patients with sideroblastic anemia often have these iron-laden granules in their circulating erythrocytes known as Pappenheimer bodies. In patients with refractory cases, iron overload becomes a complication leading to heart failure, diabetes, and endocrine dysfunction.

Etiology/Epidemiology

Sideroblasts are erythroblasts with one or more iron-containing granules within the cytoplasm and are found in normal bone marrow specimens. Ring sideroblasts, in which the erythroblasts have at least five granules covering at least one-third of the circumference of the nucleus, are not considered pathologic.[2] The iron in ring sideroblasts is stored in ferritin form in the mitochondria. Due to ineffective hemoglobin synthesis, the sideroblastic anemias are often classified as a microcytic anemia in spite of the macrocytes seen due to ineffective erythropoiesis.

Acquired sideroblastic anemias are under the classification of myelodysplastic syndromes.[2] They may arise de novo or be due to a previous insult to the marrow such as chemotherapy. (See Chapter 22.)

Pathophysiology

All cases of sideroblastic anemia, regardless of whether they are hereditary or acquired, are due to impaired synthesis of heme in the erythroid series in the bone marrow.[3] Heme is a noncovalent complex of reduced iron (ferrous Fe^{2+}) with protoporphyrin IX. Inadequate synthesis of protoporphyrin IX, failure of iron to properly couple with protoporphyrin IX, or other various mitochondrial abnormalities that affect mitochondrial iron transport will result in heme production defects. Iron utilization becomes abnormal, and hypochromia results.[4]

Hereditary Sideroblastic Anemia

The most common hereditary sideroblastic anemia is the X-linked form, which results from mutations that impair the amount of activity in mitochondrial enzyme 5-aminolevulinate synthase (ALAS).[5] ALAS is the rate-limiting catalyst of the first step in heme synthesis. While heme synthesis is impaired in deficiencies of ALAS, iron transport is not impaired, leading to mitochondrial overload.[6] Other inheritance patterns have been described associated with sideroblastic anemia; studies into these families have found various alterations with the heme synthesis pathway. Additionally, other genetic disorders have been associated with the presence of ring sideroblasts and are detailed in Table 7.1.

Acquired Sideroblastic Anemia

The most common acquired sideroblastic anemia is the myelodysplastic syndrome, refractory anemia with ringed sideroblasts. Also known as idiopathic refractory sideroblastic anemia, this disorder is due to various mutations in the RNA splicing machinery. Additionally, various drugs and metabolic derangements have been associated with acquired sideroblastic anemia, as detailed in Table 7.2.

Table 7.1 Hereditary causes of sideroblastic anemia

Nonsyndromic
- X-linked
- Autosomal dominant
- Autosomal recessive
- Erythropoietic protoporphyria
- Glutaredoxin 5 deficiency
- Mitochondrial transport defects (SLC25A38)

Syndromic
- Myopathy, lactic acidosis and sideroblastic anemia (MLASA)
- Sideroblastic anemia, B cell immunodeficiency, periodic fevers, and developmental delay (SIFD)
- X-linked with ataxia (XLSA/A)
- Pearson marrow-pancreas syndrome
- Thiamine-responsive megaloblastic anemia (TRMA)

Table 7.2 Acquired causes of sideroblastic anemia

Neoplastic/Myelodysplastic Syndromes

- Refractory anemia with ring sideroblasts (RARS)
- Refractory anemia with ring sideroblasts and thrombocytosis (RARS-T)
- Refractory cytopenia with multilineage dysplasia and ring sideroblasts (RCMD-RS)

Drugs
- Alcohol
- Chloramphenicol
- Isoniazid
- Linezolid

Copper deficiency

Zinc toxicity

Hypothermia

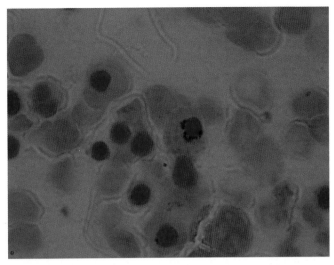

Figure 7.1 Bone marrow aspirate stained with Prussian Blue showing ring sideroblasts

Clinical Presentation (History/Physical Exam)

As is the case with all anemias, the degree of symptoms depends on the degree of anemia and the rate at which the disease is progressing. Patients may report fatigue and dyspnea on exertion. On exam, they may appear pale. While dyserythropoiesis may lead to an indirect bilirubinemia, rarely does it lead to significant jaundice. The spleen may or may not be palpable on exam depending on the degree of splenomegaly.

Patients with iron overload may exhibit signs of heart failure or have developed diabetes mellitus due to iron deposition in the heart and pancreas, respectively. Additionally, there may be bronzing of the skin, glucose intolerance, or arthropathies. Some patients may have profound hypothermia, although the association between hypothermia and ring sideroblasts is unclear. When related to certain other disorders such as porphyria or Pearson syndrome, the anemia is often a minor part of the overall clinical picture.

In the hereditary forms, patients present in late childhood or early adolescence. Some families are aware of the history of anemia but may not be aware of the ultimate diagnosis.

Diagnostic Evaluation/Lab Findings

The complete blood count is abnormal, showing some degree of anemia. However, the remainder of parameters (e.g., WBC, platelets) are variable in presentation, depending on the ultimate etiology. Hereditary sideroblastic anemia will often present as a microcytic anemia. In contrast, the acquired form, especially when present as part of a myelodysplastic syndrome, will often have an element of macrocytosis.[7]

Iron overload is common and is evidenced by increased serum iron, ferritin, and transferrin saturation along with decreased serum transferrin levels or total iron binding capacity. Imaging performed to evaluate the sequelae of iron overload may demonstrate iron deposition.[8] Given the profound iron overload sometimes seen in sideroblastic anemia,

it is important to exclude idiopathic hemochromatosis as the source. While both have evidence of iron overload and a family history of the disorder, the inheritance patterns are different, and the hematologic parameters are distinct. Patients with idiopathic hemochromatosis should have normal or high hemoglobin levels and a normal mean corpuscular volume.

Review of the red cell parameters from automated counters may show either a microcytic or normocytic cell population, but the red cell distribution width (RDW) is elevated, indicating a dimorphic population. The reticulocyte count is low, indicating a hypoproliferative marrow.

Iron studies show that patients have adequate or elevated iron stores. Ferritin is often elevated with a high transferrin saturation along with an elevated serum ferritin level. The total iron binding capacity (TIBC) is usually below or low-normal.

Review of the peripheral blood smear is crucial and may show siderotic granules, known as Pappenheimer bodies, within circulating erythrocytes.[9] The red cell population demonstrates anisocytosis and is dimorphic in line with the automated machine parameters. A detailed family history should be documented, and there may be value in examining the complete blood count and peripheral blood smear of family members if a hereditary form is suspected. If the sideroblastic anemia is due to a myelodysplastic syndrome such as refractory anemia with ring sideroblasts and thrombocytosis (RARS-T) or refractory cytopenia with multilineage dysplasia and ring sideroblasts (RCMD-RS), the peripheral blood smear may show abnormalities in other cell lines.[1]

Ultimately, all patients will require a bone marrow examination in order to confirm the diagnosis. While the trephine biopsy is useful in complete evaluation, the aspirate is of utmost importance in order to assess for the presence of ring sideroblasts (Figure 7.1). The presence of ring sideroblasts indicates pathology. The bone marrow aspirate of patients with myelodysplastic syndrome will show dyserythropoiesis. Other myeloid precursors often show dysplastic changes as well. It should be noted that ring sideroblasts may be present in a variety of conditions. While *necessary* for the diagnosis of sideroblastic anemia, their presence alone is not *sufficient* to make the diagnosis.

In those patients with an overlap between the myelodysplastic syndrome and a myeloproliferative disorder such as essential thrombocythemia or myelofibrosis, testing for JAK2 may show the V617F mutation. The presence of this mutation suggests better prognosis, although targeted therapy with a JAK2 inhibitor has not yet been studied in this population.[10]

Treatment and Prognosis

Hereditary Sideroblastic Anemia

Once a diagnosis of hereditary sideroblastic anemia is made, a trial of pyridoxine (100–200 mg/day orally) should be started and continued for at least 3 months. While only 25–50% of patients will respond to this therapy, those that do can be continued on pyridoxine indefinitely. The dose may be slowly titrated down after 3 months in order to find the lowest possible maintenance dose in order to reduce the likelihood of developing peripheral neuropathy.[11]

Acquired Sideroblastic Anemia

While pyridoxine may have therapeutic benefit in the hereditary forms of sideroblastic anemia, it is much less likely to be effective in the acquired forms. The treatment for sideroblastic anemia due to a myelodysplastic syndrome is supportive care, with use of transfusions as needed. Many patients may require long term transfusion support and are at risk of transfusional iron overload in addition to the iron overload associated with the disease. Chelation therapy should be considered in all patients with sideroblastic anemia requiring periodic transfusion.[12]

In myelodysplastic syndromes associated with ring sideroblasts, immunosuppression with corticosteroids or other agents such as cyclosporine has been used with varying amounts of success.[13] Trials of immunosuppression should be brief and discontinued if there is no evidence of benefit. Comprehensive management of the myelodysplastic syndromes is covered in Chapter 22.

If the acquired sideroblastic anemia is secondary to a behavioral factor such as alcoholism, abstinence generally results in reversal of the sideroblastic changes within several weeks, but the anemia may persist secondary to other complications of alcohol intake such as cirrhosis or splenomegaly. For sideroblastic anemia secondary to isoniazid, cessation of the drug results in complete reversibility of the condition. If isoniazid needs to be continued for treatment of tuberculosis, pyridoxine may be used to ameliorate the condition until the end of therapy. While rarely used anymore, chloramphenicol-induced

sideroblastic anemia is also completely reversible upon removal of the drug. Copper deficiency as a cause of sideroblastic anemia is reversible but may take several months.[14]

If caught early, idiopathic sideroblastic anemia has a prognosis associated with the severity of the anemia and the patient's risk of developing iron overload. Transfusion support with cautious management of iron overload extends survival.

As with other myelodysplastic syndromes, karyotype is important in myelodysplasias with sideroblastic anemia.[15,16] A normal karyotype has the most favorable prognosis, while monosomy 7 of deletion of 7p are associated with worse prognosis.

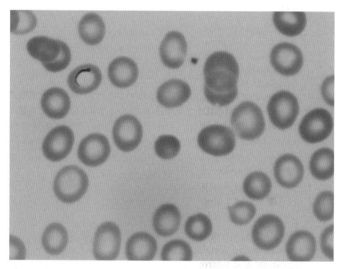

Figure 7.2 Peripheral Blood Smear

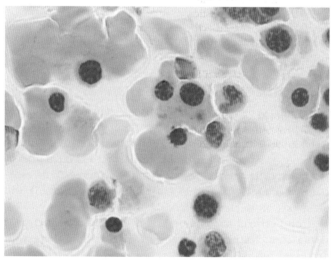

Figure 7.3 Bone marrow aspirate stained with Prussian Blue

Case Study

A 71-year-old man presents for evaluation due to fatigue. The complete blood count shows a hemoglobin of 9.1 mg/dL with a mean corpuscular volume of 101 fL. The leukocyte count, platelet count, and leukocyte differential are within the normal reference intervals. The peripheral blood smear is shown in Figure 7.2. A bone marrow examination, shown in Figure 7.3, demonstrates dyserythropoiesis and the presence of ring sideroblasts. There is no evidence of dysmyelopoiesis or dysmegakarypoiesis, and the blast count is 2%. Cytogenetics indicate a normal karyotype. The diagnosis of refractory anemia with ring sideroblasts is confirmed, and the patient is given a trial of pyridoxine without response. He requires red cell transfusion approximately every 4–6 weeks in order to prevent symptoms from his anemia.

References

1. Bottomley SS, Fleming MD. Sideroblastic anemia: diagnosis and management. *Hematology/Oncology Clinics of North America.* 2014; 28 (4):653–670. Epub 2014/07/30.

2. Mufti GJ, Bennett JM, Goasguen J, Bain BJ, Baumann I, Brunning R, et al. Diagnosis and classification of myelodysplastic syndrome: International Working Group on Morphology of Myelodysplastic Syndrome (IWGM-MDS) consensus proposals for the definition and enumeration of myeloblasts and ring sideroblasts. *Haematologica.* 2008; 93 (11):1712–1717. Epub 2008/10/08.

3. Alcindor T, Bridges KR. Sideroblastic anaemias. *British Journal of Haematology.* 2002; 116(4):733–743.

4. McLintock LA, Fitzsimons EJ. Erythroblast iron metabolism in sideroblastic and sideropenic states. *Hematology.* 2002; 7(3):189–195. Epub 2002/09/24.

5. Bottomley SS, Healy HM, Brandenburg MA, May BK. 5-Aminolevulinate synthase in sideroblastic anemias: mRNA and enzyme activity levels in bone marrow cells. *American Journal of Hematology.* 1992; 41(2):76–83.

6. Cazzola M, Invernizzi R, Bergamaschi G, Levi S, Corsi B, Travaglino E, et al. Mitochondrial ferritin expression in erythroid cells from patients with sideroblastic anemia. *Blood.* 2003; 101 (5):1996–2000. Epub 2002/10/31.

7. Rovo A, Stussi G, Meyer-Monard S, Favre G, Tsakiris D, Heim D, et al. Sideroblastic changes of the bone marrow can be predicted by the erythrogram of peripheral blood. *International Journal of Laboratory Hematology.* 2010; 32(3):329–335. Epub 2009/08/27.

8. Takagi S, Tanaka O, Origasa H, Miura Y. Prognostic significance of magnetic resonance imaging of femoral marrow in patients with myelodysplastic syndromes. *Journal of Clinical Oncology: Official Journal of the American Society of Clinical Oncology.* 1999; 17(1):277–283. Epub 1999/08/24.

9. Zarco MA, Feliu E, Rozman C, Masat T, Aymerich M, Jou JM, et al. Ultrastructural study of erythrocytes containing Pappenheimer bodies in a case of congenital sideroblastic anaemia (CSA). *British Journal of Haematology.* 1991; 78(4):577–578. Epub 1991/08/01.

10. Broseus J, Alpermann T, Wulfert M, Florensa Brichs L, Jeromin S, Lippert E, et al. Age, JAK2(V617F) and SF3B1 mutations are the main predicting factors for survival in refractory anaemia with ring sideroblasts and marked thrombocytosis. *Leukemia.* 2013; 27(9):1826–1831. Epub 2013/04/19.

11. Parry GJ, Bredesen DE. Sensory neuropathy with low-dose pyridoxine. *Neurology.* 1985; 35(10):1466–1468. Epub 1985/10/01.

12. Malcovati L. Red blood cell transfusion therapy and iron chelation in patients with myelodysplastic syndromes. *Clinical Lymphoma & Myeloma.* 2009; 9 Suppl 3:S305–311. Epub 2009/09/26.

13. Broliden PA, Dahl IM, Hast R, Johansson B, Juvonen E, Kjeldsen L, et al. Antithymocyte globulin and cyclosporine A as combination therapy for low-risk non-sideroblastic myelodysplastic syndromes. *Haematologica.* 2006; 91(5):667–770. Epub 2006/05/04.

14. Takeuchi M, Tada A, Yoshimoto S, Takahashi K. Anemia and neutropenia due to copper deficiency during long-term total parenteral nutrition. [Rinsho ketsueki] *The Japanese Journal of Clinical Hematology.* 1993; 34(2):171–176. Epub 1993/02/01.

15. Iwase O, Iwama H, Okabe S, Ando K, Yaguchi M, Miyazawa K, et al. Refractory anemia with ringed sideroblasts with a low IPSS score progressed rapidly with de novo appearance of multiple karyotypic abnormalities and into acute erythroleukemia (AML-M6A). *Leukemia Research.* 2000; 24 (7):597–600. Epub 2000/06/27.

16. Bernasconi P, Alessandrino EP, Boni M, Bonfichi M, Morra E, Lazzarino M, et al. Karyotype in myelodysplastic syndromes: relations to morphology, clinical evolution, and survival. *American Journal of Hematology.* 1994; 46(4):270–277. Epub 1994/08/01.

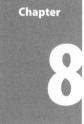

Chapter

The Thalassemia Syndromes

Madeleine M. Verhovsek, MD, FRCPC, and David H. K. Chui, MD, FRCPC

Introduction

Normal hemoglobin (Hb) is a heterotetramer comprised of two α-like and two β-like globin chains. In fetal life, HbF ($\alpha_2\gamma_2$) predominates. Beginning in the third trimester of gestation and through the first year after birth, HbF level gradually decreases to approximately 1% of the total hemoglobin. Concomitantly, HbA ($\alpha_2\beta_2$) production increases to about 95% and persists throughout adult life (Chapter 1).

Thalassemia is caused by globin gene mutations that lead to markedly decreased or absent globin chain production from the affected globin gene.[1] These mutations, now numbering more than 500, are found in all fetal and adult globin genes. However, β- and α-thalassemias affecting β- and α-globin genes, respectively, are by far the most important, and they manifest as microcytic, hypochromic anemia of varying severity.

The thalassemia syndromes are among the most common hereditary monogenic diseases and are increasingly important in global health.[2] Their high prevalence is ascribed to the carriers having a natural selective advantage against the severe form of malaria caused by *Plasmodium faciparum*. The molecular mechanisms for this protection are not yet fully understood.

Thalassemias originated in parts of the world where malaria was and may still be endemic, that is, sub-Saharan Africa, the Mediterranean Sea, the Black Sea and the Caspian Sea regions, the Middle East, Indian subcontinent, Southeast Asia, and Southern China. With population migrations during the past centuries, thalassemia syndromes are now found in every corner of the world. Their clinical severity varies from asymptomatic carriers to severe anemia in β-thalassemia, major, requiring lifelong transfusions, and to fetal demise in homozygous α^0-thalassemia.

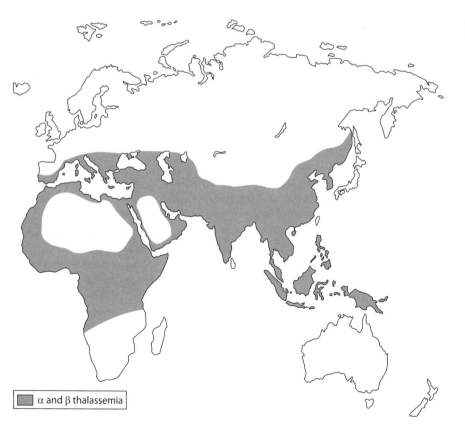

Figure 8.1 The world distribution of the origins of the α and β thalassemias[1]

α and β thalassemia

Beta-Thalassemia

Beta-Thalassemia Mutations and Pathophysiology

- There are more than 250 known β-thalassemia mutations. Most are point mutations or small insertions/deletions that interfere with either transcription, RNA splicing and polyadenylation signaling, or translation due to initiation codon, non-sense, and frame-shift mutations.[3,4] Those that result in markedly decreased β-globin chain production are known as β^+-thalassemia mutations; those that result in the absence of β-globin chain production are known as β^0-thalassemia mutations.

- There are "silent" mutations, so-called because the carriers do not have significant hematological abnormalities, which may belie their diagnosis.[4] However, in combination with other β-thalassemia mutations, they can cause moderate to severe anemia.

- Dominant β-thalassemia is caused by more than 40 mutations usually found in the second intron or third exon. A single copy of the mutated β-globin gene can lead to β-thalassemia intermedia or even more severe anemia, often with erythroid cell inclusion bodies.[4] The variant β-globin chains are characteristically extremely unstable.

- Deletions can also cause β-thalassemia, though relatively uncommon. Some deletions remove part or all of the β-globin gene. Others remove either the δ- and β-globin genes or $^A\gamma$-, δ-, and β-globin genes, known as $(\delta\beta)^0$- or $(^A\gamma\delta\beta)^0$-thalassemia deletions respectively, often with moderately elevated HbF expression but normal HbA_2 level.[4]

- There are other deletions that remove the β-locus control region (LCR), thus silencing the expression of all downstream β-like globin genes. Other large deletions remove the complete β-globin gene cluster on chromosome 11p15.4. Both cause $(\varepsilon^G\gamma^A\gamma\delta\beta)^0$-thalassemias. Heterozygotes for these deletions can present with fetal and neonatal hemolytic anemia of varying severity that evolves with age to assume a phenotype of simple β-thalassemia trait but with normal Hb A_2 level.[5]

Relatively few β-thalassemia mutations usually account for those found in most people in an area where thalassemia is common. These findings facilitate designing regional programs for population screening and family counseling.

The pathophysiology of β-thalassemia is largely due to imbalance of β- and α-globin chain synthesis, leading to excess of normally produced α-globin chains. These excess α-globin chains form precipitates, resulting in ineffective erythropoiesis and hemolysis (Figure 8.2). In addition, both chronic transfusions and ineffective erythropoiesis contribute to iron overload and subsequent organ damage.[1,6] In general, when excess α-globin chains are made worse, as by concomitant α-globin gene triplication, the β-thalassemia manifestations are more severe. Conversely, the concomitant inheritance of α-thalassemia could help improve β-thalassemia disease severity.[7]

Beta-Thalassemia Trait

Heterozygosity for β-thalassemia, also known as β-thalassemia trait or β-thalassemia minor, causes mild anemia, microcytosis, and hypochromia. These individuals are generally well. However, any superimposed causes of anemia, such as during pregnancy, might lead to more severe anemia.

Microcytosis with low mean corpuscular volume (MCV ~70 fL) or low mean corpuscular hemoglobin (MCH ~22 pg) without iron deficiency, regardless of Hb level, is the most important screening test for thalassemia carriers. Beta-thalassemia trait is usually characterized by elevated HbA_2 (above 3.5%). Rarely, β-thalassemia trait is not accompanied by elevated HbA_2, due to "silent" mutations, deletions that remove the δ-globin gene, concomitant δ-globin gene thalassemia, or missense mutations. Definitive genotyping by DNA-based diagnostics is needed for proper genetic counseling and for complicated cases.[8]

Individuals of reproductive age found to have β-thalassemia trait ought to have their partners tested in order to determine if they are at risk for conceiving offspring with clinically severe hemoglobinopathies such as β-thalassemia major, HbE/β-thalassemia, and HbS/β-thalassemia. When necessary, they ought to be referred for genetic counseling.

People with β-thalassemia trait might be mistaken to have iron deficiency and given iron replacement. Unnecessary iron supplementation should be avoided, as it can lead to iatrogenic iron overload and possible organ damage.

Clinical Vignette #1

A 54-year-old man of Italian heritage is seen by a hematologist for microcytic anemia. History of longstanding mild anemia. Denied family history of anemia. Previously on oral iron supplement for 4 years with no improvement in his hemoglobin or MCV. No history of overt bleeding. Screening colonoscopy normal. Not currently on any medications. Feels well. Negative review of systems. On examination, vital signs are normal. No overt pallor, normal cardiorespiratory exam, no splenomegaly.

His Hb is 11.8 g/dL, MCV 62 fL (Figures 8.4A and 8.4B), WBC 8,100, platelets 323,000; serum ferritin 577µg/l; normal creatinine. HbA_2 is 5.1% by high-performance liquid chromatography.

Comments: This is a classic presentation of β-thalassemia trait. The patient is from an ethnic background with high prevalence of thalassemia. Positive family history is helpful. However, lack of family history does not in any way exclude the possibility of hereditary hemoglobin disorders, because most heterozygotes are asymptomatic. He was treated with iron supplement in the past with no change in his hemoglobin or MCV. Ferritin is high. Further iron supplementation is not indicated. In fact, calculation of transferrin saturation is needed to assess for possible iron overload. He should be counseled on his diagnosis and instructed on the importance of carrier screening for

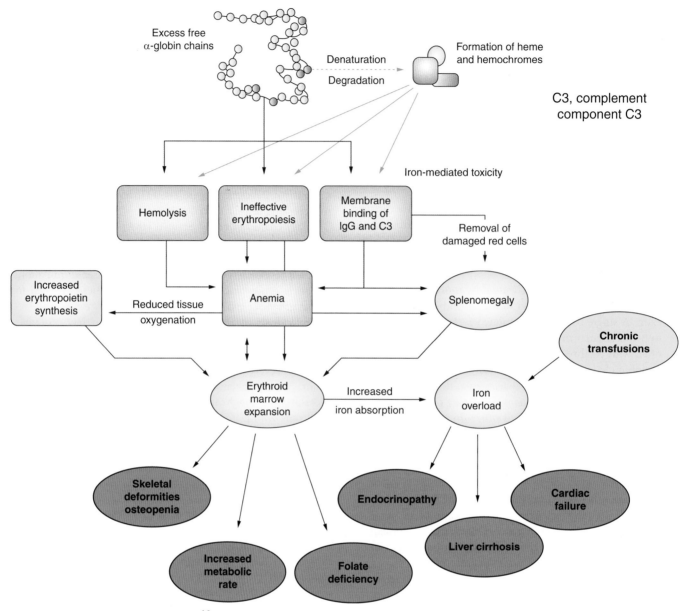

Figure 8.2 Pathophysiology of β-thalassemia[1,6]

other family members, particularly those at reproductive age, in order to assess possible risks of conceiving fetuses with β-thalassemia major.

Beta-Thalassemia Major

This severe form of thalassemia is caused by inheriting mutations in both β-globin genes. The affected neonates are well at birth but develop increasing anemia with time as "hemoglobin switching" occurs, accompanied by increasing γ-globin gene silencing and β-globin gene expression. By 4 months to 1 year old, these infants have pallor due to severe microcytic anemia, often accompanied by feeding difficulties, failure to thrive, and splenomegaly. For disease management, it is advisable to avail

oneself of the expertise and resources available at regional thalassemia treatment centers.

Complications and Management of Thalassemia Major[6,9–12]

Anemia and Transfusions

Once the diagnosis of β-thalassemia major is made, it is important to monitor these children carefully for some time in order to be certain of the severity of their baseline clinical and laboratory findings, which might warrant committing them to an extended, often lifelong, blood transfusion treatment program. Usually they are transfused every 3–4 weeks to maintain a hemoglobin level at more than 9.0–10.5 g/dL at all times. Inadequate transfusion can result in poor growth, bone

Table 8.1 Iron chelating agents – dosing, administration, and possible adverse effects

	Common starting dose and administration	Maximum daily dose	Possible adverse effects
Deferoxamine	20 mg/kg administered by subcutaneous infusion* over 8–12 hours, 5–7 nights per week	40 mg/kg	Infusion site reactions; vision or hearing abnormalities; skeletal and growth abnormalities; zinc deficiency; *Yersinia enterocolitica* infection.
Deferasirox	20–40 mg/kg by mouth daily (dispersible tablets – suspended in water). 14 mg/kg by mouth daily (film-coated tablets).	40 mg/kg (dispersible tablets). 28 mg/kg (film-coated tablets).	Rash, GI symptoms, mild elevation in transaminases, hearing impairment, nonprogressive elevation in serum creatinine.
Deferiprone	75 mg/kg/d in three divided doses by mouth daily	100 mg/kg	Agranulocytosis, arthralgias, zinc deficiency; mild GI symptoms and mild aminotransferase elevations.

* Deferoxamine can also be administered intravenously. Table adapted from Verhovsek and McFarlane (2012).[14]

marrow expansion, thalassemic facies, osteopenia, hepatosplenomegaly, and other complications.

Splenomegaly with hypersplenism manifested as increased transfusion requirement (more than 200 ml of packed red blood cells per kg of body weight per year) that is not due to other causes such as alloimmunization is an indication to consider splenectomy.[11,12] Care should be taken to guard against and treat postsplenectomy complications such as fulminant infections, thrombo-embolism, and pulmonary hypertension. In elective splenectomy, perioperative immunization should be performed according to published guidelines.[13]

Patients on a chronic transfusion program should first be vaccinated for hepatitis B virus. Risks associated with RBC transfusion include alloimmunization, transfusion-transmitted infection, and hemolytic or febrile transfusion reactions. To avoid alloimmunization, RBC phenotyping or genotyping can be undertaken on the patient in order to provide matched RBCs for transfusions.

Iron Overload and Chelation

Due to long-term transfusions and enhanced intestinal iron absorption as a result of ineffective erythropoiesis, β-thalassemia major patients invariably develop iron overload that can cause cardiac, liver, and endocrine toxicities. If untreated, iron overload is fatal, often due to heart failure in the second or third decade of life. Iron chelation is an essential therapy for disease management, usually commencing at 2–3 years of age and continuing throughout life. Currently there are three chelating agents available (Table 8.1). Deferasirox is available as dispersible or film-coated tablets.

Early in the course of a chronic transfusion regimen, the cumulative volume of RBCs transfused can be monitored in concert with trends in serum ferritin. After approximately 10--20 transfusions and when the serum ferritin level is persistently elevated >1,000 μg/ml, chelation therapy may be initiated. Liver MRI (using either R2 or R2* analysis) has now largely replaced liver biopsy to estimate liver iron concentration (LIC). Chelation should be initiated when LIC is above the normal range for

healthy volunteers. Some guidelines recommend starting chelation when LIC is >7 mg/g of dry tissue weight. Cardiac iron overload can also be accurately assessed with cardiac T2* MRI. Cardiac function should be monitored using echocardiography and ECG, although these modalities are unlikely to detect early stages of cardiac iron overload.

Growth Delay and Endocrinopathy

Short stature, delayed puberty, hypogonadotropic hypogonadism, hypothyroidism, diabetes mellitus, and hypoparathyroidism may all occur and are primarily due to endocrine gland iron overload. Routine monitoring for these complications is required, with prompt medical management and endocrine specialist consultation as necessary.

Osteoporosis

This is a common complication with multifactorial etiology. Preventative care includes adherence to appropriate transfusion thresholds and chelation therapy. Adolescent and adult patients should have routine bone density monitoring. First-line therapy for osteopenia is lifestyle modification (e.g., increase weight-bearing activities and intake of calcium-containing foods) accompanied by vitamin D and calcium supplementation. Specialist consultation is recommended for patients with osteoporosis or worsening osteopenia despite conservative management.

Extramedullary Hematopoiesis

Without adequate transfusions, extramedullary hematopoietic masses may form including in and around the spine, leading to possible neurological sequelae. Treatment must be individualized based on symptoms and size and location of the mass. Therapeutic modalities include radiation therapy and chronic RBC transfusion, often with higher target hemoglobin level to suppress ineffective erythropoiesis.

Bone Marrow Transplantation and Other Disease-Modifying Therapy

Hematopoietic stem-cell transplantation can be curative but has associated morbidity and mortality. The best outcomes are for young children without hepatomegaly and transplanted with HLA-matched sibling donor.[15,16] Pharmacological agents to increase HbF production, such as arginine butyrate, hydroxyurea, and erythropoietin, have been tried with inconsistent results.[17]

Significant progress has been made in recent years on understanding the molecular mechanisms responsible for hemoglobin switching. There are three major HbF quantitative trait loci on chromosomes 2, 6, and 11. Transcription factors KLF1, BCL11A, and MYB play pivotal roles in modulating HbF expression and are potential targets for gene editing or search for small therapeutic molecules.[18] The outlook for success in gene therapy for thalassemias is now brighter than ever.[19]

With proper medical management, β-thalassemia major has become a chronic disease. Many patients now live to be in their fifth or sixth decade, with anticipated normal life expectancy of individuals receiving attentive medical care from an early age. With proper transfusion and chelation management, many patients are able to become parents themselves.[20]

Prevention

If both parents are β-thalassemia carriers, they have a 25% risk in each pregnancy of conceiving a fetus with β-thalassemia major. Ideally, couples should be screened prior to their first pregnancy. At the least, a pregnant woman must be screened during the first trimester to find out if she is a carrier of β-thalassemias, and if so, her partner ought to be similarly tested as soon as possible.

Community education, carrier screening, genetic counseling, and antenatal diagnosis by chorionic villi biopsy or amniocentesis are essential components of a preventive program for β-thalassemia major. Noninvasive sampling of fetal DNA for antenatal diagnosis through maternal peripheral blood may soon be possible for clinical application. Preimplantation genetic diagnosis (PGD) is carried out in highly specialized centers.

This preventive program has been successfully implemented in some Mediterranean countries, resulting in many fewer affected newborns.[21] This public health initiative has also been increasingly recognized as a priority in Southeast Asia and in Southern China.[22]

Clinical Vignette #2

A 27-year-old woman with β-thalassemia major. Newly arrived to North America from Southeast Asia. She presents to her primary care provider with complaints of fatigue and shortness of breath on exertion (one flight of stairs, walking 1–2 blocks).

Thalassemia was diagnosed at 1 year of age, and she has been transfusion dependent since that time. She typically received 3 units red blood cell transfusion every 4 weeks, but her last transfusion was 6 weeks previously. She had no known history of hepatitis B, hepatitis C, or HIV; no known alloantibodies; no history of transfusion reactions. She had no surgical history (specifically no history of cholecystectomy or splenectomy). She

was amenorrheic for the past 2 or 3 years. She was known to have hepatic iron overload, having had liver biopsy performed twice in the past 15 years (results not available). She has never had hepatic or cardiac MRI. She had been on deferoxamine (age 8–15) then was switched to deferiprone 1,500 mg TID, which was stopped 2 years ago due to lack of funds. On examination, she had short stature and was pale. Normal cardiorespiratory exam. Splenomegaly (4 cm below LCM).

Her Hb was 6.2 g/dL, MCV 70, RDW 32.1, WBC 3,900, ANC 2,300, platelet count 160,000. Peripheral blood smear shows a dual population of hypochromic, microcytic, and normochromic, normocytic cells. Ferritin 6,250 μg/L, AST 120 U/L, ALT 145 U/L, GGT 52 U/L, ALP 78 U/L, total bilirubin 62 μmol/L, conjugated bilirubin 14 μmol/L, normal creatinine; blood group A+, antibody screen negative; negative hepatitis B and C serology; normal calcium; low vitamin D; normal TSH, free T4, fasting glucose; low FSH and LH; negative βHCG. Echocardiogram showed normal valves and biventricular structure; LVEF (left ventricular ejection fraction) 60%. DEXA (bone densitometry) scan showed Z-score −2.2 in femoral neck, −3.1 in spine.

R2 liver MRI showed LIC 36 mg/g dry tissue wt (normal reference range is 0.8–1.8 mg/g). Cardiac T2* MRI shows an average T2* measurement 10.3 ms (normal reference range is >20ms)

Comments: This patient had significant complications of poorly managed β-thalassemia major. Ideally, she should be referred to a regional thalassemia treatment center for consultation and recommendations.

She required reinitiation of her chronic transfusion program, with target pretransfusion hemoglobin of 9.0–10.5 g/dL. Due to the severity of her hepatic and cardiac iron overload, an intensive chelation regimen should be implemented. Options could include single-agent deferasirox, deferiprone or deferoxamine (subcutaneous or continuous intravenous), or combined chelation therapy. Close monitoring for improvement of iron overload and drug adverse effects was required.

Her symptoms of fatigue and shortness of breath were likely due to her anemia. Other cardiorespiratory evaluation should be considered. She had hypogonadotropic hypogonadism, causing amenorrhea. Endocrinology consultation would help plan treatment for the amenorrhea, low FSH/LH, and low bone mineral density. Referral to social services was needed for evaluation of her socioeconomic needs and to provide appropriate assistance. She ought to be introduced to a local thalassemia patient support group.

Beta-Thalassemia Intermedia

This refers to a group of β-thalassemia disorders with a broad spectrum of disease severity varying between that of β-thalassemia major and trait (Figure 8.4C).[23] The diagnosis often occurs after 1 year of age or older, reflecting their milder disease manifestations. Most patients require infrequent RBC transfusions. However, some patients develop increasing anemia with age and may become transfusion dependent.

Their globin genotypes are varied: (1) compound heterozygosity for a severe (β^0) and a mild (β^+) or silent β-thalassemia mutations with or without concomitant α-thalassemia mutation or hereditary propensity for elevated HbF expression; (2) compound heterozygosity for a β-thalassemia mutation with either $(\delta\beta)^0$- or $(^A\gamma\delta\beta)^0$-thalassemia deletion; (3) heterozygosity for a severe β^0-thalassemia mutation in combination with α-globin gene triplication or quadruplication; and (4) dominant β-thalassemia mutation.

These patients generally appear to be well, but they must be followed carefully because with time, they too can develop many of the complications as in β-thalassemia major. These include iron overload due to increased gastrointestinal iron absorption and intermittent transfusions and its associated complications. Others are splenomegaly, cholelithiasis, thalassemic facies, chronic leg ulcers, osteoporosis, extramedullary hematopoiesis, and heart failure.

Modest improvement to decrease the excess α-globin chains in these patients, such as by increasing γ-globin chain synthesis, can significantly improve hemoglobin level. Medications such as hydroxyurea and arginine butyrate and its oral derivatives have been tried with variable efficacy.

HbE/β-Thalassemia

HbE is a mildly unstable variant hemoglobin due to β-globin gene codon 26 GAG>AAG or glutamic acid to lysine mutation. This mutation creates a cryptic RNA splice site and is associated with a β^+-thalassemia phenotype. HbE ranks as either the second or third most common variant hemoglobin worldwide and is found mostly in Southeast Asia, Eastern half of the Indian subcontinent, and neighboring countries. In Thailand, for example, HbE/β-thalassemia is of public health importance.[24]

HbE heterozygotes are well. They have minimal anemia with 30% HbE. HbE homozygotes are also asymptomatic. They have mild anemia with microcytosis, hypochromia, many target cells, and slightly elevated HbF level (Figure 8.4D).

Patients with HbE/β-thalassemia have variable disease severity. Once the diagnosis is made, it is imperative to monitor these children for some time in order to ascertain whether they have a severe disease phenotype with severe microcytic anemia, markedly elevated HbF, and growth retardation and require regular transfusions. They are at risk for all the complications found in β-thalassemia major. A patient with transfusion-dependent HbE/β^0-thalassemia was treated by gene therapy and became transfusion independent, which has been sustained now for more than 7 years after the treatment.[25]

Other patients with HbE/β-thalassemia may be less anemic and relatively well without the need for regular transfusions. Patients who inherit a mild β^+- instead of β^0-thalassemia mutation, α-thalassemia, or HbF quantitative trait loci such as the *XmnI* site 5' to the $^G\gamma$-globin gene usually associated with increased HbF may have a milder disease course.

There are interactions between HbE and α-thalassemia or different variant hemoglobins resulting in many disease phenotypes in Southeast Asia. In particular, AEBart's disease due to coinheritance of HbH disease and heterozygous HbE and EFBart's disease due to coinheritance of HbH disease and either homozygous HbE or HbE/β-thalassemia have moderate anemia similar to the thalassemia intermedia phenotype.

Alpha-Thalassemia

The α-globin gene cluster is located on chromosome 16p13.3, consisting of an embryonic ζ- and 2 α-globin gene loci. Each person usually has four α-globin genes, two on each chromosome 16. Alpha-thalassemia is often caused by deletion of one to four α-globin genes, although single nucleotide mutations or small insertions/deletions are also found.

Alpha-Thalassemia Trait

Deletion or mutation of a single α-globin gene does not lead to abnormal clinical or laboratory findings (Table 8.2). Deletion or mutation involving two α-globin genes either *in cis* (both on the same chromosome 16) or *in trans* (one on each of the two chromosomes 16) can cause microcytosis (MCV ~70 fL) and hypochromia (MCH ~22 pg) but not severe anemia. Affected individuals might be mistaken to have iron deficiency, and care should be taken to avoid giving iron supplement unnecessarily.

HbH Disease

Patients with HbH disease have only one active α-globin gene, often due to the deletion of three α-globin genes.[26] The excess β-globin chains form β_4 homotetramer, known as HbH, which is unstable and forms intracellular precipitates, causing apoptosis, ineffective erythropoiesis, and hemolysis. Approximately 20% of HbH disease is caused by deletion of two α-globin genes *in cis* plus a nondeletional α-thalassemia mutation such as Hb Constant Spring (α2 codon 142 TAA>CAA or Term>Gln) involving one of the two remaining α-globin genes. Patients with these "nondeletional HbH diseases" are generally more anemic and need to be transfused more often.[26–28] Rarely, inheritance of nondeletional mutations involving two α-globin genes can present clinically as HbH disease.[26]

Patients with HbH disease have moderate microcytic hypochromic anemia (Table 8.2) yet are often clinically well. Ingestion of oxidative compounds or drugs, hypersplenism, pregnancy, and febrile or Parvovirus B19 infections can precipitate severe anemia and need for transfusions. Adult patients may have hepatosplenomegaly, cholelithiasis, iron overload not necessarily related to transfusions, extramedullary hematopoiesis, and thromboembolic disorders. The natural history of HbH disease has not been well studied. The optimal care for pregnant women with HbH disease[29] and the effect of the disease upon fetal, neonatal, and childhood development are two areas that still await more rigorous investigation.

Table 8.2 Hematologic data on adults with different α-globin genotype

Gender	Number of adults	α-Globin genotype	Clinical disorder	Hb (g/dL)	RBC (10^{12}/L)	MCV (fL)	MCH (pg)
Men	–	αα/αα	Normal	15.5 ± 1.0	5.2 ± 0.4	90 ± 5	30 ± 2
	81	– α/αα	Silent	14.3 ± 1.4	5.4 ± 0.6	81 ± 7	26 ± 2
	22	$α^T$α/αα	α-Thalassemia	14.5 ± 0.9	5.8 ± 0.5	76 ± 5	25 ± 2
	31	– α/– α	α-Thalassemia trait	13.9 ± 1.7	6.0 ± 0.8	72 ± 4	23 ± 1
	63	– –/αα		13.7 ± 1.1	6.3 ± 0.6	69 ± 4	22 ± 2
	6	– α/$α^T$α		12.3 ± 1.0	5.8 ± 0.8	66 ± 3	21 ± 2
	28	– –/– α	HbH disease	11.1 ± 1.1	6.1 ± 0.8	65 ± 7	19 ± 2
	6	– –/$α^T$α		10.5 ± 1.0	5.1 ± 0.3	68 ± 6	19 ± 2
Women	–	αα/αα	Normal	14.0 ± 1.0	4.6 ± 0.3	90 ± 5	30 ± 2
	106	– α/αα	Silent	12.6 ± 1.2	4.9 ± 0.5	81 ± 7	26 ± 2
	17	$α^T$α/αα	α-Thalassemia	12.5 ± 0.6	5.2 ± 0.5	76 ± 5	25 ± 2
	45	– α/– α	α-Thalassemia trait	12.0 ± 1.0	5.3 ± 0.5	72 ± 4	23 ± 1
	83	– –/αα		12.1 ± 1.1	5.6 ± 0.5	69 ± 4	22 ± 2
	6	– α/$α^T$α		10.6 ± 0.6	5.1 ± 0.4	66 ± 3	21 ± 2
	59	– –/– α	HbH disease	9.4 ± 1.2	5.1 ± 0.8	65 ± 7	19 ± 2
	5	– –/$α^T$α		8.5 ± 0.7	4.7 ± 0.7	68 ± 6	19 ± 2

Results are expressed as mean ± SD. – denote deletion of a single α-globin gene. $α^T$ denotes nondeletional α-thalassemia mutation. Table adapted from Higgs (2001).[1]

Diagnosis

Incubation of HbH disease peripheral blood with a mild oxidant dye such as brilliant cresyl blue will cause precipitation of HbH to form intraerythrocytic inclusion bodies, easily visualized by light microscopy (Figures 8.4E and 8.4F). This relatively simple test is highly diagnostic of HbH disease but unfortunately is not carried out in many clinical laboratories in the United States nowadays. HbH can be identified by high-performance liquid chromatography (HPLC) or isoelectric focusing (IEF). Patients with HbH disease who are also carriers of β-globin variants such as HbE, S, C, or β-thalassemia mutation have much less HbH, which can confound the correct diagnosis.[26] DNA-based tests are needed to provide definitive diagnosis of α-globin gene deletions and non-deletional mutations.

Treatment

Treatment is primarily supportive, including folic acid supplement, prompt treatment of infections especially in children, and transfusions to combat severe anemia when necessary. Oxidative compounds or medications are to be avoided, as is iron supplementation without proven iron deficiency.

Other HbH Disease Syndromes

The most severe form is the rare HbH hydrops fetalis syndrome, usually caused by "nondeletional HbH disease."[30] The affected fetuses have severe anemia, congenital malformation, and even fetal demise similar to the Hb Barts hydrops fetalis syndrome.

There are three other rare HbH syndromes: (1) ATR–16 syndrome, caused by extensive deletions of chromosome 16p telomere associated with mental retardation;[31] (2) ATR-X syndrome due to mutation in *ATRX* gene on chromosome Xq13, also associated with severe mental retardation;[31] (3) ATMDS is an acquired α-thalassemia associated with myelodysplastic syndrome found in elderly men and caused also by somatic mutation in *ATRX* gene.[32]

Clinical Vignette #3

A 62-year-old woman was seen in the emergency department for dyspnea and fatigue. Born in Cambodia, lived in the United States for many years, and worked in a health-related field. In the past, she reported occasional mild dyspnea on exertion but otherwise was in reasonably good health. She denied history of blood transfusions. Stopped smoking cigarettes 15 years ago. She was on iron supplement. No family history of anemia. She was afebrile and had splenomegaly (12 cm below LCM) but no hepatomegaly.

Her Hb was 8.7 g/dL; RBC 5.4×10^6/mm³, MCV 54 fL; MCH 16 pg; WBC 6,500; platelet count 185,000; serum ferritin 300. Peripheral blood smears showed microcytosis, hypochromia, polychromasia, and some degree of poikilocytosis. Bone marrow aspiration revealed erythroid hyperplasia and dyserythropoiesis. Chest X-rays and subsequent CT revealed paraspinal masses, one 3 × 5 cm from T9 to T11, and two other smaller ones. Needle biopsy revealed features consistent with extramedullary hematopoiesis.

Hemoglobin analysis by high-performance liquid chromatography was done and showed Hb A_2 1.8 %, a small early

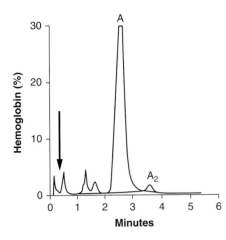

Figure 8.A
Hemoglobin analysis by high-performance liquid chromatography (HPLC), showing HbA and minor components of HbA$_2$ and HbF. There is a fast eluting (at ~0.4 minute) hemoglobin fraction that could be consistent with HbH.

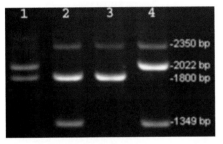

Figure 8.B Gel electrophoresis of gap-PCR amplicons. Lane 1, known (– α$^{3.7}$ / α α); Lane 2, known (– –^{SEA} / α α); Lane 3, known (α α / α α); Lane 4, patient with HbH disease (– α$^{3.7}$ / – –^{SEA}). Adapted from Benz Jr. et al. (2011).[33]

eluting (at ~ 0.4 min) hemoglobin fraction that could be consistent with HbH, and the rest being HbA (Figure 8.A). DNA-based gap-polymerase chain reaction (PCR) test was done and showed that the patient had HbH disease, with deletion of three α-globin genes – α$^{3.7}$ / – –^{SEA} (Figure 8.B).

Comments: The differential diagnoses for microcytic hypochromic anemia include iron deficiency, anemia of chronic disease, sideroblastic anemia, and thalassemia. The ethnic background, the marked microcytosis, and polychromasia would favor the diagnosis of thalassemia. This case reinforces that, while positive family history is helpful, the lack of family history does not in any way negate the possibility of thalassemia.

The differential diagnoses of thalassemias include β-thalassemia intermedia caused by β$^+$/β$^+$-thalassemia mutations, HbE/β-thalassemia mutation, or HbH disease including the "nondeletional" form. Acquired HbH disease, usually found in elderly men with myeloproliferative disease, is an unlikely possibility. Possible β-thalassemia intermedia due to β$^+$/β$^+$-thalassemia mutations was ruled out by the presence of HbA documented by HPLC. DNA-based globin genotyping provided the definitive diagnosis of HbH disease (Figure 8.B).

If symptomatic, irradiation may be necessary to avert compression complication of the extramedullary masses. Transfusions are needed to ameliorate severe anemia and to suppress endogenous ineffective erythropoiesis. Iron supplement ought not be given to HbH disease patients unless iron deficiency is documented. The patient and her family physician ought to be thoroughly informed about HbH disease and its potential complications. Screening

among family members and genetic counseling are important in order to assess and avert possible reproductive risk for the devastating Hb Barts hydrops fetalis syndrome.

Hb Barts Hydrops Fetalis Syndrome

This is the most severe form of α-thalassemia. It is caused by deletions removing all α-globin genes, but sparing either one or both embryonic ζ-globin genes.[34] The affected fetuses have Hb Barts (γ$_4$), which is incapable of oxygen delivery to tissues. These fetuses survive in utero on embryonic Hb Portland 1 (ζ$_2$γ$_2$) but invariably succumb in late second or early third trimester. The early onset of severe anemia and tissue hypoxia results in heart failure and impedes organogenesis as well as motor and cognitive development (Figure 8.3). In addition, this syndrome is accompanied by serious maternal morbidity and even mortality (Figure 8.3).

Epidemiology

The deletion of two α-globin genes *in cis* of the Southeast Asian type (– –^{SEA}) is very common in Southeast Asia and Southern China. The carrier rate in the general population varies from 4% in Southern China to 14% in Northern Thailand.[34,35] Homozygosity of (– –^{SEA}) deletion is by far the most common cause for Hb Barts hydrops fetalis syndrome there. In many areas, this devastating disease outnumbers β-thalassemia major. For example, in 1,240 antenatal diagnoses carried out in Taiwan, there were 220 fetuses with Hb Barts hydrops fetalis syndrome compared to 47 with β-thalassemia major.[36] Rarely, this syndrome has also been described among Mediterranean populations. With population migrations, this syndrome is now encountered throughout the world. Yet it is not well recognized by many health care providers because the vast majority of affected fetuses do not survive. There are reports of affected newborns who survived after either in utero or postnatal transfusions followed by regular transfusions and iron chelation thereafter. With few exceptions, many of these children had congenital, motor, and/or cognitive abnormalities.[37]

Diagnosis

Ultrasonography is highly reliable in the diagnosis of this syndrome as early as the 12th week of gestation, based on placental thickness, fetal cardiothoracic ratio, and middle cerebral artery peak systolic velocity measurements.[38]

The definitive diagnosis is by DNA-based globin genotyping of fetal genomic DNA obtained by chorionic villi biopsy or by amniocentesis. Fetal blood sample can be obtained by cordocentesis during the second trimester, but this procedure is fraught with serious complications. Hemoglobin analysis of fetal blood would yield Hb Barts (γ$_4$) and 10–20% Hb Portland 1 (ζ$_2$γ$_2$) but no Hb F or Hb A.

Prevention

If both parents have α-thalassemia trait due to deletion of two α-globin genes in cis, they have a 25% risk in each pregnancy

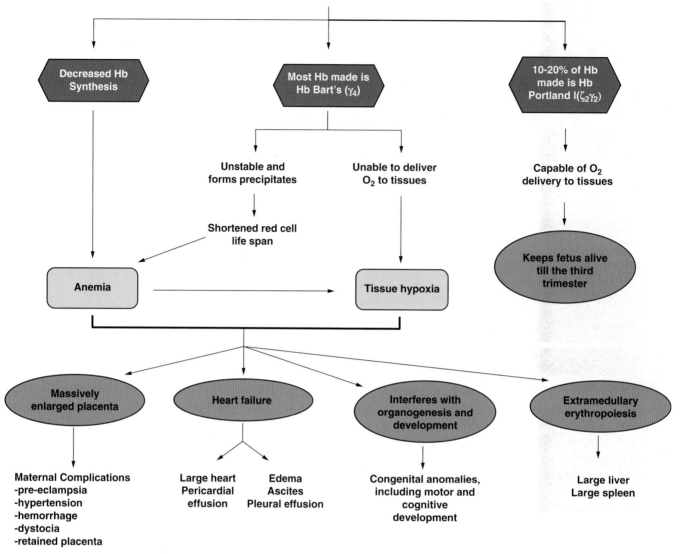

Figure 8.3 Pathophysiology of Hb Barts Hydrops Fetalis syndrome caused by deletions removing all α-globin genes.[34]

of conceiving a fetus with Hb Barts hydrops fetalis syndrome. People with α-thalassemia trait are asymptomatic but usually have borderline anemia with microcytosis and hypochromia (Table 8.2) without elevated HbA₂.

It should be noted that β-thalassemia trait carriers with elevated HbA₂ can also be concomitant carriers of α-thalassemia trait. These individuals therefore might be at risk for conceiving fetuses with either β-thalassemia major or Hb Barts hydrops fetalis syndrome, depending on their partner's globin genotype. Therefore, it is advisable to determine α-globin genotype in all β-thalassemia trait carriers in order to determine all possible reproductive risks.

Successful preventive programs will need to have government and community support in order to undertake public education, carrier screening, genetic counseling, and antenatal diagnosis.[21,22] If successfully implemented, couples at risk of

conceiving fetuses with these devastating disorders will be spared serious medical and psychological ordeals in their quest to have families with children.

a. β-Thalassemia trait with microcytosis, hypochromia, anisopoikilocytosis, teardrop cells.
b. β-Thalassemia trait with basophilic stippling.
c. β-Thalassemia intermedia with microcytosis, marked hypochromia, anisopoikilocytosis, basophilic stippling, and nucleated red blood cell.
d. Hb EE with microcytosis, hypochromia, and target cells.
e. HbH disease with microcytosis, marked hypochromia, and anisopoikilocytosis.
f. HbH disease with HbH inclusion bodies stained with brilliant cresyl blue dye.

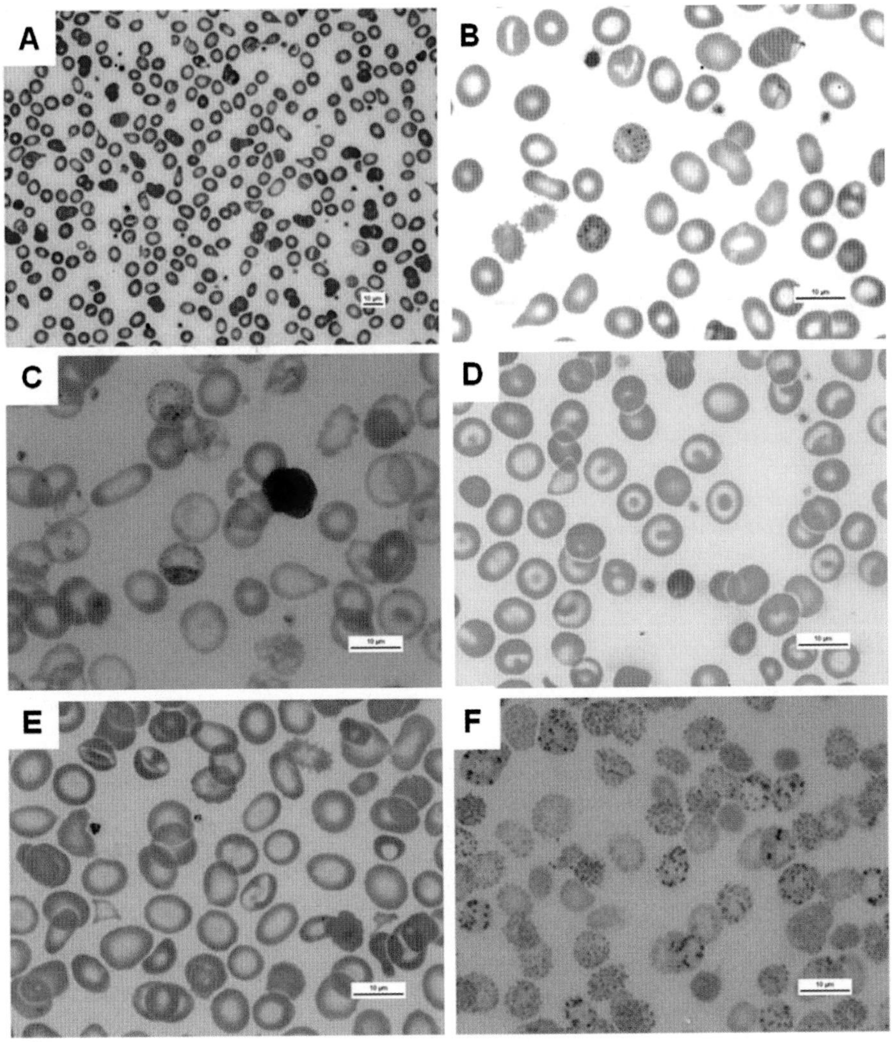

Figure 8.4 Photomicrographs of peripheral blood smears.

References

1. Weatherall DJ, Clegg JB. *The Thalassaemia Syndromes*, 4th ed. Oxford, Blackwell Science; 2001.

2. Weatherall DJ. Thalassemia as a global health problem: recent progress toward its control in the developing countries. *Ann N Y Acad Sci.* 2010; 1202:17–23.

3. Patrinos GP, Giardine B, Riemer C, et al. Improvements in the HbVar database of human hemoglobin variants and thalassemia mutations for population and sequence variation studies. *Nucl Acids Res.* 2004;32: D537–541. http://globin.cse.psu.edu/hbvar/menu.html

4. Thein SL. The molecular basis of β-thalassemia. In: Weatherall DJ, Schechter AN, Nathan DG, eds. *Hemoglobin and Its Diseases.*

Cold Spring Harbor, NY: Cold Spring Harbor Laboratory Press; 2013:159–182.

5. Verhovsek MM, Shah NR, Wilcox I, et al. Severe fetal and neonatal hemolytic anemia due to a 198 kb deletion removing the complete β-globin gene cluster. *Pediatr Blood Cancer.* 2012; 59:941–944.

6. Olivieri NF. The β-Thalassemias. *N Engl J Med.* 1999; 341:99–109.

7. Krishnamurti L, Chui DHK, Dallaire M, et al. Co-inheritance of α-thalassemia-1 and hemoglobin E/β[0]-thalassemia: important implications for neonatal screening and genetic counseling. *J Pediatr.* 1998; 132:863–865.

8. Luo H-Y, Chui DHK. Diverse haematological phenotypes of

β-thalassemia carriers. *Ann N Y Acad Sci.* 2016; 1368:49–55.

9. Cunningham MJ, Macklin EA, Neufeld EJ, et al. Complications of β-thalassemia major in North America. *Blood.* 2004; 104:34–39.

10. Rund D, Rachmilewitz EA. β-Thalassemia. *N Engl J Med.* 2005; 353:1135–1146.

11. Rachmilewitz EA, Giardina PJ. How I treat thalassemia. *Blood.* 2011; 118:3479–3488.

12. Higgs DR, Engel JD, Stamatoyannopoulos G. Thalassemia. *Lancet.* 2012; 379:373–383.

13. Centers for Disease Control and Prevention. Advisory Committee on Immunization Practices Recommended Immunization Schedules for Persons Aged 0 Through 18 Years and Adults

Aged 19 Years and Older—United States, 2013. *MMWR.* 2013; 62 (Suppl 1).

14. Verhovsek M, McFarlane A. Abnormalities in red blood cells. In: McKean S, ed. *Principles and Practice of Hospital Medicine*, 1st ed. McGraw-Hill Professional; 2012.

15. Sabloff M, Chandy M, Wang Z, et al. HLA-matched sibling bone marrow transplantation for β-thalassemia major. *Blood.* 2011; 117:1745–1750.

16. Locatelli F, Kabbara N, Ruggeri A, et al. Outcome of patients with hemoglobinopathies given either cord blood or bone marrow transplantation from an HLA-identical sibling. *Blood.* 2013; 122:1072–1078.

17. Musallam KM, Taher AT, Cappellini MD, et al. Clinical experience with fetal hemoglobin induction therapy in patients with β-thalassemia. *Blood.* 2013; 121:2199–2212.

18. Canver MC, Orkin SH. Customizing the genome as therapy for the β-hemoglobinopathies. *Blood.* 2016; 127:2536–2545.

19. Thompson AA, Kwiatkowski J, Rasko J, et al. Lentiglobin gene therapy for transfusion-dependent β-thalassemia: update from the Northstar Hgb-204 phase 1/2 clinical study. *Blood.* 2016; 128:Abstract 1175.

20. Thompson AA, Kim HY, Singer ST, et al. Pregnancy outcomes in women with thalassemia in North America and the UK. *Am J Hematol.* 2013; 88:771–773.

21. Cao A, Kan YW. The prevention of thalassemia. In: Weatherall DJ, Schechter AN, Nathan DG, eds. *Hemoglobin and Its Diseases.* Cold Spring Harbor, NY: Cold Spring

Harbor Laboratory Press; 2013:285–299.

22. Hvistendahl M. China heads off deadly blood disorder. *Science.* 2013; 340:677–678.

23. Taher AT, Musallam KM, Cappellini MD, et al. Optimal management of β thalassaemia intermedia. *Br J Haematol.* 2011; 152:512–523.

24. Fucharoen S, Weatherall DJ. The hemoglobin E thalassemias. In: *Hemoglobin and Its Diseases.* Weatherall DJ, Schechter AN, Nathan DG, eds. Cold Spring Harbor, NY: Cold Spring Harbor Laboratory Press; 2013:229–243.

25. Cavazzana-Calvo M, Payen E, Negre O, et al. Transfusion independence and HMGA2 activation after gene therapy of human β-thalassemia. *Nature.* 2010; 467:318–322.

26. Chui DHK, Fucharoen S, Chan V. Hemoglobin H disease: not necessarily a benign disorder. *Blood.* 2003; 101:791–800.

27. Chen FE, Ooi C, Ha SY, et al. Genetic and clinical features of hemoglobin H disease in Chinese patients. *N Engl J Med.* 2000; 343:544–550.

28. Lal A, Goldrich ML, Haines DA, et al. Heterogeneity of hemoglobin H disease in childhood. *N Engl J Med.* 2011; 364:710–718.

29. Tongsong T, Srisupundit K, Luewan S. Outcomes of pregnancies affected by hemoglobin H disease. *Int J Gynaecol Obstet.* 2009; 104:206–208.

30. Lorey F, Charoenkwan P, Witkowska HE, et al. Hb H hydrops foetalis syndrome: a case report and review of literature. *Br J Haematol.* 2001; 115:72–78.

31. Higgs DR, Buckle VJ, Gibbons R, Steensma D. Unusual types of α

thalassemia. In: *Disorders of Hemoglobin Genetics, Pathophysiology, and Clinical Management,* 2nd ed. Steinberg MH, Forget BG, Higgs DR, Weatherall DJ, Eds. Cambridge: Cambridge University Press; 2009:296–320.

32. Steensma DP, Gibbons RJ, Higgs DR. Acquired α-thalassemia in association with myelodysplastic syndrome and other hematologic malignancies. *Blood.* 2005; 105:443–452.

33. Benz EJ Jr., Wu CC, Sohani AR. Case records of the Massachusetts General Hospital. Case 25-2011. A 62-year-old woman with anemia and paraspinal masses. *N Engl J Med.* 2011; 365:648–658.

34. Chui DHK, Waye JS. Hydrops fetalis caused by α-thalassemia: an emerging health care problem. *Blood.* 1998; 91:2213–2222.

35. Lau Y-L, Chan L-C, Chan Y-YA, et al. Prevalence and genotypes of α- and β-thalassemias in Hong Kong: implications for population screening. *N Engl J Med.* 1997; 336:1298–1301.

36. Peng CT, Liu SC, Peng YC, et al. Distribution of thalassemias and associated hemoglobinopathies identified by prenatal diagnosis in Taiwan. *Blood Cells Mol Dis.* 2013; 51:138–141.

37. Songdej D, Babbs C, Higgs DR, et al. An international registry of survivors with Hb Bart's hydrops fetalis syndrome. *Blood.* 2017; 129:1251–1259.

38. Leung KY, Cheong KB, Lee CP, et al. Ultrasonographic prediction of homozygous α[0]-thalassemia using placental thickness, fetal cardiothoracic ratio and middle cerebral artery Doppler: alone or in combination? *Ultrasound Obstet Gynecol.* 2010; 35:149–154.

Macrocytic Anemias
Megaloblastic and Nonmegaloblastic Anemias

Peter W. Marks, MD, PhD

Macrocytosis in adults is defined as a mean corpuscular volume (MCV) above the upper limit of normal, commonly 100 fL, and is observed in 1.7–3.6% of the general population.[1] Macrocytosis associated with anemia can be subdivided into two main subcategories: (1) megaloblastic anemia, associated with impaired nucleic acid synthesis, and (2) nonmegaloblastic anemia, associated with several different etiologies. Modest elevation in the MCV (101–110 fL) may result from either cause, whereas a markedly elevated MCV (>120 fL) is usually associated with megaloblastic anemia. Review of the peripheral blood smear can contribute meaningfully to the distinction between megaloblastic and nonmegaloblastic anemia. Clinical presentation and additional diagnostic and laboratory evaluation facilitate appropriate further categorization.

Megaloblastic Anemia
Epidemiology and Etiology

Although a variety of different conditions can be associated with the development of megaloblastic anemia (Table 9.1, Figure 9.1), folate and vitamin B12 (cobalamin) deficiency are the most common entities that are clinically encountered. Depending on the population evaluated, between 6 and 28% of cases of macrocytosis are attributable to deficiency in one or both of these vitamins.[2] Whereas folate deficiency is commonly due to decreased intake, vitamin B12 deficiency most commonly results from decreased absorption from the gastrointestinal tract.

Folate is naturally present in the highest amounts per serving in beef liver and certain green vegetables such as spinach. The average daily requirement of folate is 100–200 µg, and average daily intake in a Western diet is about 400 µg. The jejunum is the primary site of absorption of dietary folate, which is generally present as polyglutamates. These are hydrolyzed to monoglutamates at the intestinal brush border then absorbed through a receptor-mediated process and converted into 5-methyltetrahydrofolate within the intestinal epithelial cells prior to being transferred into the circulation. Approximately 8–20 mg of folate is stored in the liver, so in the effective absence of intake, folate deficiency will develop in a matter of months.

Vitamin B12 is present in milk, eggs, and other animal products. The average daily requirement of vitamin B12 is 2.5 to 3 µg, and the average daily intake of vitamin B12 in a Western diet is about 5 µg. The absorption process for vitamin B12 is complex.[3] Vitamin B12 in food is generally bound to protein and is released in the stomach, where it is bound by R-binder that is present in saliva and gastric secretions. The vitamin B12-R binder complex travels to the jejunum, where in an alkaline environment pancreatic trypsin breaks down the R-binder and the vitamin B12 is bound by intrinsic factor produced by the parietal cells of the gastric mucosa. The vitamin B12-intrinsic factor is then absorbed in the terminal ileum through a receptor-mediated process involving the cubulin receptor. Very small amounts of vitamin B12 are also absorbed by passive diffusion in the gastrointestinal tract. Upon delivery into the circulation, about 80–90% of vitamin B12 is bound by transcobalamin I (haptocorin) and 10–20% by transcobalamin II. However, only transcobalamin II is capable of effectively delivering vitamin B12 to cells. Approximately 3–5 mg of vitamin B12 is stored primarily in the liver, so in the effective absence of intake, deficiency takes a few years to develop.

Folate plays an important role in nucleic acid metabolism and is involved in both purine (adenine, guanine) and pyrimidine (thymidine) synthesis. Vitamin B12 has a role in nucleic acid and protein metabolism as well as in fatty acid metabolism. The metabolic processes involving folate and vitamin B12 for nucleic acid and protein metabolism are in part linked (Figure 9.2), in that vitamin B12 is required for effective recycling of 5′-methylene tetrahydrofolate to tetrahydrofolate. However, vitamin B12 acts independently in fatty acid metabolism. It is involved in the entry of propionate, a degradation product of the branched chain amino acids isoleucine and valine, into the citric acid cycle through conversion to succinyl-CoA.

Pathophysiology

Dietary insufficiency of folate is less common now than previously, since most developed countries introduced mandatory folate fortification of flour and other grain products. It is most frequently observed in older individuals with poor

Table 9.1 Differential Diagnosis of Macrocytosis

Megaloblastic	Nonmegaloblastic
Folate deficiency	Reticulocytosis
Dietary deficiency	Recent blood loss
Malabsorption related	Hemolytic anemia
Increased requirement	Spurious
Hemolytic anemia	Cold agglutinin-induced
Pregnancy	aggregation
Increased loss	Hyperglycemia
Cobalamin (vitamin B12)	Marked leukocytosis
deficiency	Physiologic
Dietary deficiency	Pregnancy
Competition for dietary	Newborns/Infants
vitamin B12	Alcohol use
Food-cobalamin	Liver disease
malabsorption	Chronic obstructive
Associated with aging	pulmonary disease
Related to other	Hypothyroidism
conditions	Drug effects (various
From drugs or toxins	mechanisms)
(metformin, alcohol)	Stavudine
Malabsorption related	Sulfasalazine
Gastric or ileal resection	Valproic acid
Inflammatory bowel	Valacyclovir
disease	Zidovudine
Pernicious anemia	
Genetic abnormalities	
Imerslund-Gräsbeck syndrome	
Transcobalamin II deficiency	
Drug effects on folate	
metabolism	
Methotrexate	
Phenytoin	
Primadone	
Trimethoprim/	
sulfamethoxasole	
Drugs associated with	
megaloblastic marrow	
Azathioprine	
Hydroxyurea	
6-mercaptopurine	
Primary bone marrow disorders	
Aplastic anemia	
Myelodysplastic syndromes	
Erythroleukemia	
Congenital dyserythropoietic	
anemia	
Inherited defects in nucleic acid	
synthesis	

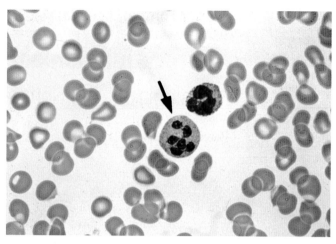

Figure 9.1 Megaloblastic peripheral blood smear. The arrow points to a six-lobed neutrophil. A megaloblastic process is indicated by the finding of just a few neutrophils with six or more lobes, 5% of neutrophils with five lobes, or more than 50% with four lobes.

pregnancy or chronic hemolytic anemia. Less commonly, increased loss may be associated with dialysis.

The pathophysiology of vitamin B12 deficiency is more complex than that of folate deficiency, and this is related, at least in part, to the greater complexity associated with its absorption. Dietary insufficiency is relatively rare and is generally only observed in strict vegans. Competition for dietary vitamin B12 may occur in the presence of the fish tapeworm *Diphyllobothrium latum*. Bacterial conversion of vitamin B12 to inactive metabolites may also occur in the presence of abnormal intestinal anatomy, such as when a blind pouch is present. However, most commonly the equivalent of dietary insufficiency results because of the impaired release of vitamin B12 in food-cobalamin malabsorption (Table 9.2).[4] In this case, impaired gastric acidity, most commonly due to gastric atrophy in older individuals, prevents the liberation of vitamin B12 from its protein-bound state so that it can be bound to R binders. The equivalent of dietary insufficiency is the result. Several drugs can interfere with vitamin B12 absorption, including aminosalicylic acid, cholestyramine, colchicine, and slow-release potassium chloride. Nitrous oxide inactivates methylcobalamin and can cause acute and chronic toxicity.

Malabsorption may occur in a manner analogous to that for folate. Resection of the terminal ileum may result in loss of the site for the absorption of the vitamin B12 intrinsic factor complex. Crohn's disease or other gastrointestinal disorders may also impair absorption. Alternatively, there may be inadequate or absent intrinsic factor present to facilitate the efficient receptor-mediated uptake of vitamin B12. Very rarely this is the result of a congenital deficiency. Much more commonly, this results from gastric resection, gastric bypass, or through the autoimmune process of pernicious anemia, in which there is a cellular and humoral reaction against the parietal cells of the stomach, leading to the absence of

diets and in individuals who chronically abuse alcohol. Insufficient absorption of ingested folate may occur in a variety of gastrointestinal disorders, including celiac disease, or may result from drug-induced malabsorption (e.g., sulfasalazine) or following jejunal resection. Folate deficiency may also result from increased requirements, such as in the setting of

Table 9.2 Diagnostic Criteria for Food-Cobalamin Malabsorption

1. Low serum vitamin B12 level

2. No evidence for dietary deficiency in vitamin B12

3. Associated with:
   - Aging **and/or**
   - Clinical conditions such as atrophic gastritis, pancreatic insufficiency, intestinal overgrowth syndromes, rheumatologic disease, **and/or**
   - Drugs or toxins such as alcohol, acid-blocking drugs (e.g., H2 blockers, proton pump inhibitors), and metformin

4. Intrinsic factor antibodies absent

5. Normal Schilling test using radiolabeled free cyanocobalamin or abnormal result of a derived Schilling test using food-bound cobalamin

The first four criteria should all be met. Since the Schilling test is not routinely available, consideration may be given to substitution of the fifth criterion with a methylmalonic acid level.

gastric acid and intrinsic factor production.[5] Occasionally, pernicious anemia may be a component of a polyglandular autoimmune syndrome.[6]

Inherited syndromes may lead to inadequate absorption or cellular update of vitamin B12. Imerslund-Gräsbeck syndrome is a rare condition in which there is a mutation in either the cubilin or amnionless gene. It is associated with deficient absorption of the vitamin B12-intrinisc factor complex as well as with proteinuria. Although quite uncommon, deficiency in transcobalamin II, which delivers vitamin B12 to cells, can be associated with signs and symptoms of vitamin B12 deficiency in the presence of normal levels.

With both folate and vitamin B12 deficiency, nucleic acid synthesis is adversely affected in rapidly dividing cells, such as those of the hematopoietic system and gastrointestinal tract. Most notable from the hematologic perspective is that the resulting defect in DNA synthesis leads to intramedullary death of abnormal appearing hematopoietic precursors. Homocytsteine levels increase in both folate and vitamin B12 deficiency, possibly increasing the risk for arterial and venous thrombosis. Methylmalonic acid levels are elevated only in vitamin B12 deficiency. However, the most important distinction between the clinical manifestations of folate and vitamin B12 deficiencies relates to the neurologic consequences of vitamin B12 deficiency. Through a mechanism that is still incompletely understood, vitamin B12 deficiency is associated with demyelination and the development of posterior column signs and cognitive deficits. Although this has been thought to relate to abnormalities in one carbon metabolism, other theories exist.[7]

Aside from deficiency in folate or vitamin B12 themselves, treatment with a number of different drugs is associated with the development of megaloblastic anemia. Some of the agents clearly act as antifolates (e.g., methotrexate), whereas others act through different mechanisms (e.g., azathioprine).

Clinical Presentation

Symptoms of fatigue and pallor, which may accompany any anemia, may be present with either folate or vitamin B12 deficiency. Symptoms and signs, such as dyspnea on exertion and flow murmurs, may occur in the presence of moderate to severe anemia. Stomatitis is a somewhat less frequently encountered symptom with either folate or vitamin B12 deficiency due to adverse effects on the gastrointestinal mucosa.

Neurologic manifestations may occur in vitamin B12 deficiency when mild to moderate macrocytosis is present, prior to the development of anemia; such neurologic manifestations are very rarely seen with folate deficiency. Paresthesias may lead individuals with vitamin B12 deficiency to seek medical attention, and posterior column signs including loss of vibratory and position sense may be found upon physical examination. Cranial nerve abnormalities or frank dementia may be observed.

Diagnostic Evaluation/Laboratory Findings

Megaloblastic anemia is within the differential diagnosis when there is macrocytosis and a low absolute or corrected reticulocyte count. Review of the peripheral blood smear may reveal a variety of morphologic abnormalities (Figure 9.1). Finding even a few neutrophils with six or more lobes, 5% with five lobes, or more than 50% with four lobes is indicative of a megaloblastic process. In the erythroid lineage, macroovalocytes may be present. As the anemia becomes more severe, additional abnormalities may become manifest, including a marked anisopoikilocytosis as well as teardrop cells. The latter morphologic abnormality results from the presence of ineffective erythropoiesis, leading to a packed bone marrow.

Both serum folate and red blood cell folate levels have been used for the diagnosis of folate deficiency. Red blood cell folate levels provide insight into folate status during the red cell lifespan and thus are felt by some to more accurately reflect body stores. However, this area is controversial, since there is greater cost associated with this test and since serum levels often suffice for establishing the diagnosis. Serum homocysteine levels may be determined and will be elevated in folate deficiency. A low serum folate level accompanied by an elevated homocysteine level is diagnostic of folate deficiency in the absence of renal insufficiency or other conditions independently associated with abnormal homocysteine levels (Table 9.3).

Assessment of vitamin B12 deficiency is sometimes not straightforward. Falsely elevated levels may be seen in the presence of high levels of transcobalamin I accompanying chronic myeloid leukemia. Levels are also generally normal in the presence of transcobalamin II deficiency. In addition, levels at the lower end of the normal range variably correlate with true deficiency. For these reasons, an elevated methylmalonic acid level is a more reliable indicator of vitamin B12 deficiency than the serum vitamin B12 level in the absence of renal insufficiency or other conditions independently associated with abnormal methylmalonic acid levels.

Table 9.3 Diagnostic Information for Folate and Vitamin B12 Deficiency

Parameter	Folate Deficiency	Vitamin B12 Deficiency
Folate level	Low	Normal or low
Vitamin B12 level	Normal	Low or normal
Homocysteine level	Elevated	Elevated
Methylmalonic acid level	Normal	Elevated

Because of the nature of the assays used, vitamin B12 levels in the low normal range may be associated with deficiency, as evidenced by symptoms, signs, and other laboratory tests. Homocysteine and methylmalonic acid levels may be elevated in certain settings such as in individuals with a reduced creatinine clearance and therefore may be uninformative in these settings for the purpose of diagnosis.

Unless it is obvious from the historical information provided, a further search for the underlying cause leading to the development of folate or vitamin B12 deficiency is in order. This is particularly true for vitamin B12 deficiency, as it is important to identify gastrointestinal malabsorption syndromes and to diagnose pernicious anemia. The latter may be associated with an increased risk of gastric cancer, and enhanced surveillance for this malignancy may be warranted.[8] Use of the Schilling test to localize the site of the absorptive lesion has become much less common due to its use of radioactive materials and the difficulty in completing the test appropriately. Diagnosis of pernicious anemia is now often based on the concomitant presence of intrinsic factor and parietal cell antibodies with vitamin B12 deficiency.[9]

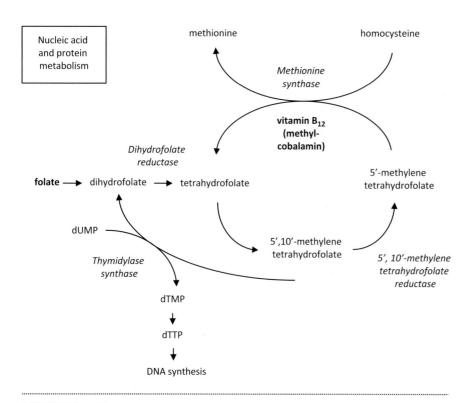

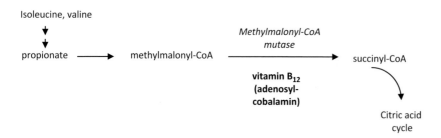

Figure 9.2 Folate and vitamin B12 (cobalamin) metabolism. Folate and vitamin B12 are both required for normal nucleic acid metabolism. However, vitamin B12 is uniquely involved in fatty acid metabolism.

Treatment and Prognosis

Folate deficiency is generally managed with the administration of folate 1–2 mg daily. Vitamin B12 deficiency may be managed with parenteral or oral repletion. It is reasonable to initially replete vitamin B12 by the parenteral route when neurologic symptoms are present. In this case, vitamin B12 1,000 µg is administered at least several times a week for the first 1–2 weeks until there is clear improvement in symptoms, followed by monthly injections. Alternatively, in the absence of neurologic symptoms or for long-term maintenance, oral vitamin B12 at high doses of 1–2 mg daily may be administered.[10]

Given the development of compensatory changes over time maximizing oxygen delivery to tissues, blood transfusion should only be administered if the patient is symptomatic and then should be given judiciously to avoid volume overload. With effective repletion of folate or vitamin B12, megaloblastic change in the marrow resolves within days, and a reticulocytosis ensues within about a week. However, complete resolution of accompanying biochemical abnormalities may take weeks. The neurologic manifestations may take even longer to resolve and, in some cases, may represent irreversible change. This highlights the need for the accurate early diagnosis of vitamin B12 deficiency.

Nonmegaloblastic Macrocytic Anemia

Epidemiology and Etiology

Nonmegaloblastic macrocytic anemia may result from a number of different causes (Table 9.1). Reticulocytosis in the setting of acute blood loss or accompanying hemolytic anemia and spurious causes account for a small portion of cases. More commonly, nonmegaloblastic macrocytic anemia is associated with liver disease, alcoholism, drugs, and endocrine effects.[11] Though only a few percent of patients with nonalcoholic liver disease are found to have macrocytosis, about half of individuals with a history of chronic alcoholism will have an MCV greater than 100 fL.[12] The macrocytosis is accompanied by anemia in fewer individuals with chronic alcoholism, and some of these individuals may have folate deficiency as a contributing cause. Next to alcohol, drugs are among the most common causes of macrocytic anemia, and several different antiviral agents and certain anticonvulsants have been associated with the development of macrocytic anemia. Chronic obstructive pulmonary disease (COPD) is associated with a mild to moderate macrocytosis in a significant fraction of those affected, regardless of whether there is concomitant hypoxia.[13] Hypothyroidism and other etiologies of nonmegaloblastic macrocytic anemia are less common causes.

Pathophysiology

Alcohol is toxic to the bone marrow, and its chronic use is associated with marrow suppression, manifest in some cases as a macrocytic anemia. Liver disease is associated with cholesterol loading of the red blood cell outer leaflet, which leads to macrocytosis and potentially to acanthocytes (spur cells). In a fraction of affected individuals, the morphologic change in the erythrocytes will be accompanied by hemolysis (spur cell anemia). The mechanisms underlying the development of macrocytic anemia to various drugs are diverse. Though COPD is believed to lead to the release of more immature red cells from the bone marrow, the precise mechanism of the macrocytosis is incompletely understood. Hypothyroidism is thought to cause macrocytosis through the deprivation of triiodothyronine and thyroxine from erythroid precursors during development. However, it should be noted that hypothyroidism may also be associated with normocytic and microcytic anemia.

Clinical Presentation

Patients with nonmegaloblastic macrocytic anemia may be asymptomatic or may exhibit symptoms and signs generally referable to anemia. Patients with hypothyroidism may present with concomitant cold intolerance, dry skin, thinning hair, and other symptoms consistent with this endocrine disorder. Individuals may present with a history of liver disease or alcohol abuse, or the latter may be elicited on careful questioning. A history of current and recent medications must be considered as well.

Diagnostic Evaluation/Laboratory Findings

In the diagnostic evaluation of nonmegaloblastic macrocytic anemia, it is important to first rule out the presence of a megaloblastic process, since serious neurologic consequences may result from missing a diagnosis of vitamin B12 deficiency (Figure 9.3). Thoughtful review of the peripheral blood count, peripheral blood smear, and the reticulocyte count is important in this regard. Macrocytosis with an elevated reticulocyte count may simply be indicative of a brisk and appropriate response to recent blood loss or to a concomitant hemolytic process. Occasionally, red cell agglutination in the absence of an elevated reticulocyte count may cause spurious macrocytosis, such as early on with development of a cold agglutinin. Liver function tests may provide supportive evidence for underlying liver disease or hepatitis due to alcohol. Thyroid function testing is indicated if there is any suspicion for endocrinopathy. In occasional cases, bone marrow examination may be necessary to distinguish macrocytic anemia due to alcoholism from other causes including bone marrow failure states. Vacuolization in hematopoietic precursors, particularly proerythroblasts, is potentially consistent with chronic alcohol use.[14]

Treatment and Prognosis

The treatment of nonmegaloblastic macrocytic anemia depends on the cause but commonly involves discontinuation of offending toxins (alcohol) or medications. In general, this results in gradual resolution of the macrocytosis and accompanying

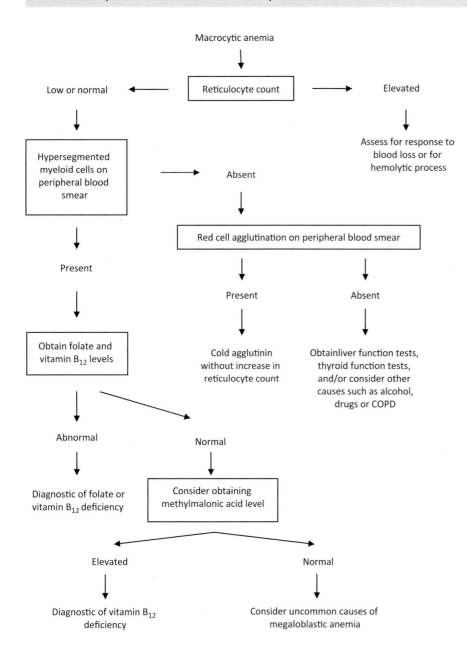

Figure 9.3 Diagnostic algorithm for macrocytic anemia. Note that checking a vitamin B12 level may be appropriate even in the absence of megaloblastic change if the clinical scenario is consistent (e.g., in the presence of neurologic symptoms such as paresthesias).

anemia. The response of macrocytic anemia to thyroid replacement therapy for hypothyroidism may take some time.[15]

Case Study: Megaloblastic Anemia

A 63-year-old woman presents to the emergency department with dyspnea on exertion. She denies any history of coronary artery disease, pulmonary disease, hypertension, or diabetes. Her medical history is only remarkable for resection of a colon cancer about 12 years prior. On physical examination, she is afebrile. The skin is without petechiae or purpura, and the sclerae are anicteric. The tongue is smooth, but there are no other oral lesions. Lungs are clear to auscultation, and tachycardia is noted with a grade I/VI systolic flow murmur. The abdomen is soft, nontender, and notable for a well-healed abdominal scar near the midline. The extremities are without edema. Neurologic examination is remarkable for decreased vibration sense in the distal lower extremities but is otherwise grossly normal.

Laboratory studies reveal WBC of 2,900/µL, hemoglobin 5.5 g/dL, hematocrit 18%, MCV 116 fL, RDW 21%, platelets 89,000/µL, reticulocyte count 0.1%. The LDH is 2,200 U/L, total bilirubin 1.9 mg/dL; direct bilirubin 0.5 mg/dL. Review of the peripheral blood smear reveals marked anisopoikilocytosis with numerous teardrop cells. The nuclei of most neutrophils have five or more lobes (see Figure 9.1).

On further questioning, she notes that shortly following her surgery, she was told to go to her primary care doctor monthly for "vitamin" shots. She reports that she continued to do so regularly until about 3 years prior, when she says that she was told by a new primary care provider that she no longer needed these injections.

The individual is hospitalized. Blood transfusion is withheld, and she is started on a course of vitamin B12 1 mg IM daily for 7 days, followed by weekly injections for 1 month. Folate 1 mg daily is also administered. On the second hospital day, vitamin B12 level is reported as 110 pg/ml and the folate level is reported as 5 ng/ml. Four days into this regimen the reticulocyte count is 4% and the LDH has decreased to 550 U/L. When seen in follow-up 1 month later, she feels well, and the dyspnea on exertion has resolved. Vibration sense is improved over presentation but is still mildly decreased in the distal lower extremities. The WBC, platelets, LDH, and bilirubin levels have normalized, and the hemoglobin is 10.5, hematocrit 33%, MCV 94 fL. The individual elects to continue on monthly vitamin B12 injections.

Case Study: Nonmegaloblastic Anemia

A 72-year-old man is referred for further evaluation of mild anemia noted at the time of his most recent routine medical evaluation. He notes that he feels well and has no complaints.

His medical history is notable for hypertension, and his only medications are atenolol and hydrochlorothiazide. He is retired, lives with his wife, and notes that he does not smoke but that he does drink a cocktail or two each evening. Review of systems is only remarkable for decreased libido. Physical examination is essentially unremarkable except for testicular atrophy.

Laboratory studies reveal WBC of 6,500/μL, hemoglobin 12.8 g/dL, hematocrit 39%, MCV 104 fL, RDW 14%, platelets 135,000/μL, reticulocyte count 1%. The serum creatinine is 1.2 mg/dL, ALT 60 U/L, AST 110 U/L. Serum testosterone is 150 ng/dL. Review of the peripheral blood smear reveals mild macrocytosis and no other abnormalities.

On further questioning about his drinking, he notes that his alcohol consumption consists of a total of about 4 to 5 ounces of liquor each evening, and this has been the case for several years. The individual is counseled to cut back significantly on his drinking. In addition, he declines intervention following a discussion of the potential risks of testosterone supplementation. When seen in follow-up 3 months later, he notes that he has cut back to 1 ounce of liquor each evening, and the hemoglobin is 13 g/dL, hematocrit 40%, and MCV 93 fL. Liver function tests are within the normal range.

References

1. Aslinia F, Mazza JJ, Yale SH. Megaloblastic anemia and other causes of macrocytosis. *Clin Med Res.* 2006; **3**:236–241.

2. Kaferle JK, Strzoda CE. Evaluation of macrocytosis. *Am Fam Phys.* 2009; **79**:203–208.

3. Quadros EV. Advances in the understanding of cobalamin assimilation and metabolism. *Br J Haematol.* 2010; **148**: 195–204.

4, Andrès E, Affenberger S, Vinzio S, et al. Food-cobalamin malabsorption in elderly patients: clinical manifestations and treatment. *Am J Med.* 2005; **118**:1154–1159.

5. Neumann WL, Coss E, Rugge M, Genta RM. Autoimmune atrophic gastritis-pathogenesis, pathology and management. *Nat Rev Gastroenterol Hepatol.* 2013; **10**:529–540.

6. Michels AW, Gottlieb PA. Autoimmune polyglandular syndromes. *Nat Rev Endocrinol.* 2010; **6**:270–277.

7. Scalabrino G, Peracchi M. New insights into the pathophysiology of cobalamin deficiency. *Trends Mol Med.* 2006; **12**:247–254.

8. Vannella L, Lahner E, Osborn J, Annibale B. Systematic review: gastric cancer incidence in pernicious anaemia. *Aliment Pharmacol Ther.* 2013; **37**:375–382.

9. Annibale B, Lahner E, Fave GD. Diagnosis and management of pernicious anemia. *Curr Gastroenterol Rep.* 2011; **13**:518–524.

10. Stabler SP. Vitamin B12 deficiency. *N Engl J Med.* 2013; **368**:149–160.

11. Kaferle J, Strzoda CE. Evaluation of macrocytosis. *Am Fam Physician.* 2009; **79**:203–208.

12. Morgan MY, Camilo ME, Luck W, et al. Macrocytosis in alcohol-related liver disease: its value for screening. *Clin Lab Haematol.* 1981; **3**:35–44.

13. Garcia-Pachon E, Padilla-Navas I. Red cell macrocytosis in COPD patients without respiratory insufficiency: a brief report. *Respir Med.* 2007; **101**:349–352.

14. Latvala J, Parkkila S, Niemelä O. Excess alcohol consumption is common in patients with cytopenia: studies in blood and bone marrow cells. *Alcohol Clin Exp Res.* 2004; **28**:619–624.

15. Sims EG. Hypothyroidism causing macrocytic anemia unresponsive to B12 and folate. *J Natl Med Assoc.* 1983; **75**:429–431.

Chapter

Sickle Cell Syndromes

10

Maureen Achebe, MD, MPH

The sickle cell syndromes are a group of disorders caused by the homozygous inheritance of the sickle gene (sickle cell anemia) or the double heterozygous inheritance of the sickle gene with another abnormal hemoglobin gene (sickle cell disease).

Etiology and Epidemiology

Worldwide, more than 200,000 babies are born annually with SCD, most in sub-Saharan Africa. In the United States, there are over 80,000 persons with SCD.[1] Sickle cell disease (SCD) is due to a point mutation at the sixth amino acid position of the beta globin gene of hemoglobin, with a switch of valine for glutamic acid, β_6 (Glu $\rightarrow$ Val), which results in sickle hemoglobin (HbS). As is true for many red blood cell (RBC) abnormalities, the sickle mutation β_6 (Glu $\rightarrow$ Val), arose under the natural selection pressure of lethal *Plasmodium falciparium* malaria.

There are four haplotypes of the sickle gene that arose independently of one another, three in sub-Saharan Africa (Benin, Senegal, Central African Republic/Bantu) and one in Asia (Arab-Indian; see Figure 10.1). The sickle gene in heterozygosity with normal hemoglobin (sickle cell trait, HbAS) is protective against malaria. Homozygous SCD (HbSS) provides no protection, and malaria is often more severe than in normal adults (HbAA).

Pathophysiology

The core pathophysiology of the sickle cell syndrome lies with the tendency of HbS to polymerize when deoxygenated. Deoxygenated HbS, and not oxy-HbS, forms 14-strand polymer fibers. The formation of the sickle polymer involves many chemical interactions involving specific contact points on the beta and alpha chains of HbS. The three amino acid positions on the hemoglobin molecule that are important in polymer formation are β_6 (Glu $\rightarrow$ Val), (the required mutation), the β-73 residue in *trans* (β_1) position, and the β-121 residue (Figure 10.2). Alignment of HbS polymer fibers induces an RBC membrane change in shape (sickle shape) to accommodate the new deoxy-HbS fibers within. The polymerized hemoglobin damages many erythrocyte components leading to the formation of dense, inflexible, adherent ("sticky") cells, which have difficulty traversing the capillaries.

The solubility of HbS is principally dependent on the state of oxygenation of HbS. The more deoxygenated the HbS, the more readily polymer is formed (Figure 10.3). Also, as the concentration of HbS increases, delay time for polymer formation decreases exponentially. Soluble oxy-HbS behaves like hemoglobin A (HbA), with a normal oxygen dissociation curve. But deoxy-HbS polymer has a low affinity for oxygen and functions as a poor respiratory pigment.[2] For this reason, HbS polymer releases oxygen to tissues quite efficiently for a given hemoglobin level.

Clinical Presentation

The severity of the clinical manifestations of SCD varies widely. The multiple phenotypic expressions of SCD are due to modifiers and genetic interactions that are not completely understood.[3] SCD in its worst form is a severe disease characterized by chronic anemia, functional asplenia, frequent painful crises, and end-organ damage. SCD can affect every organ and/or tissue in the body.

Pain in SCD

The Acute Vaso-occlusive Crisis (**VOC**) is the most prominent clinical manifestation of SCD. Acute VOCs are severe excruciating attacks of pain involving one or more parts of the body, of sudden onset and cessation. More often than not, these acute attacks are interspersed by pain-free periods of varying duration. The severity of the pain impulse and its processing through the dorsal horn of the spinal cord determine whether the pain sensation is intermittent or intractable.[4]

Acute VOCs progress through 4 sequential phases:[5]

1) a *prodromal phase* of paresthesias and aches, lasting 1–2 days, at the site of subsequent pain;

2) *an initial phase* – a time of escalation to debilitating pain, described as throbbing, sharp, pounding, stabbing, and gnawing like a generalized toothache;

3) *an established phase* of pain at peak intensity, that may last ~4–5 days, with gradual reversal of abnormalities; and

4) *a resolving phase* of pain resolution, of 1–2 days.

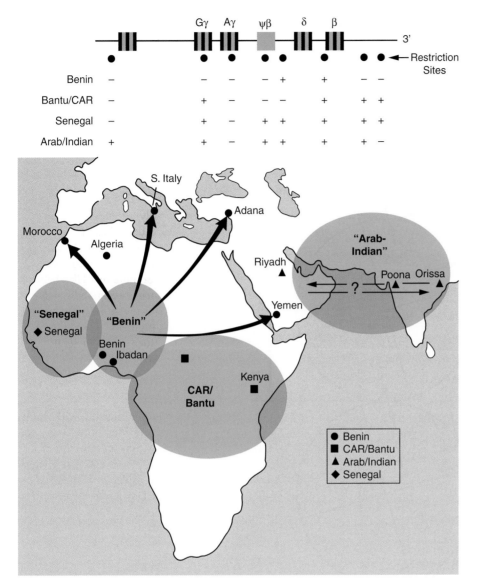

Figure 10.1 Distribution of the origin of sickle haplotypes. The haplotypes have the sickle mutation but differ in restriction endonuclease sites within the β-globin gene cluster on chromosome 11, signifying independent origins several times in evolution. The origin and spread of the four haplotypes is shown. Ragusa A, Lomabrdo M, Sortino G, et al. Beta S gene is Sicily isin linkage disequilibrium with Benin haplotype: implications for gene flow. *Am J Hematology*.1988;27:139. (From *Blood: Principles and Practice of Hematology*, edited by R.I. Handin, Samuel E. Lux, Thomas P. Stossel, with permission.)

Chronic Pain in SCD is defined as pain lasting 3 months or longer. Patients with SCD have chronic pain of two types: (1) pain from secondary pathologies such as chronic leg ulcers, avascular necrosis, osteomyelitis, and neuropathy; and (2) *intractable VOC pain,* pain with an identical *quality* as an acute VOC, albeit less severe. Intractable VOC pain is an indirect consequence of repeated severe acute pain stimuli, which exert effects on both the peripheral and central nervous systems. At the peripheral level, there is recruitment of dormant nociceptors, following which at the dorsal horn of the spinal cord, transmission of the pain impulse is modulated by activation of Na^+ gated channels (α-amino-3-hydroxy-5-methyl-4-isoxazolepropioinc acid (AMPA) and N-methyl-D-aspartic acid (NMDA) receptors), which facilitate the transmission of painful stimuli to the central nervous system. Excessive nociceptive signals from the periphery can flood the brain and spinal cord, causing continuous amplification of pain. This presents clinically as areduced pain threshold, expanded fields of pain,

chronicity of pain allodynia (pain due to a stimulus which does not normally provoke pain) and is referred to as *central sensitization.*[6,7] The brain also undergoes functional and structural changes that cause altered perceptual processing and the perpetuation of pain (neuroplasticity). In addition, *glial activation* (activation of oligodendrocytes, astrocytes, and microglia) with microglial release of proinflammatory cytokines and glutamate accentuates the perception of pain. Studies in sickle cell mice demonstrate nociceptor and glial activation in mice with pain patterns similar to patients.[8]

Neuropathic pain is described as numbness, shooting, lancinating pain in SCD associated with hyperalgesia and allodynia. Neuropathic pain may be isolated, such as in mental nerve neuropathy, trigeminal neuralgia, and spinal cord infarction, or be generalized in the course of a painful crisis.[5] Neuropathic pain in SCD is thought, anecdotally, to be due to ischemia of the vasa nevorum (vessels supplying nerves), causing tissue damage of nerves. This is yet to be proven.

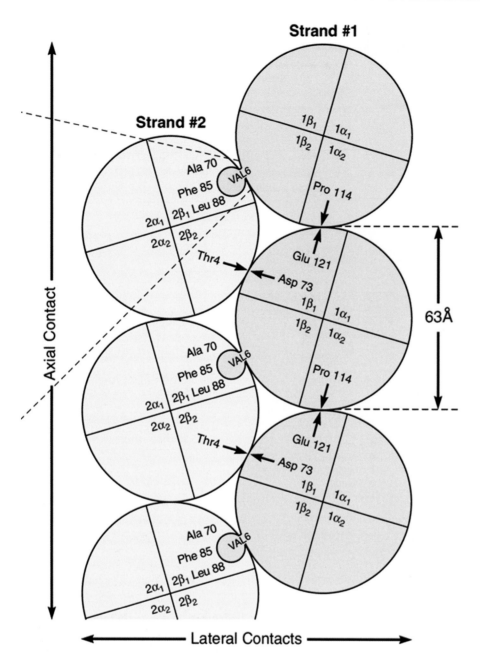

Figure 10.2 Wishner-Love Double strand showing key intermolecular contacts between neighboring Hb S molecules. Wishner BC, Ward KB, Lattman EE, et al. Crystal structure of sickle cell deoxyhemoglobin at 5 Å resolution. *J Mol Biol*.1975; 98:179. (From *Blood: Principles and Practice of Hematology*, edited by R.I. Handin, Samuel E. Lux, Thomas P. Stossel, with permission.)

Respiratory System

Acute chest syndrome (ACS) refers to the appearance of a new infiltrate on the radiograph of a patient with chest pain, hypoxia, fever, tachypnea, and/or cough. After pain crises, ACS is the next most common complication of SCD, affecting 12.8 cases/100 patient years. ACS is three times more common in young children but more severe in adults. Only 36% of patients have an abnormal radiograph at presentation, underscoring the need for vigilance in managing hospitalized patients, who may develop ACS in hospital.[9] In a multicenter randomized trial of 671 ACS episodes, pulmonary fat embolism and respiratory infection with chlamydia, mycoplasma, or virus were the main etiologies.[10] Prognosis was worse if patients had platelet count <200,000, extensive pulmonary infiltrates, or underlying cardiac disease.

Pulmonary Hypertension (Pulm HTN) is a severe complication in SCD that negatively impacts morbidity and mortality.[11,12] Gladwin et al. reported that an abnormal systolic pulmonary artery pressure (tricuspid regurgitant jet [TRJ] velocity >2.5 m/s) correlated with increased risk of death.[11] The predictive value of TRJ velocity in defining pulmonary HTN in adults is only about 25–33%[13] and in children is not easily reproducible. Pulmonary HTN by right heart catheterization is also associated with a poor survival.[13] Factors implicated in pulmonary HTN in SCD include endothelial dysfunction, vascular remodeling and pulmonary

O$_2$ Saturation

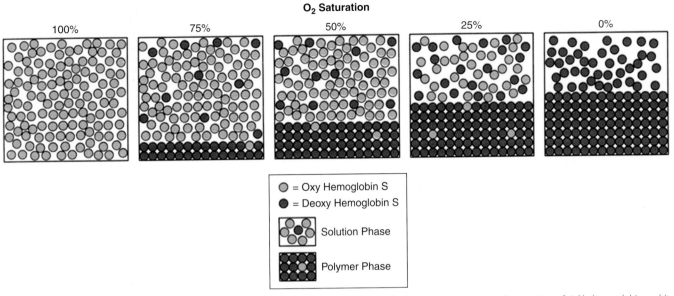

○ = Oxy Hemoglobin S

● = Deoxy Hemoglobin S

Solution Phase

Polymer Phase

Figure 10.3 Sickle hemoglobin at equilibrium at various oxygen saturations. Noguchi CT, Schechter AN. Intracellular polymerization of sickle hemoglobin and its relevance to SCD. *Blood.*1981;58:1057. (From *Blood: Principles and Practice of Hematology*, edited by R.I. Handin, Samuel E. Lux, Thomas P. Stossel, with permission.)

vasoconstriction mediated by reduced levels of nitric oxide, a pulmonary vasodilator, and increased endothelin-1, a pulmonary vasoconstrictor.[14] Surveillance echocardiography detects pulmonary HTN in the usually asymptomatic patient.

Central Nervous System

The Brain

The effects of SCD on the brain range from being clinically 'silent' infarcts to causing significant morbidity and/or mortality.

Silent Cerebral Infarcts were first described in the Cooperative Study of Sickle Cell Disease (CSSCD) from brain magnetic resonance imaging (MRI) findings in children who had no neurological event or findings.[15] These lesions were associated with neuro-cognitive impairment and an increased risk for overt stroke.[16] In the CSSCD, stroke occurred in 8% of children with silent infarcts and in 1% of those without.

Neurocognitive Impairment is defined in areas of executive function, attention, verbal performance, and memory in patients with and without lesions on MRI.[17] Anemic hypoxia may explain cognitive changes in children with SCD. Several studies have demonstrated a correlation between biomarkers of anemia and neurocognitive functioning in children with SCD.[18–20] Hypoxia and inflammation are systemic consequences of SCD that have been shown to impact the brain and cognitive functioning in patients without SCD and may account for cognitive difficulties in individuals with SCD.[21]

Strokes occur in 11% of children with HbSS (age < 20) and in 24% of adults by age 45.[22] The majority of strokes in adults are hemorrhagic and in children are infarctive. Subarachnoid bleeding is the most common. Patients present with severe headache, meningismus and photophobia, and typical localizing neurological deficits. High systolic blood pressure, leukocytosis, and severe anemia are correlated with hemorrhagic strokes in children.[23] Overall mortality may be as high as 50%. Diffusion-weighted intensity MRI detects acute ischemia. Magnetic resonance angiography shows obstruction of blood flow in large intracranial vessels and abnormal vessel wall formation, including Moyamoya syndrome. Moyamoya syndrome denotes a collateral circulation of neovasculature, prone to aneurysmal dilatation and hemorrhage, that develops to compensate for the impaired function of occluded vessels.

The Eye

Ophthalmologic changes due to SCD are relatively common. No vascular bed is exempt from possible derangement.

The Conjunctiva in patients with SCD have comma-shaped dilatations of vessels that are full of sickled RBCs. The implicated vessels show endothelial proliferation, RBC aggregation in the distal capillaries, and dilatation of the proximal segments of the vessels. These lesions do not cause blindness.

Retinopathy

Nonproliferative retinopathy is due to retinal hemorrhage and invariably does not lead to blindness. *Salmon patch hemorrhage* is an area of hemorrhage within the superficial retina. Resorption of the salmon patch results in a *Retinoschisis cavity*. If the retinoschisis cavity contains refractile, copper-colored hemosiderin-laden macrophages, it is called an *Iridescent spot*. When a retinal hemorrhage tracks to the subretinal space, a round-to-oval stellate hyperpigmented lesion, a *Black Sunburst* is formed.

Proliferative retinopathy progresses through five stages (24), the last two of which are vitreous hemorrhage and retinal detachment. These may result in blindness.Stage I is arteriolar occlusion, which instigates the local release of angiogenic substances and development of "sea-fan" arteriovenous anastomoses and hairpin loops (Stage 2) at the junction of the perfused central retina and nonperfused peripheral retina. Neovascularization (Stage 3) is a precursor to stages that affect vision. Abnormalities tend to be located peripherally and are easy to miss on ophthalmologic exam.

Cardiovascular System

To maintain adequate tissue oxygenation, cardiac output in SCD is increased, and cardiomegaly results. In spite of the high oxygen extraction of the coronary circulation, blood in the coronary sinus exhibits no more sickling than blood elsewhere in the circulation, atherosclerosis is rare,and classic myocardial infarction is uncommon. *Arrhythmias* are common during pain crises, though they are usually of little clinical significance. Blood pressure in SCD patients is lower than in the normal population, but relative hypertension is a risk factor for stroke and early mortality.[25] Ventricular function is normal, but left ventricular diastolic filling pressure is increased.

Multiple red cell transfusions cause severe *cardiac hemosiderosis* characterized by diastolic dysfunction, increased susceptibility to arrhythmias, and late-stage dilated cardiomyopathy. Baseline EKG and echocardiograms are done to evaluate cardiac status. No specific recommendations exist for the frequency of surveillance.

Gastrointestinal System

Chronic hemolysis, recurrent ischemia, and reperfusion injury from SCD affect the liver and biliary tree.

Pigmented (bilirubin) gallstones are seen in 12% of patients by age 4 and 42% of patients between ages 15 and 18.[26]

Right Upper Quadrant Syndrome refers to acute pain in the right upper quadrant and encompasses different etiologies. *Intrahepatic cholestasis* is a life-threatening condition marked by severe hyperbilirubinemia (>50 mg/dL), direct bilirubin making up > 50%. Prothrombin time is often elevated, and patients may develop hepatorenal syndrome. Transaminases are relatively unaffected. Acute, rapid liver enlargement with worsening anemia indicates hepatic congestion and *hepatic sequestration*. *Hepatitis B and C* in SCD is related to blood product exposure. All patients should be screened for hepatitis A, B, and C. *Hepatic siderosis* is of increasing importance as the indications for RBC exchange transfusions broaden. T2* MRI quantifies tissue iron burden.

Functional Asplenia from recurrent splenic microinfarction varies in severity according to genotype, most severe in HbSS and S/β⁰-thalassemia, then S/β⁺-thalassemia, and least HbSC. Patients are thus predisposed to encapsulated organisms, most importantly *Streptococcus pneumoniae*.

Genitourinary System

Hyposthenuria (the inability to concentrate urine)develops in early childhood and is probably due to decreased medullary blood flow and a disturbed countercurrent multiplier system. Nocturia and enuresis are common. The water loss promotes dehydration and sickling.

Hematuria results mostly from renal papillary necrosis in SCD. It also occurs in sickle cell trait.

Priapism is a persistent, painful, purposeless penile erection. The exact pathogenesis is not well understood, but priapism is perpetuated by a vicious cycle of high local tissue oxygen extraction and impaired venous blood outflow by sickled cells. The median age at onset is 22. Priapism in adults is a marker for severe disease and the development of other SCD-related complications. Priapism is more frequent in patients with thrombocytosis, low HbF, and severe hemolysis.[27]

Sickle nephropathy in SCD is progressive over years. The most common glomerular lesion is focal and segmental glomerulosclerosis, but the exact cause is unknown. Microalbuminuria, macroalbuminuria, or nephrotic syndrome may be due to glomerular capillary hypertension.

Musculoskeletal System and Skin

Dactylitis is the painful inflammation of the soft tissues of the hands and feet. Peak incidence is between 6 months and 2 years of age. Bone and marrow ischemia and infarction with increased erythropoiesis and bone marrow expansion are implicated in the pathogenesis. Prolonged ischemia leads to bony destruction of metacarpal and phalangeal bones and irregular shortening of digits.

Chronic leg ulcers are most frequently located around the medial malleolus but may develop anywhere on the distal lower extremity. Histopathology of leg ulcers shows intimal proliferation, neovascularization, and perivascular proliferation at the ulcer base. Ulcers are seen almost exclusively in patients with HbSS. The ulcers start small and shallow, with central necrosis, are very painful, produce copious slough, and may widen and deepen to expose underlying muscle. Complications include chronic osteomyelitis, local adenitis, and chronic cellulitis.Ulcers can persist for years, and the recurrence rate is 25–50%.

Avascular necrosis (AVN) results from decreased blood supply to the articular surfaces and ends of long bones, primarily the femur and humerus. The prevalence of AVN amongst HbSS children is over 25% and in adults is over 40%.[28] AVN most commonly affects the hip, shoulder and spine. Patients present with pain and loss of function of the affected joint. The progression of AVN from first symptoms to joint collapse is rapid (3–5 years) without intervention. Radiographs or MRI make the diagnosis.

Osteopenia/Osteoporosis affects 30–80% of patients with SCD. Increased iron deposition in the marrow causes chronic inflammation, which impedes osteoblast activity and increases osteoclast function.

Diagnostic Evaluation

Inheritance of the sickle cell gene can be identified by the presence of HbS on hemoglobin electrophoresis or high-performance liquid chromatography (HPLC).

Hemoglobin electrophoresis is based on the differential mobility of different hemoglobins in an electric field. HbS, with its higher negative charge, has slower mobility toward the anode in an aqueous medium than HbA. (Figure 10.4) HbSS shows >90% HbS on electrophoresis. (Table 10.1).

HPLC works based on charge and column retention times. Each hemoglobin has a specific column retention time, but some variants overlap. Hemoglobin electrophoresis, and not HPLC, is FDAapproved for the definitive diagnosis of sickle cell syndromes.

DNA analysis of the specific globin gene by polymerase chain reaction or Southern blot may be required in unusual or challenging cases.

Sickle prep and sickle solubility tests are less reliable tests for diagnosing SCD. In the sickle prep, RBCs containing HbS change shape in response to hypoxia (2% metabisulphite solution). In the sickle solubility test, deoxy-HbS shows decreased solubility in a high-phosphate buffer compared to other hemoglobins such as HbG and HbD. These tests are rapid, inexpensive, and useful in resource-poor settings but are not 100% sensitive.

Laboratory data in SCD include anemia with/without leukocytosis and thrombocytosis, microcytosis (if coinherited with a thalassemia gene), and evidence of hemolysis. The peripheral smear shows irreversibly sickled cells, Howell-Jolly bodies, polychromasia, and target cells (Figure 10.5).

Table 10.1 Hemoglobin Electrophoresis Patterns and Clinical Features of Sickle Cell Syndromes. (Modified from *Blood: Principles and Practice of Hematology: Sickle Syndromes*, Orah S. Platt, edited by Robert I. Handin, Samuel E. Lux, Thomas P. Stossel, with permission.)

| | Hemoglobin Electrophoresis | | | | | Clinical Features | | | | |
| | | | | | | | | Morphology | | |
Diagnosis	S	A	F	A2	Other	Hematocrit	Reticulocytes	ISC	Targets	Vaso-occlusive features
SS	80–98	0	2–20	2–4		18–30	>10	4+	3+	Marked
SC	~50				~50% C	30–35	<10	2+	4+	Mild to moderate
S trait	35–40	50–60	<2	< 3.5		Normal	Normal	Normal	Normal	
SD Los Angeles	~50				~50% D	20–30	>10	4+	3+	Moderate to marked
S/β⁰ thal	80–98	0	1–15	3–6		25–40	>10	3+	4+	Moderate to marked
S/β⁺ thal	55–75	10–30	1–15	3–6		25–38	<5	2+	4+	Mild to moderate
S/HPFH	70–80	0	20–30	< 3.5		35–45	<5	0	3+	Mild

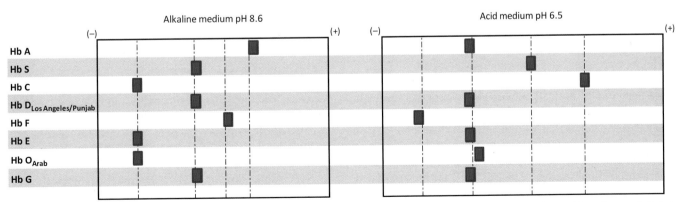

Figure 10.4 Electrophoresis of hemoglobins in cellulose (alkaline) and citrate (acid) media. Citrate agar is useful in distinguishing hemoglobins that run similarly in cellulose media, such as Hb C, E and O$_{Arab}$, and HbS from D$_{Punjab}$ or G.

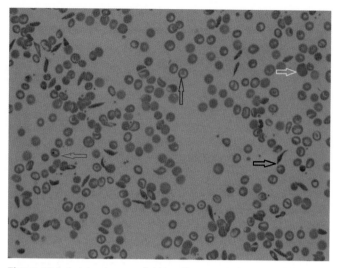

Figure 10.5 Peripheral smear of sickle cell anemia. Red arrow – Howell Jolly body; blue arrow – target cell; yellow arrow – polychromasia (a reticulocyte); black arrow – irreversible sickle cell.

Table 10.2 Newborn Screening Result Interpretations

Electrophoretic Pattern	Interpretation
FA	Normal pattern
FS	Sickle cell anemia (or less commonly Hb S/β⁰-thalassemia or Hb S/HPFH)
FAS	Sickle cell trait (or less commonly Hb S/β⁺-thalassemia)
FSC	Hemoglobin SC disease
FAC	Hemoglobin C trait
Bart's hemoglobin	α-thalassemia

Newborn Screening

All 50 United States and the District of Columbia now perform universal newborn screening for SCD in *all* newborns. Detection is by thin-layer isoelectric focusing or HPLC performed ideally within 48 hours of birth and before any blood transfusions. Table 10.2.

Prenatal Diagnosis

Chorionic villous biopsy is used to obtain fetal DNA for diagnosis in the first trimester. Preimplantation diagnosis and retrieving fetal cells from the maternal circulation are currently under investigation.

Management of SCD

Hydroxyurea

Fetal hemoglobin interrupts HbS polymer formation. The only FDA-approved medication specifically indicated for SCD is hydroxyurea, which induces fetal hemoglobin and is taken chronically (daily) to increase HbF and thereby decrease symptoms of SCD.[29]

Pain

Pain is the hallmark manifestation of SCD and the reason for more than 90% of hospitalizations. Twenty% of SCD patients have weekly to monthly episodes that warrant medical attention, 50% have occasional episodes, and 30% of patients have rare or no pain episodes.[30] Pain management is a significant portion of care. Pain management in SCD lags behind our present knowledge of the pathophysiology of pain in SCD[4] and is extrapolated from recommendations in patients with other pain states.

Opioids are the most frequently used medications for the inpatient management of SCD pain. Many patients will not derive adequate pain relief with standard doses of opioids, and the variability in opioid responsiveness is partly related to genetic factors affecting drug metabolism. The best dose range and opioid choice for a particular patient is one that has been effective in the past. Therefore, employing a historical perspective to management is essential. Providers who are familiar with the patient or a pain service team's guidance is invaluable in SCD pain management. Patients may derive better pain control from one agent over another. There are no controlled trials comparing the safety and efficacy of different opioids in SCD pain management. Morphine is most commonly used. Meperidine (Demerol) use is discouraged because of neurotoxic effects of its major metabolite, nor-meperidine.[31] Chronic opioid use causes glial activation that accentuates the perception of pain.[4]

For acute painful VOCs, intravenous opioids are given, titrating to pain relief. Dose-limiting toxicities include respiratory depression and hypotension that should be assessed for frequently, especially during initiation and dose escalation. Opioids are often combined with nonopioid "adjuvant" medications (nonsteroidal anti-inflammatory drugs, anxiolytics, selective serotonin reuptake inhibitors, antihistaminergics). These serve to increase analgesic effect and reduce chances of side effects of primary medications and manage associated symptoms such as anxiety.[32]

For chronic intractable VOC pain, opioid rotation, methadone,[33] and ketamine[35,36] may break the cycle of pain by blocking Na+ channel activation in the dorsal horn of the spinal cord and limiting central sensitization. Chronic intractable VOC is difficult to manage.

For chronic pain syndromes from leg ulcers, avascular necrosis, osteomyelitis, neuropathy, long-acting opioids are used, with short-acting opioids for breakthrough pain. A detailed description of pain management in SCD is outside the scope of this chapter. Principles of current pharmacological pain management in SCD are detailed in an NIH publication on SCD.[32] Nonpharmacological strategies include hot/cold packs, relaxation, hypnosis, massage, vibration acupuncture, and biofeedback, tailored to be patient specific.

Acute Chest Syndrome

Emergency RBC exchange transfusion to achieve a HbS fraction of 30% and a hematocrit ~30% is indicated. The goal is to reduce sickling and provide maximal oxygenation to tissues, as well as to provide empiric antibiotic coverage for atypical organisms.

Pulmonary Hypertension

There is little data on specific therapy of pulmonary HTN in SCD. Studies examining sildenafil to improve nitric oxide availability and using an endothelin-1 receptor blocker were inconclusive.

Stroke

Infarctive stroke in SCD is an indication for an immediate RBC exchange transfusion. Patients undergo immediate brain computer tomography to rule out hemorrhage. Then emergent RBC exchange transfusion is needed to achieve an HbS fraction of ≤30% and a hematocrit of 30% (hemoglobin ≤11 g/dL). This reverses acute neurological deficits and prevents recurrent strokes in the acute setting. Secondary prevention involves routine RBC transfusions to maintain HbS fraction between 30 and 50% indefinitely.[37] Routine prophylactic blood transfusions to children at high risk (transcranial Doppler distal carotid artery velocities >200 cm/sec) has reduced the incidence of strokes in children from 11%[22] to 2–3%.[38]

Retinopathy

The goal is to prevent hemorrhage and retinal detachment. Regression of neovasculature is achieved by laser photocoagulation, cryotherapy, and diathermy.

Gastrointestinal Tract

Acute cholecystitis is treated conservatively, with elective cholecystectomy performed weeks afterward. Intrahepatic cholestasis may benefit from RBC exchange transfusion. Vaccinations against hepatitis A and B should be given to all patients. Appropriate patients with hepatitis C show favorable outcomes with interferon and ribavirin.[39] For hemosiderosis, chelation is accomplished with parenteral deferoxamine, or oral agents, deferasirox, or deferiprone.

Functional Asplenia

For prophylaxis against *Streptococcus pneumoniae* (and other encapsulated organisms), newborns (from age 2 to 3 months) are given penicillin prophylaxis up to age 5. Adults are vaccinated against *S. pnemoniae*. All patients should be vaccinated against *Neisseria meningitidis* and *Haemophilus influenzae type B*.

Hematuria

Management entails bed rest, maintaining high urinary flow, and cautious use of aminocaproic acid for refractory bleeding.

Priapism

Management is geared toward pain control and prevention of impotence. Episodes lasting up to 4 hours are an emergency. If intravenous hydration and pain medication are ineffective, penile aspiration and epinephrine irrigation will cause detumescense in the majority of cases. If priapism lasts 24 hours, RBC exchange transfusion while maintaining hematocrit close to the patient's baseline is indicated. Exchanging to a hematocrit well above patients' baseline can cause neurological complications.[40] Shunting procedures between the cavernosa and the spongiosum may be needed to achieve detumescense. Penile implants are used to manage impotence.

Nephropathy

Whether angiotensin-converting enzyme inhibitors reduce proteinuria in SCD remains unclear.[41] Hemodialysis, peritoneal dialysis, and renal transplant are used for end-stage renal disease.

Dactylitis

Management involves aggressive hydration, surveillance for secondary infection, and nonsteroidal anti-inflammatory drug and other pain relief. Hydroxycarbamide (hydroxyurea) use significantly reduces rates of dactylitis.[42]

Leg Ulcers

Primary prevention of leg ulcers (avoiding trauma, insect bites) is a major component of care. Ulcer management entails frequent debridement, prevention and control of local edema, prevention of infection, and treatment of systemic disease. Skin grafts and flaps are variably successful.

Avascular Necrosis

In the early stages, non–weight-bearing exercises and physical therapy maintain joint use. With progression, core decompression is used. However, in a randomized trial, the addition of core decompression was not superior to intensive physical therapy alone.[43]

Total joint replacement is standard therapy for advanced AVN. Limb length discrepancy and muscle imbalance are potential problems in growing children. New therapies under investigation include extracorporal shock wave therapy and the use of vascularized bone grafts to facilitate bone regeneration after core decompression. Hydroxyurea use has not been shown to reduce the risk of AVN.

Hematopoietic Stem Cell Transplantation and Gene Therapy

Hematopoietic stem cell transplant is considered the only curative treatment for SCD. Worldwide, over 1000 patients with severe SCD have received HLA-identical sibling transplants with a 5-yr event free survival and a 5-yr overall survival of 91.4% and 92.9% respectively (Gluckman 2017).

Gene therapy for SCD is based on transplantation of genetically modified autologous hematopoietic stem cells with a lentiviral vector expressing a globin gene variant under the control of globin transcriptional regulatory elements (Lidonnici 2017). The successful case of a 13 year old boy with severe SCD who received βA-T87Q-globin variant which disrupts the formation of axial and lateral contacts between HbS tetramers (polymerization) was recently reported (Ribeil 2017) and clinical trials are underway.

Prognosis

By 1994, only 50% of patients with sickle cell anemia survived beyond the fifth decade. The average life expectancy of HbSS patients was reported as 42 years in males and 48 years in females and in patients with HbSC disease as 60 years in males and 68 years in females.[44] With the use of hydroxyurea and better supportive care, the median survival of HbSS is estimated at 58 years (Elmariah 2014).

References

1. Hassell KL. Population estimates of sickle cell disease in the U.S. *American Journal of Preventive Medicine*. 2010;38 (4 Suppl):S512–521.

2. Hofrichter J. Kinetics of sickle hemoglobin polymerization. III. Nucleation rates determined from stochastic fluctuations in polymerization progress curves. *Journal of Molecular Biology*. 1986;189 (3):553–571.

3. Steinberg MH. Genetic etiologies for phenotypic diversity in sickle cell anemia. *The Scientific World Journal*. 2009;9:46–67.

4. Ballas SK. Pathophysiology and principles of management of the many faces of the acute vaso-occlusive crisis in patients with sickle cell disease. *European Journal of Haematology*. 2014.

5. Ballas SK, Gupta K, Adams-Graves P. Sickle cell pain: a critical reappraisal. *Blood*. 2012;120(18):3647–3656.

6. Latremoliere A, Woolf CJ. Central sensitization: a generator of pain hypersensitivity by central neural plasticity. *The Journal of Pain: Official Journal of the American Pain Society*. 2009;10(9):895–926.

7. Woolf CJ. Central sensitization: uncovering the relation between pain and plasticity. *Anesthesiology*. 2007;106 (4):864–867.

8. Kohli DR, Li Y, Khasabov SG, Gupta P, Kehl LJ, Ericson ME, et al. Pain-related behaviors and neurochemical alterations in mice expressing sickle hemoglobin: modulation by cannabinoids. *Blood*. 2010;116 (3):456–465.

9. Davies SC, Luce PJ, Win AA, Riordan JF, Brozovic M. Acute chest syndrome in sickle-cell disease. *Lancet*. 1984;1 (8367):36–38.

10. Vichinsky EP, Styles LA, Colangelo LH, Wright EC, Castro O, Nickerson B. Acute chest syndrome in sickle cell disease: clinical presentation and course. Cooperative study of sickle cell disease. *Blood*. 1997;89(5):1787–1792.

11. Gladwin MT, Sachdev V, Jison ML, Shizukuda Y, Plehn JF, Minter K, et al. Pulmonary hypertension as a risk factor for death in patients with sickle cell disease. *The New England Journal of Medicine*. 2004;350(9):886–895.

12. Ataga KI, Moore CG, Jones S, Olajide O, Strayhorn D, Hinderliter A, et al. Pulmonary hypertension in patients with sickle cell disease: a longitudinal study. *British Journal of Haematology*. 2006;134(1):109–115.

13. Fonseca GH, Souza R, Salemi VM, Jardim CV, Gualandro SF. Pulmonary hypertension diagnosed by right heart catheterisation in sickle cell disease. *The European Respiratory Journal*. 2012;39 (1):112–118.

14. Kato GJ, Martyr S, Blackwelder WC, Nichols JS, Coles WA, Hunter LA, et al. Levels of soluble endothelium-derived adhesion molecules in patients with sickle cell disease are associated with pulmonary hypertension, organ dysfunction, and mortality. *British Journal of Haematology*. 2005;130 (6):943–953.

15. Moser FG, Miller ST, Bello JA, Pegelow CH, Zimmerman RA, Wang WC, et al. The spectrum of brain MR abnormalities in sickle-cell disease: a report from the Cooperative Study of Sickle Cell Disease. *AJNR American Journal of Neuroradiology*. 1996;17 (5):965–972.

16. Pegelow CH, Macklin EA, Moser FG, Wang WC, Bello JA, Miller ST, et al. Longitudinal changes in brain magnetic resonance imaging findings in children with sickle cell disease. *Blood*. 2002;99 (8):3014–3018.

17. Berkelhammer LD, Williamson AL, Sanford SD, Dirksen CL, Sharp WG, Margulies AS, et al. Neurocognitive sequelae of pediatric sickle cell disease: a review of the literature. *Child Neuropsychology: A Journal on Normal and Abnormal Development in Childhood and Adolescence*. 2007;13 (2):120–131.

18. Kral MC, Brown RT, Connelly M, Cure JK, Besenski N, Jackson SM, et al. Radiographic predictors of neurocognitive functioning in pediatric sickle cell disease. *Journal of Child Neurology*. 2006;21(1):37–44.

19. Steen RG, Xiong X, Mulhern RK, Langston JW, Wang WC. Subtle brain abnormalities in children with sickle cell disease: relationship to blood hematocrit. *Annals of Neurology*. 1999;45(3):279–286.

20. Steen RG, Miles MA, Helton KJ, Strawn S, Wang W, Xiong X, et al. Cognitive impairment in children with hemoglobin SS sickle cell disease: relationship to MR imaging findings and hematocrit. *AJNR American Journal of Neuroradiology*. 2003;24 (3):382–389.

21. Iampietro M, Giovannetti T, Tarazi R. Hypoxia and inflammation in children with sickle cell disease: implications for hippocampal functioning and episodic memory. *Neuropsychology Review*. 2014;24(2):252–265.

22. Ohene-Frempong K, Weiner SJ, Sleeper LA, Miller ST, Embury S, Moohr JW, et al. Cerebrovascular accidents in sickle cell disease: rates and risk factors. *Blood*. 1998;91(1):288–294.

23. Lebensburger JD, Miller ST, Howard TH, Casella JF, Brown RC, Lu M, et al. Influence of severity of anemia on clinical findings in infants with sickle cell anemia: analyses from the BABY HUG study. *Pediatric Blood & Cancer*. 2012;59(4):675–678.

24. Goldberg MF. Natural history of untreated proliferative sickle retinopathy. *Archives of Ophthalmology*. 1971;85(4):428–437.

25. Pegelow CH, Colangelo L, Steinberg M, Wright EC, Smith J, Phillips G, et al. Natural history of blood pressure in sickle cell disease: risks for stroke and death associated with relative hypertension in sickle cell anemia. *The American Journal of Medicine.* 1997;102 (2):171–177.

26. Sarnaik S, Slovis TL, Corbett DP, Emami A, Whitten CF. Incidence of cholelithiasis in sickle cell anemia using the ultrasonic gray-scale technique. *The Journal of Pediatrics.* 1980;96 (6):1005–1008.

27. Emond AM, Holman R, Hayes RJ, Serjeant GR. Priapism and impotence in homozygous sickle cell disease. *Archives of Internal Medicine.* 1980;140 (11):1434–1437.

28. Marouf R, Gupta R, Haider MZ, Al-Wazzan H, Adekile AD. Avascular necrosis of the femoral head in adult Kuwaiti sickle cell disease patients. *Acta Haematologica* 2003;110(1):11–15.

29. Charache S, Terrin ML, Moore RD, Dover GJ, Barton FB, Eckert SV, et al. Effect of hydroxyurea on the frequency of painful crises in sickle cell anemia. Investigators of the Multicenter Study of Hydroxyurea in Sickle Cell Anemia. *The New England Journal of Medicine.* 1995;332(20):1317–1322.

30. Vichinsky EP, Johnson R, Lubin BH. Multidisciplinary approach to pain management in sickle cell disease. *The American Journal of Pediatric Hematology/Oncology.* 1982;4 (3):328–333.

31. Hagmeyer KO, Mauro LS, Mauro VF. Meperidine-related seizures associated with patient-controlled analgesia pumps. *The Annals of Pharmacotherapy.* 1993;27(1):29–32.

32. The Management of Sickle Cell Disease. In: USDoHaH, ed. *Services.* 4th edition. National Institutes of Health, Bethesda, MD; 2004:59–74.

33. Inturrisi CE. Pharmacology of methadone and its isomers. *Minerva Anestesiologica.* 2005;71(7–8):435–437.

34. McCance-Katz EF. (R)-methadone versus racemic methadone: what is best for patient care? *Addiction.* 2011;106 (4):687–688.

35. Uprety D, Baber A, Foy M. Ketamine infusion for sickle cell pain crisis refractory to opioids: a case report and review of literature. *Annals of Hematology.* 2014;93(5):769–771.

36. Tawfic QA, Faris AS, Kausalya R. The role of a low-dose ketamine-midazolam regimen in the management of severe painful crisis in patients with sickle cell disease. *Journal of Pain and Symptom Management.* 2014;47(2):334–340.

37. Aygun B, McMurray MA, Schultz WH, Kwiatkowski JL, Hilliard L, Alvarez O, et al. Chronic transfusion practice for children with sickle cell anaemia and stroke. *British Journal of haematology.* 2009;145(4):524–528.

38. Enninful-Eghan H, Moore RH, Ichord R, Smith-Whitley K, Kwiatkowski JL. Transcranial Doppler ultrasonography and prophylactic transfusion program is effective in preventing overt stroke in children with sickle cell disease. *The Journal of Pediatrics.* 2010;157 (3):479–484.

39. Ancel D, Amiot X, Chaslin-Ferbus D, Hagege I, Garioud A, Girot R, et al. Treatment of chronic hepatitis C in sickle cell disease and thalassaemic patients with interferon and ribavirin. *European Journal of Gastroenterology & Hepatology.* 2009; 21(7):726–729.

40. Siegel JF, Rich MA, Brock WA. Association of sickle cell disease, priapism, exchange transfusion and neurological events: ASPEN syndrome. *The Journal of Urology.* 1993;150 (5 Pt 1):1480–1482.

41. Roy NB et al. Interventions for chronic kidney disease in people with sickle cell disease. *Cochrane Database Syst Rev.* 2017, https://www.ncbi.nlm.nih.gov/pubmed/28672087.

42. Wang WC, Ware RE, Miller ST, Iyer RV, Casella JF, Minniti CP, et al. Hydroxycarbamide in very young children with sickle-cell anaemia: a multicentre, randomised, controlled trial (BABY HUG). *Lancet.* 2011;377 (9778):1663–1672.

43. Neumayr LD, Aguilar C, Earles AN, Jergesen HE, Haberkern CM, Kammen BF, et al. Physical therapy alone compared with core decompression and physical therapy for femoral head osteonecrosis in sickle cell disease. Results of a multicenter study at a mean of three years after treatment. *Journal of Bone and Joint Surgery.* 2006;88(12):2573–2582.

44. Platt OS, Brambilla DJ, Rosse WF, Milner PF, Castro O, Steinberg MH, et al. Mortality in sickle cell disease. Life expectancy and risk factors for early death. *The New England Journal of Medicine.* 1994;330(23):1639–1644.

Structural Hemoglobinopathies

Edward J. Benz, Jr., MD

Sickle cell anemia (Chapter 10) and the thalassemia syndromes (Chapter 8) are by far the most commonly encountered hemoglobinopathies. They account for the vast majority of morbidity and mortality attributable to abnormalities of the hemoglobin molecule. However, there are a number of other inherited or acquired alterations of hemoglobin that can derange the physiological behavior of hemoglobin and produce distinctive clinical syndromes. While rare on an individual basis, these conditions, in the aggregate, are sufficiently common that patients with one form or another are likely to be encountered by most hematologists. For the purposes of this chapter, we shall refer to these conditions as "structural" hemoglobinopathies.

Hemoglobin is perhaps the most thoroughly studied of all human proteins at both the genetic and protein levels. Well over 1,000 mutations have been described that alter the structure and/or function of human hemoglobins. Only a handful of these actually derange function sufficiently to produce clinical abnormalities or morbidity. Those that achieve clinical significance invariably impair one or both of two fundamental properties of hemoglobin: its extraordinary solubility and its ability to acquire, transport, and deliver oxygen in a reversible manner over the normal physiological range of oxygen tensions. Hemoglobinopathies that result from reduced solubility of hemoglobin are called "unstable hemoglobins" while hemoglobinopathies are rising from altered oxygen affinity can be subclassified as "high-affinity" hemoglobins, "low-affinity" hemoglobins, and the important special case of methemoglobinemia. The latter can arise from mutations but results more often from exposure to toxins.

Table 11.1 provides a classification of hemoglobinopathies and places the structural hemoglobinopathies in context of the sickle cell syndromes, the thalassemia syndromes, and other less common inherited and acquired abnormalities. In contrast to the distinctively higher geographical incidence of thalassemia and sickle cell anemia in malaria-endemic regions, structural hemoglobinopathies tend to occur sporadically in all populations. A general diagnostic caution about these structural hemoglobinopathies is that they arise not infrequently by spontaneous mutation; thus, while heritable, they may arise in patients without a positive family history.

Hemoglobins with Reduced Solubility – "Unstable Hemoglobins"

As noted in Chapter 1, hemoglobin must be extraordinarily soluble in order to achieve the very high cytoplasmic concentrations needed to provide for adequate oxygen transport. For present purposes, this solubility can be thought to depend on three exquisitely evolved structural features of the normal hemoglobins (Figure 11.1): first, the placement of numerous highly charged (hydrophilic) amino acid residues on the outer surfaces of the tetramer. These are exposed to the aqueous environment. Second, internal hydrogen bonds and weak forces that hold the otherwise insoluble globin subunits together to form the highly soluble tetramer. Third, the concentration of suitable hydrophobic surfaces in the interior core that provide for stable attachments that sequester the insoluble heme moiety within the interior of the molecule. Mutations that disrupt any of these structural features tend to reduce the solubility of the molecule, causing it to precipitate and form cytoplasmic inclusion bodies containing heme and insoluble protein. More than 100 unique mutations are known to impair solubility. Only a few create sufficient impairments to produce clinical symptomatology (see Figure 11.1).

Pathophysiology of Unstable Hemoglobin Disorders

The biochemical consequences of the aforementioned disruptions have been reasonably well characterized. These mutated hemoglobins tend to dissociate into subunits, often with loss of the heme moiety. The resultant subfragments of hemoglobin, called hemipyrroles, precipitate, forming inclusion bodies ("Heinz" bodies). These highly reactive inclusions disrupt the redox homeostasis of the cell. They oxidize the delicate red cell membrane and its cytoskeleton and overwhelm the antioxidant capacity of the affected erythrocytes. The consequent metabolic and cell surface anomalies cause premature destruction of the damaged cells within the reticuloendothelial cells of the spleen and liver. When sufficiently pronounced, this shortened red cell life span produces a hemolytic anemia of variable severity. Patients afflicted with these conditions exhibit typical stigmata of hemolytic anemia, usually, but not

Table 11.1 Classification of the hemoglobinopathies

I. Biosynthetic Abnormalities
  A. The Thalassemia Syndromes – deficient production or one of more globin chains:
    1. α thalassemia – reduced or absent α globin synthesis
    2. β thalassemia – reduced or absent β globin synthesis
    3. $\delta\beta$, $\gamma\delta\beta$ thalassemias – reduced or absent synthesis of multiple globin chains
  B. Hereditary Persistence of Fetal Hemoglobin. Persistence of high levels of HbF in postnatal life
    1. Pancellular – high HbF in all RBC populations
    2. Heterocellular – high Hb restricted to increased subpopulations of "F" cells
  C. "Mixed": Structurally Abnormal Hemoglobins Exhibiting a Thalassemia Phenotype due to Pleomorhic Mutations that alter function as well as production
    1. Unequal crossover and rearrangements of globin genes producing "fused" hemoglobins that are underproduced:
      Hb Lepore, Hb Kenya
    2. Mutations altering coding properties of one or more codons, producing a globin structural variant, but also impairing mRNA metabolism, e.g., splicing, translation stability, etc.
      HbE, Hb Knossos, Hb Constant Spring
    3. Mutations resulting in exceptionally unstable hemoglobins that fail to accumulate.
      Hb Quonze, Hb Indianapolis

II. Structurally Abnormal Hemoglobins – due to Mutations Altering Hb Function or Stability
  A. Abnormal Hb Polymerization:
    1. HbS – sickle cell syndromes
  B. Hemoglobins that oxidize or precipitate readily
    1. "Unstable" hemoglobins – due to mutations that render hemoglobin less soluble – Hb Köln, Hb Terre Haut
    2. "M" Hemoglobins – mutations that render the heme iron moiety more susceptible to oxidation to the Fe^{+++} state, producing methemoglobinemia – HbM Iwate, HbM Milwaukee
  C. High-Affinity Hemoglobins – Mutations that tighten binding of Hb for O_2 and reduce release from Hb to tissues, producing polycythemia
    Hb Kempsey
  D. Low-Affinity Hemoglobins – Mutations causing Hb to bind "less tightly" to O_2, increasing O_2 delivery to tissues, producing pseudocyanosis, pseudoanemia
    Hb Kansas, Hb Titusville

III. Acquired Modification of Hb Structure and/or Synthesis
  A. Methemoglobins, Methemoglobinemia – due to toxins oxidizing heme iron to Fe^{+++} ferric state – Met Hb has a bluish-brown color, useless for O_2 transport, causes pseudo cyanosis, O_2 deprivation syndromes
  B. Carbonmonoxy hemoglobin – Hb bound to carbon monoxide via exposure to auto exhaust, uncombusted hydrocarbon fuels, etc. Cannot bind O_2 – causes tissue asphyxia
  C. Sulfhemoglobin – usually not clinically significant
  D. Acquired alterations of Hb synthesis
    HbH (alpha thalassemia) in erythroleukemia
    Elevated HbF during stress erythropoiesis and bone marrow dysplasias, recovery postchemotherapy, post–bone marrow transplant, myelodysplasias, etc.

always, apparent in childhood: jaundice due to indirect hyperbilirubinemia, premature biliary tract disease with gall stones; hepatosplenomegaly; elevations in LDH; and, in more severe cases, inanition, growth retardation, high-output congestive heart failure, leg ulcers, and secondary megaloblastosis due to folate depletion.

Clinical manifestations are highly variable and depend on several factors. First among these is the degree to which the mutation reduces solubility. A second variable is the nature of the affected globin chain. Because of the duplication of the α globin genes, mutations in only one α locus will only affect 25–35% of the hemoglobin produced; β chain mutations, on the other hand, arise from a single locus, and 50% of the hemoglobin produced will be abnormal in the heterozygous state. Homozygotes for any of these mutations will clearly have the greatest severity, but they are exceedingly rare. Most of β chain mutants, when symptomatic, are symptomatic in the heterozygous state. Alpha chain mutants tend to be less severe unless more than one α locus is affected. A third important variable is the milieu in which these abnormal hemoglobins circulate. In some cases, symptoms are seen only when other oxidative stresses increase the likelihood that the hemoglobin will precipitate, for example during infection or exposure to drugs producing oxidative stress (Table 11.2). In this regard, unstable hemoglobins exhibit variable clinical behavior within a single patient in ways somewhat analogous to patients with the most common form of glucose-6 dehydrogenase (G6PD) deficiency. One interesting example of the modifying effect of the milieu is Hb Zurich. It has a higher-than-normal affinity for carbon monoxide. When bound to carbon monoxide, Hb Zurich is less likely to precipitate, for obscure reasons. Thus, smokers with Hb Zurich, who have above-normal carbon monoxide levels, tend to fare better than their nonsmoking counterparts. Conversely, Hb Hammersmith is both unstable and possesses a lower-than-normal oxygen affinity. As described later in this chapter, this results in significantly improved oxygen delivery at the capillary tissue level, thus allowing patients to fare better clinically despite a lower hematocrit.

Diagnosis of Unstable Hemoglobins

Given the aforementioned sources of molecular and cellular variability, it is not surprising that signs and symptoms can also vary widely. In general, unstable hemoglobin should be in the differential diagnosis of patients who exhibit otherwise unexplained stigmata of hemolysis or frank hemolytic anemia, with a negative workup for autoimmune hemolysis. These signs can be as subtle as unexplained reticulocytosis, occasional passage of dark urine or transient jaundice, or as obvious as severe hemolytic anemia with its attendant stigmata. A positive family history is helpful, but a negative history does not rule out any of the structural hemoglobinopathies, because spontaneous mutations *in utero* are fairly common. The clinical presentation can resemble that of patients with inherited red cell enzymopathies or membrane disorders; the distinctive differences in red cell morphology characterizing each of these disorders are helpful means of discriminating among these.

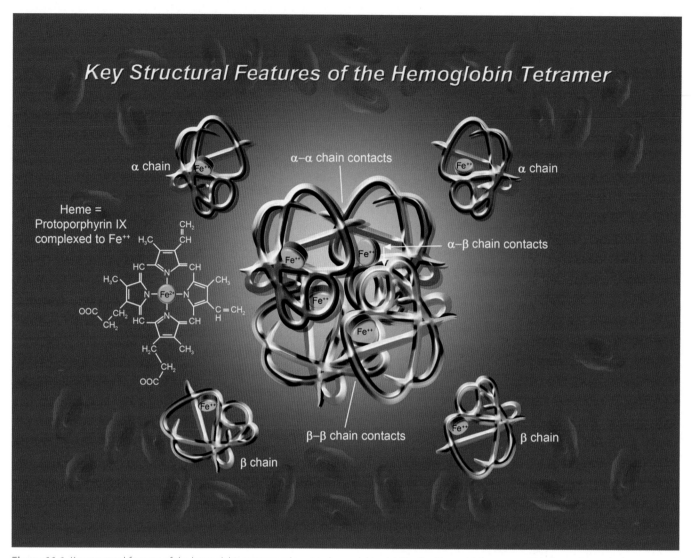

Figure 11.1 Key structural features of the hemoglobin tetramer relevant to hemoglobin stability. See Figure 1.1 for context. This figure shows the key points of contact in which mutations occur producing unstable hemoglobins.

The primary laboratory diagnostic findings, when present, will include a peripheral blood smear exhibiting striking anisocytosis and poikilocytosis with polychromasia, indicative of a high reticulocyte count, indirect hyperbilirubinemia, and, when present, splenomegaly. Anemia will most frequently present in childhood, but mutations having milder affects on solubility may not appear until the growth spurts of adolescence or in adult life as a result of exposure to the various oxidative stresses mentioned earlier. An unstable hemoglobin disorder can also present as the underlying cause of biliary tract disease and should be considered in patients who present with biliary tract symptoms at an early age or without obvious risk factors.

Only mutations affecting the alpha globin gene will exhibit phenotypic manifestations *in utero*. However, manifestations may be minimal because of the smaller fraction of hemoglobin arising from the affected locus. Nonetheless, a structurally abnormal hemoglobin should be considered if there are no other explanations for hemolytic anemia detected *in utero* or during the perinatal period.

The pathognomonic sign of unstable hemoglobin disorder is the Heinz body, the inclusion body of precipitated hemoglobin and hemoglobin fragments. These are not seen in membrane disorders or enzymopathies. They can be detected by supravital staining of red cells with brilliant cresyl blue, a test available at standard clinical laboratories. While the presence of Heinz bodies is a strong indicator of an unstable hemoglobin disorder, their absence may simply indicate that the process is sufficiently mild that splenic polishing has eliminated Heinz bodies from the circulating red cells.

The most direct diagnostic tools are direct studies of hemoglobin solubility, hemoglobin protein analysis, and globin gene sequencing. For the former, the isopropanol stability test is useful. Unstable hemoglobins tend to be significantly less soluble in solutions containing isopropyl alcohol. If the index of suspicion is sufficiently high, it is also recommended that one perform direct hemoglobin analysis by mass spectrometry or direct globin gene sequencing. Both are readily available in reference laboratories. The use of more traditional hemoglobin electrophoresis methods is also helpful if an abnormal

Table 11.2 Some mutations producing abnormal hemoglobin molecules*

Residue	Mutation	Common Name(s)	Molecular Pathology
ABNORMAL SOLUBILITY			
β6	Glu→Val	S	Polymerization
β6	Glu→Lys	C	Crystallization
β121	Glu→Gln	D-Los Angeles, D-Punjab	Increases polymer in S/D heterozygote
β121	Glu→Lys	O-Arab	Increases polymer in S/O heterozygote
INCREASED OXYGEN AFFINITY			
α92	Arg→Gln	J-Capetown	Stabilizes O_2 bound state
α141	Arg→His	Suresnes	Eliminate bond to Asn 126 O_2 bound state
β89	Ser→Asn	Creteil	Weakens bonds in T O_2 bound state
β99	Asp→Asn	Kempsey	Breaks O_2 bound intersubunit bonds
DECREASED OXYGEN AFFINITY			
α94	Asp→Asn	Titusville	Alters R deoxy state intersubunit bonds
β102	Asn→Thr	Kansas	Breaks deoxy state intersubunit bonds
β102	Asn→Ser	Beth Israel	Breaks deoxy state intersubunit bonds
METHEMOGLOBIN			
α58	His→Tyr	M-Boston, M-Osaka	Heme liganded to Tyr not His
α87	His→Tyr	M-Iwate	Heme liganded to both His and Tyr
β28	Leu→Gln	St. Louis	Opens heme pocket
β63	His→Tyr	M-Saskatoon	Tyr ligand stabilizes ferriheme
β67	Val→Glu	M-Milwaukee-I	Negative charge stabilizes ferriheme
β92	His→Tyr	M-Hyde Park	Bond of His to heme disrupted
Residue	**Mutation**	**Common Name(s)**	**Molecular Pathology**
UNSTABLE			
α43	Phe→Val	Torino	Loss of heme contact
v94	Asp→Tyr	Setif	Weakens subunit contacts
β28	Leu→Gln	St. Louis	Inserts polar group in heme pocket
β35	Tyr→Phe	Philadelphia	Loss of dimer bond favors precipitation
β42	Phe→Ser	Hammersmith	Loss of heme
β63	His→Arg	Zurich	Opens heme pocket
β88	Leu→Pro	Santa Ana	Disrupts helix

Table 11.2 Partial List of Structurally Abnormal Hemoglobins Organized by Their Primary Pathophysiologic Behavior

The structurally abnormal hemoglobins, as discussed in the text, generally produce four primary kinds of abnormalities leading to disruptions in red cell structure, function, or survival. Hemoglobins that exhibit abnormal solubility and tend to polymerize create intracellular viscosity and a variety of other abnormalities. Sickle hemoglobin (HbS) is the prototype. High-affinity hemoglobins bind oxygen more efficiently but deliver it less efficiently to tissues, producing polycythemia. Low-affinity hemoglobins bind oxygen less efficiently but acquire adequate supplies of oxygen in the normal lung and deliver oxygen far more efficiently to tissues, producing mild "pseudoanemia" and occasionally psyanosis, which is not associated with any life-threatening abnormalities. Methemoglobins have amino acid substitutions that render heme iron more susceptible to oxidation to the ferric (Fe^{+++}) state, producing a useless pigment, which, when present in sufficient quantities, deprives tissue of oxygen and can produce life-threatening hypoxia. Unstable hemoglobins have mutations that render the hemoglobin likely to precipitate in an oxidized form and damage delicate intracellular components, producing hemolytic anemia.

hemoglobin band is detected. However, many of these mutations are charge neutral, particularly those altering chain–chain interactions or the heme pocket, and therefore will not necessarily alter electrophoretic mobility. Electrophoresis is thus a useful "rule-in" test but not definitive for ruling out the disorder.

Treatment

Many patients with unstable hemoglobin disorders can be managed adequately by avoiding oxidative stresses, judicious use of transfusions during exacerbation of hemolysis, and supportive care including close monitoring for biliary tract disease and iron overload due to increased red cell and iron turnover. In severe cases, the only currently definitive therapy is splenectomy. Clearly, splenectomy should be avoided in children until at least the age of 3 or 4 in order to allow maturation of the immune system. Indeed, it is advisable to delay or to avoid splenectomy all together whenever possible because of the long-term consequences for splenectomized patients. These include susceptibility to overwhelming sepsis, requiring close monitoring for exposure to bacterial infection and use when appropriate of antibiotic prophylaxis (see Chapter 32). There is also increasing concern about the hypercoagulable state that occurs in a number of patients following splenectomy, particularly those in whom above normal levels of red cell turnover continue to occur. That said, splenectomy is often effective in reducing or eliminating transfusion dependency in these patients and in reducing secondary stigmata resulting from red cell turnover. In the future, these are disorders that should be susceptible to correction by evolving strategies of gene editing. For the most severe and treatment-refractory conditions, allogeneic bone marrow transplantation can be considered, but only as a last resort.

Hemoglobinopathies Due to Altered Oxygen Affinity

"High-Affinity" Hemoglobins

While not, strictly speaking, a cause of anemia, high-affinity hemoglobins are worth at least brief mention in this volume because they are instructive with regard to the impact hemoglobin can have on the regulation of red cell mass. High-affinity hemoglobins arise from mutations that increase the affinity of the hemoglobin molecule for oxygen (see Figure 11.2). Two major mechanisms have been described: the first arises from mutations that alter the amino acids responsible for forming the hydrogen bonds, salt bridges, or hydrophobic interactions that position heme for optimal binding to oxygen; the second involves mutations that reduce the affinity of hemoglobin for bi-phosphoglycerate (2,3-BPG). As described in Chapter 1, binding of 2,3 BPG to hemoglobin lowers its oxygen affinity; a significant fraction of the major adult hemoglobin, HbA, is bound to 2,3 BPG under physiologic conditions. When unable to bind 2,3 BPG, the mutant

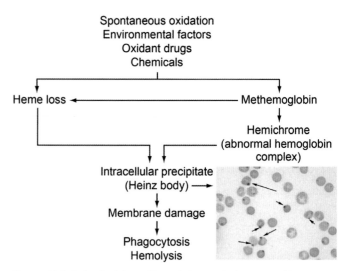

Figure 11.2 Pathophysiology of hemolytic anemia due to unstable hemoglobin disorders. Note the presence of Heinz bodies in the red cells bearing unstable hemoglobins, detected by supravital dyes.

hemoglobin has a higher oxygen affinity even in the presence of abundant 2,3 BPG.

Pathophysiology

As shown in Figure 11.3, the vast majority of oxygen acquired in the lungs and subsequently dispensed to the tissues is provided by the "top" of the sigmoidal oxygen dissociation curve. Note that, at a pO_2 of 60, normal HbA is nearly fully saturated with oxygen. It thus acquires relatively little additional oxygen at the normal pulmonary pO_2 of nearly 100. Mutations that "shift the oxygen curve to the left," that is, possess a higher affinity for oxygen, thus offer essentially no advantage in terms of acquiring more oxygen during normal respiration. Rather (see Figure 11.1), there is a significant disadvantage at the lower pO_2 of mixed capillary venous blood in the tissues because, at that pO_2, less oxygen is delivered to the tissues. The juxtaglomerular cells in the kidney, sensing this relative tissue hypoxia, produce and release higher levels of erythropoietin, driving the bone marrow to produce more red cells. The result is erythrocytosis and polycythemia. An example of a high-affinity hemoglobin is hemoglobin Kempsey ($\beta^{99Asp->Asn}$), in which the mutation disrupts the normal salt bridges that limit the modulation of the heme group for oxygen.

Diagnosis

High-affinity hemoglobin should be included in the differential diagnosis of erythrocytosis. In contrast to polycythemia vera rubra, the white cell and platelet counts are usually normal, and splenomegaly is rare unless the hemoglobin is also unstable. In the latter situation, stigmata of hemolytic anemia also should be apparent, and polycythemia would thus be unlikely to be encountered in any event. Hemoglobin electrophoresis may or may not be informative, because many of the relevant amino acids substitutions are charge neutral.

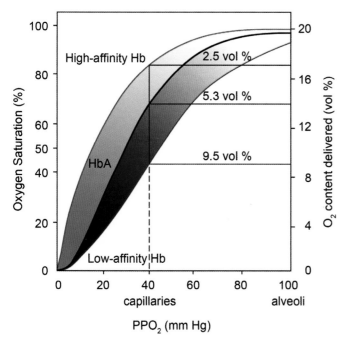

Figure 11.3 Oxygen delivery by structurally abnormal hemoglobins with altered oxygen affinity. The figure illustrates the amount of oxygen delivered as the p0₂ drops from 100 in the lungs to 40 in the capillaries (5.3 volume percent for normal HbA). High-affinity hemoglobins acquire relatively little additional oxygen in the lungs because normal hemoglobin is almost fully saturated at that point. Conversely, high-affinity hemoglobins deliver relatively little hemoglobin to tissues at capillary p0₂ (2.5 volumes percent). In contrast, low-affinity hemoglobins become well saturated in the lungs and deliver very large quantities of oxygen to the tissues (9.5 volume percent).

However, mass spectroscopy analysis or direct globin gene sequencing analysis can provide definitive diagnosis.

Treatment

The management of high-affinity hemoglobin disorders is frequently expectant. Patients are often asymptomatic and simply need reassurance that their high hematocrit is not due to a bone marrow dyscrasia. In patients in whom the hematocrit rises to symptomatic levels (usually > 55), symptoms are similar to those seen on other forms of polycythemia including mental sluggishness, hypertension, chest pain, rubor, and so forth. Judicious phlebotomy can often improve symptoms. In extreme cases, exchange transfusion may be necessary. Usually, however, cautious management with phlebotomy is sufficient. Patients with high-affinity hemoglobins and hematocrit above 55 may also be at increased risk for thrombosis. There is little evidence to support the long term use of anticoagulants; however, avoidance of situations increasing the risk of thrombosis should be provided, such as elastic stockings, frequent mild exercise during long trips, and the like.

Low-Affinity Hemoglobins

Pathophysiology

Rare mutations can disrupt the relationship between globin, heme, and oxygen in such a way as to *lower* the affinity of the hemoglobin molecule for oxygen. The best-known example is hemoglobin Kansas ($\beta^{102\ asn->thr}$). As indicated in Figure 11.1, the pathophysiology of low-affinity hemoglobins represents the mirror image of the situation with high-affinity hemoglobins. In individuals with normal pulmonary function, these hemoglobins can become almost fully saturated because, at a pO₂ of 100, even hemoglobins with reduced affinity can acquire abundant amounts of oxygen. In contrast to high-affinity hemoglobins, however, these hemoglobins deliver normal or even elevated amounts of oxygens at the mixed capillary bed (i.e., tissue) level of pO₂. Therefore, the erythropoietin levels in these individuals tend to be low. The hematocrit can thus be below normal levels, even though the patient, in terms of oxygen delivery, is perfectly normal. Moreover, since cyanosis becomes clinically apparent at a level of unsaturated hemoglobin of 5 gm/cc, these patients can exhibit "pseudo" cyanosis. Once again, however, they are physiologically healthy.

Diagnosis

Diagnosis of these disorders should be suspected when there is no other obvious cause for cyanosis or a mild anemia, especially if the patient's overall state of well-being is not compatible with these otherwise dire physical findings. Analysis of the hemoglobin by electrophoresis, mass spectroscopy, and/or globin gene sequencing will provide a definitive diagnosis in most cases.

Treatment

Reassurance is usually sufficient treatment for these disorders. However, if cyanosis is pronounced, concerns about cosmetic issues can be significant and require supportive care. It is critically important to be sure the patient is aware of the hemoglobin disorder and understands that it, not some major illness, is the basis of the abnormalities. This can forestall well-meaning but inappropriate workup of symptoms that otherwise have ominous implications.

Methemoglobinemia

Methemoglobins are structurally abnormal hemoglobins in which the abnormality resides in the iron moiety. Normal hemoglobins maintain the iron ion within each heme group in the reduced (Fe^{++}) ferrous state. In methemoglobins, the iron is in the oxidized (Fe^{+++}) ferric state. The oxidized heme groups in methemoglobin bind oxygen poorly. Paradoxically, if only some of the iron moieties are in the oxidized state within the tetramer, the remaining heme molecules have a greatly increased oxygen affinity. In either case, because of the lack of oxygen binding or the failure to release oxygen to the tissues, methemoglobin is essentially useless as a respiratory pigment.

Methemoglobin has a characteristic bluish-brown color. Patients with more than about 10–20% methemoglobin thus appear to be cyanotic and can experience symptoms of tissue hypoxia. The major distinction between these patients and patients with true cyanosis is, of course, that the arterial pO_2 is normal unless respiratory function is independently compromised or depressed as a result of obtundation.

Pathophysiology

During the normal cycle of oxygen binding and release, the oxygen-binding iron moieties within heme are transiently oxidized so that, at any given time, a small amount of normal circulating hemoglobin can be detected as methemoglobin. These amounts should never exceed 1–3%. Three basic mechanisms are known to cause clinically significant increases in methemoglobinemia:

First, exposure to toxins capable of oxidizing the iron moieties in normal hemoglobins directly or indirectly, of which nitrite or nitrate-containing compounds are the most well appreciated. A table of agents associated with clinically significant methemoglobinemia is shown in Table 11.3. This is by far the most common etiology of methemoglobinemia.

Second, mutations in the globin chains that alter the association of amino acid side chains with heme, thereby facilitating oxidation of the iron moiety. These are called hemoglobins M (HbM). These changes, such as the replacement of a histidine by a tyrosine in hemoglobin M Iwate ($\beta^{87 \text{ his->tyr}}$) tends to stabilize the oxidized state of the iron and also to render it relatively resistant to enzymatic reduction by the methemoglobin reductase system (see below).

Third, hereditary defects in an enzyme system that, under normal conditions, reduces methemoglobin to hemoglobin. This system is called the cytochrome b5 reductase system. So-called type 1 mutations in this system produce congenital cyanosis with minimal symptomatology. However, so-called type 2 mutations produce a series of systemic affects, including severe mental retardation, probably because the defect affects a spliceoform of the key enzyme that is expressed in many tissues.

Diagnosis

Methemoglobinemia should be suspected in anyone presenting with a cyanotic appearance and/or symptoms of oxygen deprivation including mental obtundation, dizziness, disorientation, or respiratory depression. The characteristic appearance of the blood should be looked for when blood is drawn and a methemoglobin level requested from the laboratory. These analyses are available stat in an emergency situation in most clinical labs. While family history can be helpful in establishing a congenital cause, spontaneous mutations are not unusual, particularly for hemoglobins M. Hemoglobin analysis will show characteristic bands on electrophoresis. Mass spectroscopy or gene sequencing provides definitive diagnosis.

Wherever possible, a careful drug history or evidence of a potential toxin ingestion should be obtained from the patient, loved ones, or companions. Individuals who live with the patient should be examined for milder signs of cyanosis, since

Table 11.3 Major agents causing methemoglobinemia (can also aggravate unstable hemoglobin oxidation)

Agent
Nitrates (metabolized to nitrites)
Nitrites (including amyl, sodium, potassium, nitroglycerin) Nitrite, nitrate-containing medications (e.g., nitrous oxide)
Trinitrotoluene, nitrobenzene, phenacetin, acetanilide
Aniline, hydroxylamine dimethylamine
Sulfanilamide
p-Aminosalicylic acid
Dapsone
Primaquine, chloroquine
Prilocaine, benzocaine, lidocaine
Menadione, naphthoquinone
Naphthalene
Resorcinol
Phenylhydrazine
Infection, Inflammation

nitrates and nitrites can be commonly found as contaminants of well water and foodstuffs. Clearly a history of ingestion of any of the medications or compounds listed in Table 11.2 should be sought. Healthcare and laboratory workers have access to nitrite and nitrate-containing compounds in laboratories or pharmacies and have been known to use them as suicide attempts.

Treatment

Methemoglobinemia is a medical emergency when methemoglobin levels exceed 20–30%. It is a life-threatening condition because of the near impossibility for methemoglobin to deliver any oxygen to the tissues. It should be noted that, even when 100% of the hemoglobin present is methemoglobin, pulse oximetry yields an oxygen saturation of 85% because the absorption spectrum of methemoglobin gives a falsely high reading. Thus, at lethal or near-lethal levels of methemoglobin (30–50%), the pulse oximetry results can appear deceptively normal. Suspicion for methemoglobinemia should be high when the patient appears cyanotic in the face of a normal or near-normal pO_2 or O_2 saturation by pulse oximetry. Use of sophisticated co-oximetry testing will detect methemoglobin levels directly.

Emergency treatment of methemoglobinemia is accomplished by eliminating further exposure to the toxic agent and by reducing the methemoglobin with intravenous methylene blue, 1–2 mg/kg as a 1% solution in normal saline. It can be rapidly infused over about 3–5 minutes and repeated every 30 minutes as needed. Methylene blue promotes the reduction of the nicotinamide adenine dinucleotide

(NADPH) reductase system, thereby generating sufficient reducing power to convert methemoglobin back into hemoglobin. Of note is the fact that this reductase requires the activity of glucose-6 phosphate dehydrogenase (G6PD) and will be much less effective in patients who also have G6PD deficiency. These latter patients might require emergency exchange transfusion. The addition of emergency exchange transfusion to methylene blue therapy may also be indicated in patients who are *in extremis* as a result of their methylene blue ingestion. Once the urgent situation is resolved, oral methylene blue (100–300 mg/day) should be administered until all of the hemoglobin is restored to normal and the toxin has left the body.

Oral riboflavin therapy (20 mg/day) has also been recommended for the treatment of methemoglobinemia. It is important, however, to recognize that riboflavin acts slowly and will not be helpful in patients requiring emergency therapy. It can, however, be used in follow-up to remove residual methemoglobin and does not carry the unpleasant side effect of discoloring the urine blue.

Patients with Hb M or deficiency of the cytochrome b reductase system usually do not require therapy directed specifically at the methemoglobinemia. The patients with so-called type 2 deficiency of cytochrome b reductase do require complex medical management. These patients invariably present with significant symptomatology in the pediatric years.

Further Reading

Bunn HF. Sickle hemoglobin and other hemoglobin mutants. In: Stamatoyannopoulos G, Nienhuis AW, Majerus, PO, et al., eds. *The Molecular Basis of Blood Disease*. 2nd ed. Philadelphia: WB Saunders; 1993: __.

Bunn HF, Forget BG. *Hemoglobin: Molecular, Cellular and Clinical Aspects*. Philadelphia: WB Saunders; 1985.

Cortazzo JA, Lichtman AD. Methemoglobinemia: A review and recommendations for management. *J Cardiothorac Vasc Anesth*. 2014; 28:1043.

Dickerson RE, Geis I. *Hemoglobin: Structure, Function, Evolution, and Pathology*. Menlo Park, CA: Benjamin-Cummings; 1983.

Ho C, ed. *Hemoglobin and Oxygen Binding*. New York: Elsevier Biomedical; 1982.

Perutz MF. Molecular anatomy, physiology, and pathology of hemoglobin. In:

Stamatoyannopoulos G, Nienhuis AW, Leder P, et al., eds. *The Molecular Basis of Blood Diseases*. Philadelphia: WB Saunders; 1987:127.

Smith RP, Olson MV. Drug-induced methemoglobinemia. *Semin Hematol*. 1973; 10:253.

Wright RO, Lewander WJ, Woolf AD. Methemoglobinemia: Etiology, pharmacology, and clinical management. *Ann Emerg Med*. 1999; 34:646.

Chapter

12

Autoimmune Hemolytic Anemia

Mark A. Murakami, MD, Edward J. Benz, Jr., MD, and Nancy Berliner, MD

Introduction

Autoimmune hemolytic anemia (AIHA) is a heterogeneous group of disorders characterized by premature clearance of circulating erythrocytes mediated by autoantibodies targeting erythrocyte surface antigens.

Epidemiology

AIHA affects 0.8 persons per 100,000 annually, with an age-related incidence and a female predilection (M:F ratio 1.0:1.3).[1] Paroxysmal cold hemoglobinuria, an acquired cold hemolytic syndrome, provides an exception to this pattern (Figure 12.1).

Classification

AIHA can be classified into warm and cold subtypes according to the temperature at which the pathogenic autoantibody

reacts with target antigens. Warm autoantibodies, causing 80% of cases, bind erythrocyte antigens at core body temperature. Cold autoantibodies react only at cooler temperatures. Both warm and cold AIHA have primary and secondary forms based on associations with putative pharmacologic or disease culprits. Commonly implicated entities include medications, infections, immunological derangements, and hematologic malignancies (Table 12.1).

Warm AIHA
Clinical Features

Warm AIHA (WAIHA) manifests with nonspecific symptoms of anemia, chiefly fatigue, exertional dyspnea, and pallor. Jaundice and splenomegaly occur in more severe cases. Symptoms may emerge insidiously in idiopathic cases and secondary cases arising from chronic autoimmune or lymphoproliferative disorders and more acutely when related to certain drugs or acute hematologic malignancies.

Laboratory Findings

Laboratory hallmarks include anemia, with evidence of hemolysis including elevations in lactate dehydrogenase (LDH) and indirect bilirubin, reductions in serum haptoglobin, and a positive Coombs test. A brisk reticulocytosis is the rule, although exceptions occur when erythrocyte progenitors express the target antigen. The peripheral blood smear demonstrates microspherocytes in nonsplenectomized individuals and polychromasia, reflecting the reticulocytosis (Figure 12.2). The microspherocytosis raises the mean corpuscular hemoglobin concentration, while the concomitant reticulocytosis increases the red cell distribution width and mean corpuscular volume.

Coombs Test

The direct antiglobulin or Coombs test measures immunoglobulin and/or complement bound to the surface of red blood cells (RBCs). It is performed by incubating washed patient erythrocytes with antibodies against IgG and the C3d fragment of complement factor 3 and evaluating for agglutination. The characteristic pattern for a warm-reacting autoantibody is

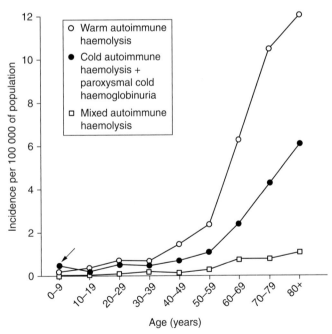

Figure 12.1 Incidence of AIHA per 100,000 population at risk by age at presentation.
From [1]. Reproduced with permission of BMJ Publishing Group Ltd. in the format republish in a book via Copyright Clearance Center.

Table 12.1 Prevalence of secondary autoimmune hemolytic anemia and the type of autoantibody implicated in various associated disorders (adapted from[1 and 11])

Associated Disorder or Exposure	Prevalence of Auto-Immune Hemolytic Anaemia	Warm Auto-Immune Hemolytic Anaemia	Cold Agglutinin Disease	Paroxysmal Cold Hemoglobinuria
Idiopathic	N/A	Most	Less common	Rare
Drug-induced		All	None	None
Drug-induced in CLL	2.9–10.5%	Nearly all	Rare	None
Interferon alpha	Incidence: 11.5/100,000 patient-years	All	None	None
Lymphoid neoplasms				
Chronic lymphocytic leukemia	2.3–4.3%	87%	7%	
Non-Hodgkin lymphoma (except CLL)	2.6%	More common	Less common	None
Angioimmunoblastic T-cell lymphoma	13%	One-third	Two-thirds	None
Hodgkin lymphoma	0.19–1.7%	Nearly all	Rare	None
Plasma cell dyscrasias				
Myeloma	Rare	Yes	Yes	None
IgM gammopathy	1.1%	Rare	Nearly all	None
Myeloid neoplasms				
Chronic myelogenous leukemia	Very rare	All	None	None
Myelodysplastic syndrome	Rare	47%	27%	None
Myelofibrosis	Very rare	Most	Less common	None
Acute myelogenous leukemia	Very rare	Most	Less common	None
Solid Tumors				
Carcinoma (nonovarian)	Very rare	70%	30%	None
Thymoma	Very rare	Yes	No	No
Ovarian tumors	Very rare	All	None	None
Infection				
Mycoplasma pneumoniae	17%	None	All	None
Infectious mononucleosis	24%	None	Nearly all	Very rare
Viral hepatitis	Very rare	Most	Less common	None
Tuberculosis	Very rare	Yes	Yes	None
Syphilis	11%	None	None	All
Rheumatologic Disease				
Systemic lupus erythematosus	6.1%	Nearly all	Rare	None
Sjögren syndrome	Very rare	Most	Less common	None
Rheumatoid arthritis	Rare	Most	Less common	None
Polyarteritis nodosa	Very rare	All	None	None
Other Immunological Derangements				
Ulcerative colitis	1.7%	All	None	None
Chronic hepatitis	Very rare	All	None	None
Pernicious anemia	Very rare	All	None	None
Thyrotoxicosis	Very rare	Nearly all	Less common	None
Myxedema	Very rare	All	None	None
Myasthenia gravis	Very rare	All	None	None
Common variable immune deficiency	5.5%	All	None	None
Autoimmune lymphoproliferative disorder	50%	All	None	None
Post–solid organ transplant	5.6% (pancreas)	All	None	None
Post–allogeneic hematopoietic stem cell transplant	4.4%	Yes	Yes	None
Adult-onset Still's disease	Very rare	Most	Less common	None
Rosai-Dorfman	Very rare	All	None	None
Pregnancy	Very rare	Most	Less common	None

Table 12.2 Clinical-serologic associations with the direct Coombs test (adapted from[48 and 49])

Anti-IgG	Anti-C3d	Antibody Isotype	Clinical Syndrome	Examples
+	−	IgG	Warm Auto Immune Hemolytic Anaemia Drug Induced Immune Hemolytic Anemia (penicillin type haptene reaction)	Penicillin
+	+	IgG	WAIHA DIIHA	Methyldopa, fludarabine
−	+	Typically IgM Less commonly IgG of low quantity or affinity Very rarely IgA	Cold Agglutinin Disease WAIHA DIIHA (ternary complex type haptene reaction) Paroxysmal Cold Hemoglobinuria	Ceftriaxone

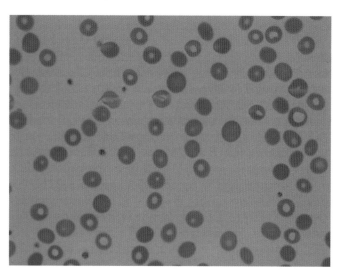

Figure 12.2 Peripheral blood smear from a nonsplenectomized patient with warm AIHA exhibiting microspherocytes and polychromasia. Image courtesy of Dr. Pavan K. Bendapudi.

agglutination with both IgG and C3d antibodies (Table 12.2). The sensitivity of the test approaches 97%.[2] Reasons for false negatives include autoantibodies of low quantity or affinity and rare warm-reacting IgM or IgA autoantibodies. While sensitive, the Coombs test is nonspecific. Rates of hemolysis in patients with erythrocyte-bound IgG are 29–58%.[3] Explanations for false positives include nonspecific immunoglobulin binding, binding of IgG and/or complement in quantities insufficient to overcome complement-regulatory proteins, cold-reacting IgG antibodies, and transfused allogeneic erythrocytes. (Figure 12.3).

Warm-Reacting Antibodies

Warm-reacting autoantibodies are usually polyclonal IgG antibodies targeting Rh complex and glycophorin blood group antigens.[4]

Associated Conditions

Most cases of WAIHA are idiopathic. A sizable minority are associated with rheumatologic diseases, viral infections, immune deficiency states, and lymphoid neoplasms.[3] An important but rare subset, with an incidence of 10^{-6}/year, is drug-induced immune hemolytic anemia (DIIHA). At least 125 drugs have been implicated to date, of which cephalosporins, piperacillin, fludarabine, and oxaliplatin are among the most common culprits in modern practice (Table 12.3).[5]

Mechanism of Hemolysis

The primary mechanisms of hemolysis in AIHA are direct complement-mediated lysis and phagocytosis by splenic macrophages. The latter predominates in WAIHA. Briefly, IgG-coated erythrocytes are trapped by splenic macrophages and to a lesser extent hepatic Kupffer cells via interaction with their FcγRI receptors, resulting in phagocytosis and extravascular hemolysis. Partial phagocytosis produces microspherocytes, the morphologic hallmark of this disorder. Direct complement-mediated lysis is uncommon in WAIHA since IgG fixes complement inefficiently, partly because the distribution of Rh complex proteins is not conducive to complement fixation by adjacent Fc moieties. IgG autoantibodies, therefore, rarely overcome complement regulatory proteins, activate the terminal complement cascade, and trigger intravascular hemolysis.

Drug-Induced Immune Hemolytic Anemia

Drugs induce hemolytic autoantibodies by multiple mechanisms. The first, exemplified by methyldopa, involves modification of an erythrocyte surface antigen by a drug, rendering it immunogenic and stimulating autoantibody formation.[6] Because only erythrocytes directly exposed to the drug bear the pathogenic epitope, hemolysis abates within 100–120 days of drug withdrawal.

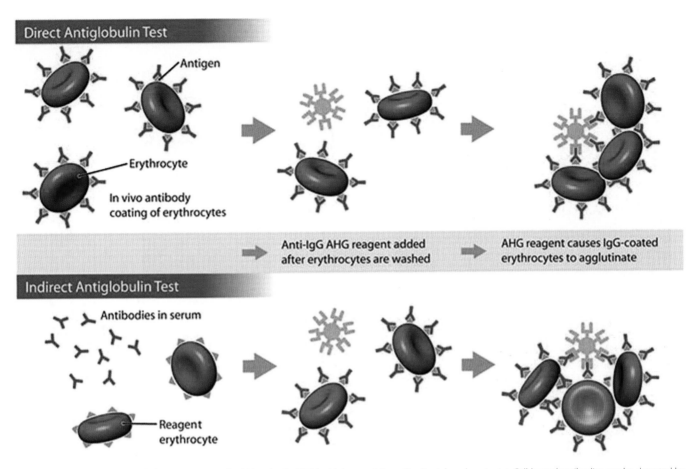

Figure 12.3 In **direct method**, the sensitization of red blood cells (RBCs) with incomplete antibodies takes place *in vivo*. Cell-bound antibodies can be detected by this test in which antiserum against human immunoglobulin is used to agglutinate patient's RBC. In **indirect method**, the sensitization of RBCs with incomplete antibodies takes place *in vitro*. Patient's serum is mixed with normal red cells and antiserum to human immunoglobulin. Agglutination occurs if antibodies are present in serum. **Coombs test is used for detection of anti-Rh antibodies and incomplete antibodies in brucellosis and other diseases**. Image from Immunologynotes.com and reproduced with permission of Dr. Sagar Aryal.

A more common mechanism involves a haptenic reaction, which requires binding of a drug (hapten) to an erythrocyte surface antigen (carrier) to elicit autoantibodies, and of which there are two primary subtypes. In the penicillin type, drugs bind erythrocyte antigens with high affinity, such that antidrug antibodies effectively coat erythrocytes and induce Fc-mediated phagocytosis. In the faudin or ternary complex type, antibodies bind free drug in plasma, forming immune complexes that can bind erythrocyte surface antigens, fix complement, and induce intravascular hemolysis.[7] An alternative model holds that drugs bound to erythrocyte membrane proteins form neo-antigens that stimulate autoantibody production.[8] In either subtype, hemolysis resolves rapidly upon discontinuation of the drug.

Finally, a drug may modify the erythrocyte membrane such that immunoglobulin and even complement adhere nonimmunologically – a process termed nonimmune protein adsorption (NIPA) – leading to phagocytosis and extravascular hemolysis.[9] Beta-lactamase inhibitors and platinum agents have been implicated in this mechanism.

Management

The first and occasionally only step required to suppress autoantibody production in secondary WAIHA is treatment of the underlying disorder. In fact, most cases of DIIHA resolve upon discontinuation of the offending drug.

Transfusion

Patients with severe anemia may require RBC transfusions. Cross-matching can be difficult, though, since many warm autoantibodies recognize blood group antigens and react broadly on antibody screening tests. Nonetheless, safe transfusions without hemolysis remain possible if clinically relevant alloantibodies can be excluded.[10,11] This requires collaboration with blood bank specialists.

Corticosteroids

First-line pharmacologic therapy consists of corticosteroids. Prednisone at 1 mg/kg/day ameliorates hemolysis in most cases in 1–3 weeks. If the hemoglobin recovers to 10 g/dL within this

Table 12.3 Drugs implicated in drug-induced immune hemolysis (adapted from)[5]

Drug-Dependent Antibodies			Drug-Independent Antibodies	Nonimmune Protein Adsorption
Catechin	Amphotericin B	Aceclofenac	Fludarabine	Cefotetan
Cefotetan	Antazoline	Acyclovir	Interferon	Cephalothin
Ceftriaxone	Azapropazone	Aminopyrine	Levodopa	Oxaliplatin
Cephalothin	Carbimazole	Amoxicillin	Mefenamic acid	Cisplatin
Diclofenac	Carboplatin	Aspirin	Methyldopa	Clavulanate potassium
Nomifensine	Cefotaxime	Buthiazide	Cimetidine	Diglycoaldehyde
Oxaliplatin	Ceftizoxime	Carbromal	Cladribine	Sulbactam
Penicillin G	Cefuroxime	Cefamandole	Nalidixic acid	Tazobactam
Phenacetin	Cephalexin	Cefixime	Procainamide	Suramin
Quinidine	Chloramphenicol	Cefpirome	Captopril	
Rifampin	Cyclofenil	Cloxacillin	Interleukin-2	
Tolmetin	Cyclosporin	Dexchlorpheniramine maleate	Tacrolimus	
	Diethylstilbestrol	Etodolac	Chaparral	
Acetaminophen	Dipyrone	Ethambutol	Fenfluramine	
Ampicillin	Erythromycin	Fenoprofen	Ketoconazole	
Cefazolin	Fluorouracil	Fluconazole	Lenalidomide	
Cefoxitin	Furosemide	Fluorescein	Mesantoin	
Ceftazidime	Glafenine	Hydralazine		
Chlorinated hydrocarbons	9-Hydroxy-methyl-ellipticinium	Latamoxef		
Chlorpromazine	Ibuprofen	Melphalan		
Chlorpropamide	Imatinib mesylate	6-Mercaptopurine		
Ciprofloxacin	Insulin	Minocycline		
Cisplatin	Levofloxacin	Nabumetone analgesic		
Hydrochlorothiazide	Mefloquine	Nitrofurantoin		
Isoniazid	Methadone	Norfloxacin		
Nafcillin	Methotrexate	Phenytoin		
p-Aminosalicylic acid	Metrizoate-based radiocontrast media	Propyphenazone		
Piperacillin	Naproxen	Pyrazinamide		
Quinine	Probenecid	Rifabutin		
Streptomycin	Pyrimethamine	Streptokinase		
Sulindac	Ranitidine	Sulfisoxazole		
Tetracycline	Stilbophen	Suprofen		
	Sulfasalazine	Tartrazine		
	Temofloxacin	Teicoplanin		
	Ticarcillin	Teniposide		
	Tolbutamide	Thiopental sodium		
	Triamterene	Trimellitic anhydride		
	Trimethoprim-sulfamethoxazole	Vancomycin		
		Zomepirac		

Number of References	
≥10	
5–9	
2–4	
1	

time, steroids can be tapered slowly and eventually discontinued if the response is maintained. Standardized criteria are lacking, but complete remissions (CRs) are generally defined as recovery of hemoglobin to baseline levels and resolution of hemolysis off all therapy for at least 4 weeks. Partial remissions (PRs) are usually defined as smaller increases in hemoglobin that are stable for several weeks off therapy. By these criteria, 80% of patients achieve a CR or PR with steroids.[12] A minority (<20%) experience long-term CRs and even cures.[12,13] Most require maintenance steroids to suppress hemolysis; of these, 40–50% require prednisone at doses up to 15 mg/day (the maximum tolerated long-term dose), while 15–20% require higher doses.[11]

Second-Line Therapy

Patients unresponsive to steroids by 3 weeks are considered refractory.[12] Those who are refractory or require high maintenance doses of prednisone ($\geq$15 mg/day) should proceed to second-line therapy. Patients requiring maintenance doses between 0.1 mg/kg/day and 15 mg/day may benefit from second-line therapy depending on their degree of steroid toxicity. Those requiring doses below 0.1 mg/kg/day can generally continue steroids with minimal toxicity. The only second-line therapies for which there are extensive data demonstrating efficacy are splenectomy and rituximab.

Splenectomy

By removing the primary site of phagocytosis, splenectomy ameliorates hemolysis in at least two-thirds of patients, with superior response rates in idiopathic cases.[14] Anemia usually improves within 2 weeks. Splenectomy may not eliminate the need for maintenance steroids, as hepatic Kuppfer cells also contribute to phagocytosis, but it typically enhances steroid sensitivity.[15] Responses are often durable, and cure rates approach 20%.[11] Splenectomy for WAIHA is well tolerated, with minimal morbidity and mortality.[16] However, risk factors for complications include morbid obesity[16] and hypercoagulable states given the risk of peri-operative DVTs with laparoscopic splenectomy.[17] Preoperative vaccinations are essential to reduce the long-term risk of sepsis with encapsulated bacteria.[18] (See Chapter 32.)

Rituximab

The anti-CD20 chimeric antibody rituximab suppresses autoantibody production via B-lymphocyte depletion and is frequently used off-label as second-line therapy for WAIHA. The standard regimen is 375 mg/m^2/week for four doses. Steroids are continued until a response to rituximab is observed, then tapered. Overall response rates (ORRs) are 64–100%; about half are CRs.[19–22] As with splenectomy, response rates are higher in idiopathic WAIHA. The median time to response is 6 weeks,[20] and responses are very durable, on the order of years.[19–22] Rituximab is generally well tolerated. The most common adverse reactions are infusion reactions, most of which are mild. Rare reports of severe infections or progressive multifocal leukoencephalopathy (PML) are confounded by immune dysregulation from underlying diseases as well as prior immune suppressive therapies.[20,22] Chronic hepatitis B is a relative contraindication given the risk of reactivation.

Salvage Therapy

Relapses after splenectomy may respond to additional courses of steroids or rituximab. For patients treated with second-line rituximab, late relapses can be treated with additional rituximab or splenectomy. IVIG induces transient responses in up to 40% of patients but requires intensive dosing (1,000 mg/kg/day for 5 days up to every 3 weeks).[23] Other therapies with activity in small series include danazol, cyclophosphamide, mycophenolate mofetil (MMF), cyclosporine, and allogeneic hematopoietic stem cell transplantation (SCT).[11] However, steroids, splenectomy, and rituximab remain the only agents with substantial evidence of lasting efficacy and should therefore be exhausted before other treatments are considered (Figure 12.4, Table 12.4).

Cold Agglutinin Disease
Clinical Features

Cold AIHA, commonly termed cold agglutinin disease (CAD) due to the ability of cold-reacting autoantibodies to agglutinate erythrocytes at low temperature, manifests with symptoms of anemia, such as fatigue and exertional dyspnea, with splenomegaly, jaundice, and hemoglobinuria in severe cases (Table 12.5). Acral cyanosis and livedo reticularis may reflect microvascular circulatory impairment due to agglutinated erythrocytes (Figure 12.5).

Laboratory Features

CAD causes anemia with evidence of hemolysis (indirect hyperbilirubinemia and elevated LDH), a reticulocytosis, a positive Coombs test, and an elevated cold agglutinin titer.[24] The peripheral smear exhibits spherocytosis and erythrocyte agglutination (Figure 12.6). Of note, blood should be warmed prior to analysis since *ex vivo* agglutination of erythrocytes can exaggerate the anemia and cause artifactual macrocytosis.[25] The highest temperature at which erythrocyte agglutination is seen *in vitro* is termed the thermal amplitude. Autoantibodies with higher thermal amplitudes tend to be more clinically significant.[26] The cold agglutinin titer is also important, since a sufficient density of autoantibodies on the erythrocyte surface is required to overcome the effect of complement regulatory proteins.

Coombs Test

The Coombs test is generally positive for complement but negative for IgG, since most cold-reacting autoantibodies are IgM.

Cold Agglutinins

Most cold agglutinins target I/i blood group antigens, universally expressed and developmentally regulated components of the polysaccharide chains bearing ABH and Lewis antigens. Strong expression of anti-i or anti-I autoantibodies often indicates a cold agglutinin. Other cold agglutinins target

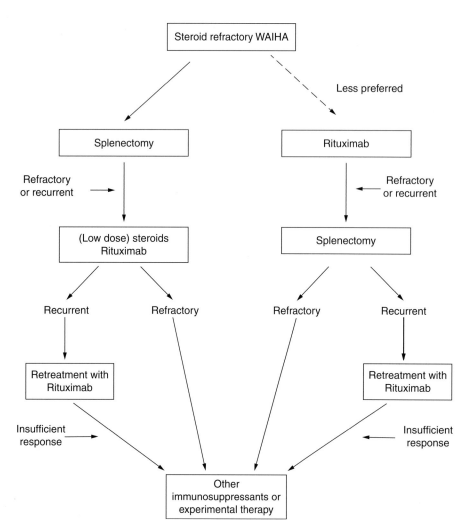

Figure 12.4 Treatment algorithm for steroid-refractory WAIHA.
From[11] in *Blood: Journal of the American Society of Hematology* by American Society of Hematology; Highwire Press. Reproduced with permission of the American Society of Hematology in the format republish in book via Copyright Clearance Center.

erythrocyte antigens that are eliminated by treatment with protease or sialidase and are termed anti-Pr and anti-Sia antibodies, respectively. IgM autoantibodies have a capacity for agglutination, because the spatial distribution of IgM Fab moieties permits bridging of adjacent erythrocytes.

Associated Conditions

Cold agglutinins often result from infections or clonal hematologic disorders. For example, acute CAD mediated by anti-I antibodies may arise after infection with *Mycoplasma pneumoniae*.[27] Infectious mononucleosis can produce CAD with anti-i antibodies.[28] Postinfectious cold agglutinins are usually low titer, oligoclonal, and kappa skewed. Hemolysis develops about two weeks after the onset of infection, peaks within a week, and resolves over several weeks following clearance of the infection. Detectable autoantibodies may persist for 2–3 months. Chronic CAD often results from an underlying lymphoproliferative or plasma cell disorder.[29] Cold agglutinins related to benign monoclonal gammopathies are typically monoclonal, kappa restricted, anti-I IgM autoantibodies. Those associated with malignant hematologic disorders are typically anti-i. In some cases, a cold agglutinin can herald an incipient lymphoproliferative disorder, for which it can later serve as a tumor marker.

Mechanism of Hemolysis

Direct complement-mediated hemolysis is the primary mechanism of CAD. Cold agglutinins bind erythrocyte target antigens in cooler regions of the peripheral circulation corresponding to their thermal amplitudes and fix C3 and C4, which in turn recruit components of the membrane attack complex (MAC) and precipitate intravascular hemolysis.[30] Fixation of complement by immune complexes on the erythrocyte membrane can, to a lesser extent, mediate phagocytosis and extravascular hemolysis, primarily in the liver.[26,31] However, this process is inefficient and plays a small role in most cases, since phagocytic cells lack IgM receptors analogous to the Fcγ receptor for IgG. For this reason, rare IgG cold agglutinins cause more severe hemolysis.[32]

Management
Cold Avoidance

The first step in management is cold avoidance, which can often ameliorate symptoms and prevent severe exacerbations of CAD.

Table 12.4 Suggested therapies for warm and cold AIHA (from[11] in *Blood: Journal of the American Society of Hematology* by American Society of Hematology; Highwire Press). Reproduced with permission of the American Society of Hematology in the format republish in a book via Copyright Clearance Center.

Disease or Condition	First Line	Second Line	Later Line	Last Resort
Primary WAIHA	Steroids	Splenectomy, rituximab	Azathioprine, MMF, cyclosporine, cyclophosphamide	High-dose cyclophosphamide, alemtuzumab
B- and T-cell non-Hodgkin lymphoma	Steroids	Chemotherapy ± rituximab (splenectomy in splenic marginal zone lymphoma)		
Hodgkin lymphoma	Steroids	Chemotherapy (radiation therapy)		
Solid tumors	Steroids, surgery			
Ovarian dermoid cyst	Oophorectomy			
SLE	Steroids	Azathioprine	MMF	Rituximab, autologous SCT
Ulcerative colitis	Steroids	Azathioprine		Total colectomy
Common variable immune deficiency	Steroids + IgG	Splenectomy		
Autoimmune lymphoproliferative disorder	Steroids	MMF	Sirolimus	
Allogeneic SCT	Steroids	Rituximab	Splenectomy, T-cell infusion	
Organ transplantation (pancreas)	Discontinuation of immune suppression	Splenectomy		
Interferon α	Withdrawal	Steroids		
Primary CAD	Cold avoidance	Rituximab, chlorambucil		Eculizumab, bortezomib
Paroxysmal cold hemoglobinuria	Supportive therapy	Rituximab		

This requires minimizing exposure to cold ambient temperatures, warming IV fluids and blood products, and avoiding surgical hypothermia. In secondary CAD, treatment of the underlying condition, such as an infection, is also essential.

Transfusion

RBC transfusions may be required for severe anemia. Unlike warm autoantibodies, cold agglutinins rarely confound alloantibody screening panels when performed at 37°C, so compatible units are usually readily identified. Transfused cells should be washed to minimize residual plasma, particularly in chronic CAD where complement is often depleted, since a complement load may exacerbate hemolysis.[33]

Pharmacologic Treatment

Pharmacologic therapy may be indicated depending on the magnitude and acuity of the anemia, the severity of associated symptoms, and the degree of transfusion dependence.[34] Standard therapy consists of rituximab, often in combination with a purine analogue.

Rituximab reduces autoantibody production via suppression of CD20 positive B-lymphocytes. Conventional dosing is 375 mg/m^2/week for 4 weeks. Rituximab monotherapy induces responses, which are essentially all PRs, in about half of patients (ORR 45–58%).[35–37] Anemia improves within weeks, with a median time to maximal response of 1.5–3.0 months. While responses are relatively short-lived (median duration 6.5–11.0 months), additional responses may be seen with second and even third courses. Rituximab is well tolerated, as discussed previously, with little toxicity and a low incidence of infectious complications even with repeated dosing.[38]

Combination of the purine analogue fludarabine with rituximab confers significant additional activity. Conventional dosing is rituximab 375 mg/m^2/week for 4 weeks plus oral fludarabine 40 mg/m^2/day on days 1–5 of four 28-day cycles. Overall response rates of 76% were reported in the largest series of patients, many of whom had previously been treated with single-agent rituximab.[34] Unlike rituximab monotherapy, a fifth of patients treated with combination therapy achieve CRs. These

Table 12.5 Clinical features of cold agglutinin disease among a published series of 89 patients (from[29] in *Blood: Journal of the American Society of Hematology* by American Society of Hematology; Highwire Press). Reproduced with permission of the American Society of Hematology in the format republish in a book via Copyright Clearance Center.

Characteristic	Number	%
Time from symptoms to diagnosis (months)		
Median	37.4	
Range	0–374.2	
Chief concern at diagnosis		
Anemia of undetermined origin	31	35
Acrocyanosis	21	24
Fatigue	19	21
Weakness	4	4
Exertional dyspnea	3	3
Hemoglobinuria	3	3
Symptoms during disease course		
Acrocyanosis	39	44
Fatigue	36	40
Exertional dyspnea	19	21
Hemoglobinuria	13	15
Weakness	9	10
Weight loss	9	10
Identification of triggers		
Cold	35	39
Other	20	22
Received drug therapy	73	82
Received transfusion	36	40
Overall survival (years)		
Median	10.6	
Range	0.0–29.9	
Five-year survival after diagnosis	68	76

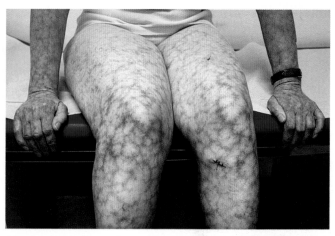

Figure 12.5 Livedo reticularis in a patient with CAD (image from[50]) Reproduced with the permission of Massachusetts Medical Society in the format republish in a book via Copyright Clearance Center.

responses are more durable as well (median duration of response 66 months). However, hematologic toxicity is common, with grade 3–4 cytopenias in 41% and grade 4 neutropenia in 14%. Nearly two-thirds experience grade 1–3 infections. Transient exacerbations of hemolysis occur in about 10%, usually in the context of a febrile illness. While trials with lower doses of fludarabine and/or rituximab have been proposed, prospective data have yet to be published.

Clinical responses with steroids – particularly as monotherapy – are uncommon and require high doses that are poorly tolerated with prolonged administration.[29,30,36] Splenectomy has no role for CAD due to an IgM autoantibody, since the spleen is not the site of extravascular hemolysis in such cases, as corroborated by retrospective series.[36] Neither IVIG nor plasmapheresis inhibit autoantibody production, but they may have limited roles such as temporizing severe or complicated cases in which definitive therapy is also deployed.[39,40]

Taken together, these data support a strategy in which young and healthy older patients are treated with combination therapy, given its superior response rates and potential for complete and more durable remissions. For older patients and those with multiple comorbidities, rituximab monotherapy may be advisable due to its tolerability, at the expense of the depth and duration of response. For relapses following rituximab monotherapy, options include retreatment with rituximab monotherapy or escalation to combination therapy.[41]

Paroxysmal Cold Hemoglobinuria

Clinical Features

Paroxysmal cold hemoglobinuria (PCH) is an acquired cold hemolytic syndrome whose hallmark symptom is hemoglobinuria after cold exposure. Others include fever, chills, abdominal cramping, back pain, Raynaud's phenomenon, and urticaria.

Laboratory Findings

Laboratory testing during acute episodes demonstrates intravascular hemolysis, with an indirect hyperbilirubinemia, elevated LDH, low haptoglobin, complement depletion, hemosiderinuria, and occasionally neutropenia.

Coombs Test

While negative at baseline, the Coombs test during acute episodes is positive for C3d but negative for IgG. Cold agglutinins are negative.

Autoantibodies

The pathogenic autoantibody in PCH is a polyclonal cold-reacting IgG with biphasic hemolytic activity, termed a Donath-Landsteiner antibody. These antibodies target the P antigen, a nearly universal erythrocyte polysaccharide that is also the binding site for parvovirus. In the post-infectious setting, they become detectable 7–10 days after the onset of fevers and persist for 6–12 weeks.[42]

Associated Conditions

While PCH was originally described in congenital syphilis, contemporary cases often arise in children following a viral infection or a bacterial upper respiratory infection. In such cases hemolysis develops acutely but resolves in a delayed

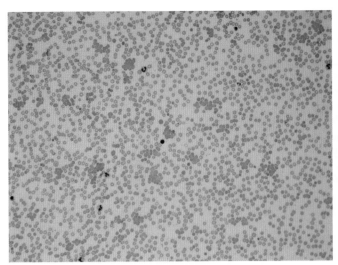
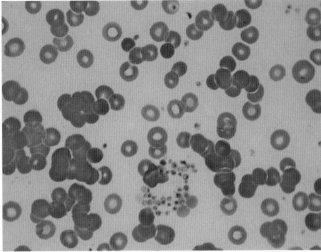

Figure 12.6 Agglutinated erythrocytes seen on the peripheral smear of a patient with cold agglutinin disease. at 40x (top panel) and 100x (bottom panel) magnification. Of note, in this instance agglutination of erythrocytes as well as platelets is seen. Image courtesy of Dr. Pavan K. Bendapudi.

fashion after clearance of the infection. PCH in adults is usually associated with rheumatologic or lymphoproliferative disorders[43] and exhibits a chronic course.

Mechanisms of Hemolysis

Donath-Landsteiner antibodies bind P antigens and fix initial components of the complement cascade at cold temperatures in the peripheral circulation. Upon return to core body temperature, the complement cascade is propagated, culminating in recruitment of the MAC and intravascular hemolysis.

Management

Treatment of acute PCH is generally supportive and relies on strict cold avoidance to minimize hemolysis.[24,44] Severe anemia may warrant transfusions, in which case blood products must be prewarmed, and rare pp or Tj(a) units lacking the P antigen should be used if available.[45] Donath-Landsteiner antibodies and their hematologic sequelae usually disappear several weeks after clearance of the underlying infection.[24] While steroids have been administered as adjunctive therapy, data supporting their use are anecdotal.[44]

Chronic PCH also requires aggressive cold avoidance and in some cases transfusions. While data are limited, a reasonable first-line pharmacologic therapy is prednisone at a dose of 1 mg/kg/day, slowly tapered once a hematologic response has been obtained to the lowest dose necessary to maintain the response.[44] For steroid-refractory adults, immune suppression with rituximab, cyclophosphamide, or azathioprine can be considered.[46] Eculizumab has not exhibited activity in chronic PCH.[47] Nor is splenectomy beneficial given the absence of extravascular hemolysis. Even with effective immune suppression, prolonged maintenance therapy is often required.

References

1. Sokol RJ, Booker DJ, Stamps R. The pathology of autoimmune haemolytic anaemia. *J Clin Pathol.* 1992; **45**(12): 1047–1052.

2. Sachs UJ, et al. Does a negative direct antiglobulin test exclude warm autoimmune haemolytic anaemia? A prospective study of 504 cases. *Br J Haematol.* 2006; **132**(5): 655–656.

3. Wheeler CA, Calhoun L, Blackall DP. Warm reactive autoantibodies: clinical and serologic correlations. *Am J Clin Pathol.* 2004; **122**(5): 680–685.

4. Vos GH, Petz L, Fudenberg HH. Specificity of acquired haemolytic anaemia autoantibodies and their serological characteristics. *Br J Haematol.* 1970; **19**(1): 57–66.

5. Garratty G, Arndt PA. An update on drug-induced immune hemolytic anemia. *Immunohematology.* 2007; **23**(3): 105–119.

6. Worlledge SM, Carstairs KC, Dacie JV. Autoimmune haemolytic anaemia associated with alpha-methyldopa therapy. *Lancet.* 1966; **2**(7455): 135–139.

7. Garratty G, Petz LD. Drug-induced immune hemolytic anemia. *Am J Med.* 1975; **58**(3): 398–407.

8. Mueller-Eckhardt C, Salama A. Drug-induced immune cytopenias: a unifying pathogenetic concept with special emphasis on the role of drug metabolites. *Transfus Med Rev.* 1990; **4**(1): 69–77.

9. Garratty G, Arndt PA. Positive direct antiglobulin tests and haemolytic anaemia following therapy with beta-lactamase inhibitor containing drugs may be associated with nonimmunologic adsorption of protein onto red blood cells. *Br J Haematol.* 1998; **100**(4): 777–783.

10. Leger, RM, Garratty G. Evaluation of methods for detecting alloantibodies underlying warm autoantibodies. *Transfusion.* 1999; **39**(1): 11–16.

11. Lechner K, Jäger U. How I treat autoimmune hemolytic anemias in adults. *Blood.* 2010; **116**(11): 1831–1838.

12. Murphy S, LoBuglio AF. Drug therapy of autoimmune hemolytic anemia. *Semin Hematol.* 1976; **13**(4): 323–334.

13. Gehrs BC, Friedberg RC. Autoimmune hemolytic anemia. *Am J Hematol.* 2002; **69**(4): 258–271.

14. Akpek G, McAneny D, Weintraub L. Comparative response to splenectomy

in Coombs-positive autoimmune hemolytic anemia with or without associated disease. *Am J Hematol.* 1999; **61**(2): 98–102.

15. Atkinson JP, Schreiber AD, Frank MM. Effects of corticosteroids and splenectomy on the immune clearance and destruction of erythrocytes. *J Clin Invest.* 1973; **52**(6): 1509–1517.

16. Casaccia M, et al. Laparoscopic splenectomy for hematologic diseases: a preliminary analysis performed on the Italian Registry of Laparoscopic Surgery of the Spleen (IRLSS). *Surg Endosc.* 2006; **20**(8): 1214–1220.

17. Ikeda M, et al. High incidence of thrombosis of the portal venous system after laparoscopic splenectomy: a prospective study with contrast-enhanced CT scan. *Ann Surg.* 2005; **241**(2): 208–216.

18. *Advisory Committee on Immunization Practices (ACIP) recommended immunization schedules for persons aged 0 through 18 years and adults aged 19 years and older–United States,* 2013. MMWR Surveill Summ. 2013(62 Suppl 1): 1.

19. D'Arena G, et al. Rituximab therapy for chronic lymphocytic leukemia-associated autoimmune hemolytic anemia. *Am J Hematol.* 2006; **81**(8): 598–602.

20. Bussone G, et al. Efficacy and safety of rituximab in adults' warm antibody autoimmune haemolytic anemia: retrospective analysis of 27 cases. *Am J Hematol.* 2009; **84**(3): 153–157.

21. Dierickx, D, et al. Rituximab in auto-immune haemolytic anaemia and immune thrombocytopenic purpura: a Belgian retrospective multicentric study. *J Intern Med.* 2009; **266** (5):484–491.

22. Narat S, et al. Rituximab in the treatment of refractory autoimmune cytopenias in adults. *Haematologica.* 2005; **90**(9):1273–1274.

23. Anderson D, et al. Guidelines on the use of intravenous immune globulin for hematologic conditions. *Transfus Med Rev.* 2007; **21**(2 Suppl 1): S9–56.

24. Gertz MA. Cold agglutinin disease and cryoglobulinemia. *Clin Lymphoma.* 2005; **5**(4):290–293.

25. Bessman JD, Banks D. Spurious macrocytosis, a common clue to erythrocyte cold agglutinins. *Am J Clin Pathol.* 1980; **74**(6):797–800.

26. Rosse WF, Adams JP. The variability of hemolysis in the cold agglutinin syndrome. *Blood.* 1980; **56**(3):409–16.

27. Feizi T. Monotypic cold agglutinins in infection by mycoplasma pneumoniae. *Nature.* 1967; **215** (5100):540–542.

28. Horwitz CA, et al. Cold agglutinins in infectious mononucleosis and heterophil-antibody-negative mononucleosis-like syndromes. *Blood.* 1977; **50**(2):195–202.

29. Swiecicki PL, Hegerova LT, Gertz MA. Cold agglutinin disease. *Blood.* 2013; **122**(7):1114–1121.

30. Nydegger UE, Kazatchkine MD, Miescher PA. Immunopathologic and clinical features of hemolytic anemia due to cold agglutinins. *Semin Hematol.* 1991; **28**(1):66–77.

31. Jaffe CJ, Atkinson JP, Frank MM. The role of complement in the clearance of cold agglutinin-sensitized erythrocytes in man. *J Clin Invest.* 1976; **58**(4):942–949.

32. Mickley H, Sorensen PG. Immune haemolytic anaemia associated with ampicillin dependent warm antibodies and high titre cold agglutinins in a patient with Mycoplasma pneumonia. *Scand J Haematol.* 1984; **32**(3):323–326.

33. Ulvestad E. Paradoxical haemolysis in a patient with cold agglutinin disease. *Eur J Haematol.* 1998; **60** (2):93–100.

34. Berentsen S, et al. High response rate and durable remissions following fludarabine and rituximab combination therapy for chronic cold agglutinin disease. *Blood.* 2010; **116** (17):3180–3184.

35. Berentsen S, et al. Rituximab for primary chronic cold agglutinin disease: a prospective study of 37 courses of therapy in 27 patients. *Blood.* 2004; **103**(8):2925–2928.

36. Berentsen S, et al. Primary chronic cold agglutinin disease: a population based clinical study of 86 patients. *Haematologica.* 2006; **91**(4):460–466.

37. Schollkopf C, et al. Rituximab in chronic cold agglutinin disease: a prospective study of 20 patients. *Leuk Lymphoma.* 2006; **47**(2):253–260.

38. Ghielmini M, et al. Effect of single-agent rituximab given at the standard schedule or as prolonged treatment in patients with mantle cell lymphoma: a study of the Swiss Group for Clinical Cancer Research (SAKK). *J Clin Oncol.* 2005; **23**(4):705–711.

39. Hoppe B, et al. Response to intravenous immunoglobulin G in an infant with immunoglobulin A-associated autoimmune haemolytic anaemia. *Vox Sang.* 2004; **86**(2):151–153.

40. Geurs F, et al. Successful plasmapheresis in corticosteroid-resistant hemolysis in infectious mononucleosis: role of autoantibodies against triosephosphate isomerase. *Acta Haematol.* 1992; **88**(2–3):142–146.

41. Berentsen S. How I manage cold agglutinin disease. *Br J Haematol.* 2011; **153**(3):309–317.

42. Heddle NM. Acute paroxysmal cold hemoglobinuria. *Transfus Med Rev.* 1989; **3**(3):219–229.

43. Sivakumaran M, et al. Paroxysmal cold haemoglobinuria caused by non-Hodgkin's lymphoma. *Br J Haematol.* 1999; **105**(1):278–279.

44. Ries CA, et al. Paroxysmal cold hemoglobinuria: report of a case with an exceptionally high thermal range Donath-Landsteiner antibody. *Blood.* 1971; **38**(4):491–499.

45. Rausen AR, et al. Compatible transfusion therapy for paroxysmal cold hemoglobinuria. *Pediatrics.* 1975; **55** (2):275–278.

46. Koppel A, et al. Rituximab as successful therapy in a patient with refractory paroxysmal cold hemoglobinuria. *Transfusion.* 2007; **47** (10):1902–1904.

47. Gregory GP, et al. Failure of eculizumab to correct paroxysmal cold hemoglobinuria. *Ann Hematol.* 2011; **90**(8):989–990.

48. Schrier SL. *Clinical Features and Diagnosis of Autoimmune Hemolytic Anemia: Warm Agglutinins.* UpToDate; 2013. Retrieved April 7, 2014, from www.uptodate.com/contents/clinical-features-and-diagnosis-of-autoimmune-hemolytic-anemia-warm-agglutinins?source=search_result&search=autoimmune+hemolytic+anemia&selectedTitle=1~128.

49. Lichtman MA, Williams WJ. *Williams hematology.* 7th ed. New York: McGraw-Hill, Medical Pub. Division; 2006.

50. Kauke T, Reininger AJ. Images in clinical medicine. Livedo reticularis and cold agglutinins. *N Engl J Med.* 2007; **356**(3):284.

Chapter

13

Drug-Induced Hemolytic Anemia

Oreofe O. Odejide, MD, MPH

Etiology and Epidemiology

Drug-induced hemolytic anemia (DIHA) is an uncommon but important diagnosis. It is characterized by immune-mediated destruction of red blood cells (RBC), resulting in an abrupt drop in hemoglobin levels after exposure to the implicated drug. It has an estimated incidence of one case per million of the population.[1] The true incidence is likely higher, as mild cases are probably not fully investigated, and it can be frequently mistaken for warm autoimmune hemolytic anemia.[2,3] Since the earliest reports of DIHA in the 1950s, more than a hundred drugs have been implicated as causes of immune hemolysis.[4] As the landscape of drugs causing hemolytic anemia has grown, the drugs commonly associated with hemolytic anemia have also changed. Methyldopa, a frequently used antihypertensive medication in the 1960s and 1970s, was the most common drug causing hemolytic anemia, representing about 67 percent of cases in a series.[5] Currently, antimicrobials, specifically, second- and third-generation cephalosporins, are the most common causes of DIHA.[5]

Pathophysiology

There are two widely accepted mechanisms of immune destruction of RBCs in DIHA. These are based on the type of antibodies induced by the putative drug, namely[1] drug-dependent antibody mechanism and[2] drug-independent antibody mechanism. The antibodies involved in DIHA are of the IgM and IgG classes. A third mechanism of drug-induced hemolysis recently described is nonimmune protein adsorption Examples of drugs that have been reported to cause DIHA through the three mechanisms are displayed in Table 13.1 (See Chapter 12, Table 12.3 for a more comprehensive list).

Drug-Dependent Antibody Mechanism

Immune hemolysis by drug-dependent antibodies is the most common mechanism of DIHA. Drug-dependent antibodies require the implicated drug to be present to demonstrate reactivity against RBCs *in vitro*. Drugs may bind firmly to RBC membrane proteins forming covalent bonds, may be loosely bound to the RBC membrane, or may exist free in plasma. These associations result in immunogenicity and generation of antibodies that are directed against epitopes on drugs and/or their metabolites[6] or a combination of drug and RBC membrane proteins, ultimately resulting in hemolysis.

A population of drug-dependent antibodies reacts with drug alone. These antibodies can be detected *in vitro*, using drug-coated RBCs. This has been well-described with penicillin and cefotetan.[7,8] When cefotetan is administered to some patients, it covalently binds to proteins on the RBC membrane, resulting in formation of IgG antibodies directed only against the drug epitope. The immunoglobin-coated RBCs then undergo Fc-mediated extravascular hemolysis by splenic macrophages.

Another population of antibodies reacts with neoantigens, variably composed of part drug and part RBC membrane. These antibodies react *in vitro* when the serum of a patient with DIHA by this mechanism is mixed with the implicated

Table 13.1 Examples of drugs that have been reported to cause DIHA

Drug-dependent antibody mechanism	Drug-independent antibody mechanism	Nonimmune protein adsorption mechanism
Acetaminophen	Cladribine	Carboplatin
Acyclovir	Fludarabine	Cephalothin
Amphotericin B	Levodopa	Cisplatin
Cefazolin	Mefenamic acid	Clavulanate
Cefotetan	Methyldopa	Oxaliplatin
Cefoxitin	Procainamide	Sulbactam
Ceftazidime		Tazobactam
Ceftriaxone		
Cefuroxime		
Cephalexin		
Ciprofloxacin		
Diclofenac		
Penicillin		
Piperacillin		

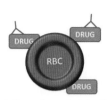

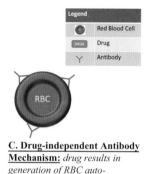

Figure 13.1 Drug induced hemolytic anemia mechanisms

A. Drug-dependent Antibody Mechanism: *drug is bound to RBC and antibody is directed against drug epitope e.g. penicillin*

B. Drug-dependent Antibody Mechanism: *antibody is directed against neoantigen variably composed of drug and RBC membrane proteins e.g. ceftriaxone*

C. Drug-independent Antibody Mechanism: *drug results in generation of RBC auto-antibodies e.g. methyldopa*

drug and RBCs. Ceftriaxone is an example of a drug that has been shown to result in generation of this population of drug-dependent antibodies.[8] Unlike penicillin, which forms firm covalent bonds with RBC membrane proteins, ceftriaxone attaches loosely to the RBC membrane, forming a neoantigen composed of both drug and membrane proteins. The neoantigen then results in generation of antibodies, which can fix complement, resulting in intravascular hemolysis.

Drug-Independent Antibody Mechanism

In this mechanism, antibodies are capable of reactivity *in vitro* without addition of any drug. Therefore, this is identical to the generation of RBC autoantibodies. The clinical findings are indistinguishable from idiopathic warm autoimmune hemolytic anemia, except for resolution of hemolysis associated with discontinuation of the implicated drug. The exact mechanism by which drug-independent antibodies are formed is poorly understood. Some of the proposed mechanisms include molecular mimicry, immune dysregulation, and drug adsorption causing altered RBC membrane antigens.[9,10] It is noteworthy that not every patient who forms drug-independent antibodies eventually develops immune hemolytic anemia. Examples of drugs in this category are methyldopa and fludarabine. Methyldopa results in the production of RBC autoantibodies in about 20 percent of patients receiving the drug, but only about 1 percent of patients go on to develop hemolytic anemia.[11]

Nonimmune Protein Adsorption

It has been described as far back as the 1970s that administration of some drugs may result in proteins binding to RBC membranes nonimmunologically.[12] This was initially thought to be an exclusively *in vitro* process causing positive direct antiglobulin tests, with no *in vivo* implication of hemolysis. Recent evidence, however, suggests that a few cases of non-immunological adsorption of IgG to RBC membranes result in hemolytic anemia.[13,14] Positive monocyte monolayer assay testing, indicative of shortened RBC survival *in vivo*, in non-immunological protein adsorption has also provided further evidence that this mechanism results in hemolysis.[15] Examples of drugs in this category include cephalothin, tazobactam, and oxaliplatin.

Clinical Presentation

Patients with DIHA present with symptoms related to anemia and hemolysis. The severity of symptoms varies with the degree of anemia and the rapidity with which it develops. Patients develop symptoms within minutes to days after exposure to the implicated drug. Associated symptoms include pallor, fatigue, and dyspnea. In more severe cases, patients may develop lethargy, confusion, hypotension, syncope, and death. Jaundice and scleral icterus may also be present secondary to circulating unconjugated bilirubin from hemolyzed RBCs. In cases with massive intravascular hemolysis, patients will develop dark-colored urine due to hemoglobinuria and may also develop oliguria or anuria indicative of renal failure.

There are key differences in DIHA between pediatric and adult populations. Children often develop symptoms very shortly after receiving the offending drug. The majority of children develop acute intravascular hemolysis in less than 1 hour after receipt of the offending drug. There is a steep decline in hemoglobin concentration, with a nadir ≤ 5 g/dL reported in more than 70 percent of children.[16] Accordingly, severe symptoms and fatalities are quite common. Several cases exemplifying this have been described in ceftriaxone-induced hemolytic anemia.[16–18] Conversely, in adults, hemolysis often develops hours to days after receiving the offending drug, and decline in hemoglobin and resultant symptoms tend to be milder. Consequently, there are fewer fatalities.

Most patients with hemolysis secondary to DIHA have had prior exposure to the offending drug without symptoms. The prior exposure to the drug induces the development of circulating antibodies, which then result in hemolysis during subsequent exposure to the drug. An important exception to this is cefotetan, which is the most common cause of DIHA. In a review of 85 cases of cefotetan-induced hemolytic anemia by the Food and Drug Administration, only 18 percent of patients had a history of prior receipt of cefotetan.[19] In addition, cefotetan antibodies have been identified in the plasma of individuals *without* prior exposure to cefotetan.[7] This phenomenon has been explained by the postulation that extensive use of prophylactic antibiotics in cattle and chicken feed in the United States may result in primary immunization of individuals who consume these animals or their products as part of their diet, with subsequent development of anticefotetan antibodies.[7]

Diagnostic Evaluation/Laboratory Findings

Accurate diagnosis of DIHA requires the documentation of hemolysis associated with drug therapy and confirmation by serologic testing. It is essential to obtain a detailed history of all medications received 2 weeks before the evidence of hemolysis. It is particularly important to pay attention to medications administered as prophylaxis prior to surgeries, as these medications may be overlooked even though they play a significant role in DIHA. For example, many cases of cefotetan-induced hemolytic anemia are associated with prophylaxis for surgery.

Laboratory Findings

The laboratory findings are consistent with evidence of hemolytic anemia, with a mean hemoglobin drop of 6.65 g/dL and a mean nadir of 5.2 g/dL reported in 85 cases.[19] The reticulocyte count is elevated, as well as levels of lactate dehydrogenase, total and indirect bilirubin, while the serum haptoglobin is decreased. Peripheral blood smear usually demonstrates spherocytosis in severe cases. Red blood cell indices may reveal an elevated mean corpuscular volume, reflective of the degree of reticulocytosis and an elevated mean corpuscular hemoglobin concentration, indicative of spherocytosis. In cases of drug-dependent antibodies against part-membrane and part-drug (e.g., ceftriaxone), massive intravascular hemolysis can occur because of complement fixation. Laboratory studies in these situations may show hemoglobinuria and elevated blood urea nitrogen and creatinine, reflecting acute renal failure.

Direct Antiglobulin Test (DAT) also called Direct Coombs test: This should be positive in all cases of DIHA. It is the most reliable laboratory finding in DIHA. If this is negative, a diagnosis of DIHA is highly unlikely. In drug-dependent antibody-mediated cases, where antibodies react only with drug-treated RBCs (e.g., penicillin or cefotetan), immunoglobulin (IgG) is detected on patients' RBCs, with or without complement (C3). On the other hand, for cases in which drug-dependent antibodies react with neoantigens composed of part-RBC membrane and part-drug (e.g., ceftriaxone), DAT testing detects C3, with or without IgG on the RBCs. Although IgG is the most common immunoglobulin class associated with DIHA, IgM can also be involved. Quinine has been shown to induce IgM antibody production, which readily activates the complement pathway resulting in intravascular hemolysis.[20] DAT testing in this situation typically detects only C3 and not IgM on the surface of RBCs. While DAT is a very sensitive test in diagnosing DIHA, it has limited specificity. Other immune processes such as autoimmune hemolytic anemia and acute and delayed hemolytic transfusion reactions are also characterized by positive DATs (See Chapter 12, figure 12.3).

Indirect Antiglobulin Test (IAT) also called Indirect Coombs test: In drug-dependent antibody-mediated DIHA, the IAT could either be positive or negative. The serum of patients with drug-dependent antibodies may test positive with reagent RBCs because significant amounts of residual drug or drug-antibody complexes may still be present at the time of testing. DIHA through the drug–independent antibody mechanism results in positive IAT, as the antibodies present in the patient's serum should be reactive with reagent RBCs regardless of whether there is residual drug present (See Chapter 12, figure 12.3).

Elution: An elution is commonly performed after a positive DAT to identify the antibody-coating RBCs. The antibodies are characterized by testing the eluate against reagent RBCs. The eluted antibodies fail to react with reagent RBCs in cases of drug-dependent DIHA because the offending drug is not present. This is an important distinguishing feature from warm autoimmune hemolytic anemia, where a positive DAT is typically accompanied by a positive elution reaction. Further testing of the eluate with drug-coated RBCs or reagent RBCs in the presence of the offending drug demonstrates reactivity, confirming the diagnosis of hemolytic anemia mediated by drug-dependent antibodies. In cases of drug-independent DIHA, the eluate demonstrates reactivity against reagent RBCs despite absence of the offending drug because the mechanism of hemolysis involves true autoantibodies.

Treatment and Prognosis

Discontinuation of the implicated drug is the primary treatment for DIHA. Due to rapid clearance of drugs from the plasma, drug-dependent antibodies can cause no further harm. Therefore, the hemolytic anemia usually resolves soon after stopping the drug. Despite resolution of symptoms, patients may have a persistently positive DAT for months following the hemolytic episode. Steroids are not indicated for treatment except in cases of drug-independent antibody-mediated DIHA (e.g., methyldopa, fludarabine), in which generated antibodies are true autoantibodies. In situations in which hemolysis is severe and persistent despite discontinuation of the drug and steroid administration, other treatments used in warm autoimmune hemolytic anemia such as intravenous immunoglobulin (IVIG) or immunosuppressive agents (e.g., rituximab, azathioprine, cyclophosphamide) should be considered. Supportive management such as transfusion of RBCs and intravenous fluid infusion are often necessary depending on the degree of anemia and decrease in circulatory volume. Dialysis may be required in the event of renal failure. Exposure to the implicated drug must be avoided in the future, as repeated exposure could result in severe, potentially fatal hemolysis.

Case Study

A 70-year-old man with recently diagnosed colon adenocarcinoma was admitted for a right hemicolectomy. The patient received perioperative prophylaxis with 2 g of cefotetan intravenously. The surgical procedure was uncomplicated. On postoperative day 4, he was noted to be jaundiced. He also complained of fatigue and dizziness on attempts of trying to get up from his bed. Laboratory workup revealed a five-point drop in his hemoglobin (6.2 g/dL from a preoperative value of 11 g/dL). Reticulocyte count was elevated at 8.5 percent, lactate dehydrogenase was 1291 IU/L, total bilirubin was 14.6 mg/dL (direct bilirubin 5.9 mg/dL), and haptoglobin was less than 8 mg/dL. Physical exam revealed jaundice, scleral icterus, and an abdominal incision with no evidence of bleeding. A peripheral blood smear was obtained and displayed in Figure 13.2. DAT was positive and demonstrated both anti-IgG and anti-C3. The eluate did not demonstrate reactivity with reagent RBCs. It however demonstrated anti-cefotetan reactivity when incubated with cefotetan-coated RBCs.

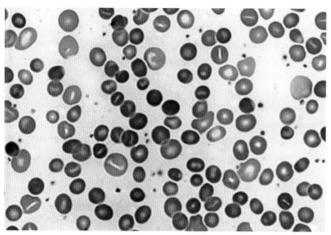

Source : Lichtman MA, Shafer MS, Felgar RE, Wang N:
Lichtman's Atlas of Hematology: http://www.accessmedicine.com

Copyright © The McGraw-Hill Companies, Inc. All rights reserved.

Figure 13.2

1. What is the most likely cause of the patient's anemia?
2. What is the specific mechanism through which the patient's anemia occurred?
3. What is the appropriate management of the patient's anemia?

Answers

1. The patient has cefotetan-induced hemolytic anemia. He received cefotetan 4 days prior to the clinical detection of his hemolytic anemia. The patient's laboratory indices of anemia, reticulocytosis, elevated lactate dehydrogenase, indirect hyperbilirubinemia, and low haptoglobin all indicate that he has hemolytic anemia. The peripheral blood smear shows spherocytosis and polychromasia. His positive DAT and lack of reactivity of the eluate with reagent RBCs are highly suggestive of DIHA. The reactivity of the eluate with cefotetan-coated RBCs confirms the diagnosis of cefotetan-induced hemolytic anemia.

2. There are several mechanisms of DIHA. The mechanism outlined in this case study is most consistent with drug-dependent antibody-mediated hemolytic anemia. Drug-dependent antibodies classically result in positive DAT, while the eluate does not react with reagent RBCs. The eluate will, however, react when drug is present. In this case, the eluate demonstrated reactivity when incubated with cefotetan-coated RBCs, confirming that the antibodies were indeed drug-dependent.

3. The most important management of this patient is to discontinue cefotetan (if still being administered) and avoid further exposure to cefotetan. Given the severity of the patient's anemia and symptoms, supportive management with RBC transfusions is also necessary. Steroid administration is not required because this is not a case of DIHA mediated by drug-independent antibodies.

References

1. Petz LD GG. *Immune Hemolytic Anemias.* 2nd ed. Philadelphia: Churchill Livingstone; 2004.

2. Ahrens N, Genth R, Kiesewetter H, Salama A. Misdiagnosis in patients with diclofenac-induced hemolysis: new cases and a concise review. *Am J Hematol.* 2006; 81(2):128–131.

3. Ahrens N, Genth R, Salama A. Belated diagnosis in three patients with rifampicin-induced immune haemolytic anaemia. *Brit J Haematol.* 2002; 117(2): 441–443.

4. Snapper I, Marks D, Schwartz L, Hollander L. Hemolytic anemia secondary to mesantoin. *Ann Intern Med.* 1953; 39(3):619–623.

5. Arndt PA, Garratty G. The changing spectrum of drug-induced immune hemolytic anemia. *Semin Hematol.* 2005; 42(3):137–144.

6. Salama A, Mueller-Eckhardt C. The role of metabolite-specific antibodies in nomifensine-dependent immune hemolytic anemia. *N Engl J Med.* 1985; 313 (8):469–474.

7. Garratty G. Immune hemolytic anemia associated with drug therapy. *Blood Rev.* 2010; 24(4–5):143–150.

8. Johnson ST, Fueger JT, Gottschall JL. One center's experience: the serology and drugs associated with drug-induced immune hemolytic anemia—a new paradigm. *Transfusion.* 2007; 47(4):697–702.

9. Kirtland HH, Mohler DN, Horwitz DA. Methyldopa inhibition of suppressor-lymphocyte function. *N Engl J Med.* 1980; 302(15):825–832.

10. Pierce A, Nester T. Pathology consultation on drug-induced hemolytic anemia. *Am J Clin Pathol.* 2011; 136(1):7–12.

11. Carstairs KC, Breckenridge A, Dollery CT, Worlledge S. Incidence of a positive direct Coombs test in patients on α-methyldopa. *Lancet.* 1966; 288 (7455):133–135.

12. Spath P, Garratty G, Petz L. Studies on the immune response to penicillin and cephalothin in humans: ii. immunohematologic reactions to cephalothin administration. *J Immunol.* 1971; 107(3):860–869.

13. Broadberry RE, Farren TW, Bevin SV, Kohler JA, Yates S, Skidmore I, et al. Tazobactam-induced haemolytic anaemia, possibly caused by non-immunological adsorption of IgG onto patient's red cells. *Transf Med.* 2004; 14(1):53–57.

14. Arndt PA, Leger RM, Garratty G. Positive direct antiglobulin tests and haemolytic anaemia following therapy with the beta-lactamase inhibitor, tazobactam, may also be associated with non-immunologic adsorption of protein onto red blood cells. *Vox Sanguinis.* 2003; 85(1):53.

15. Arndt P, Garratty G, Isaak E, Bolger M, Lu Q. Positive direct and indirect antiglobulin tests associated with oxaliplatin can be due to drug antibody and/or drug-induced nonimmunologic protein adsorption. *Transfusion.* 2009; 49(4):711–718.

16. Arndt PA, Leger RM, Garratty G. Serologic characteristics of ceftriaxone antibodies in 25 patients

with drug-induced immune hemolytic anemia. *Transfusion*. 2012; 52(3):602–612.

17. Kapur G, Valentini RP, Mattoo TK, Warrier I, Imam AA. Ceftriaxone induced hemolysis complicated by acute renal failure. *Pediatr Blood Cancer*. 2008; 50(1):139–142.

18. Garratty G. Drug-induced immune hemolytic anemia. *Hematology Am Soc Hematol Educ Program*. 2009:73–79.

19. Viraraghavan R, Chakravarty AG, Soreth J. Cefotetan-induced haemolytic anaemia. A review of 85 cases. *Adverse Drug Reac Toxicol Rev*. 2002; 21(1–2):101–107.

20. Croft JD, Jr., Swisher SN, Jr., Gilliland BC, Bakemeier RF, Leddy JP, Weed RI. Coombs'-test positivity induced by drugs. Mechanisms of immunologic reactions and red cell destruction. *Ann Intern Med*. 1968; 68(1):176–187.

Chapter

Red Cell Membrane Defects

14

Patrick G. Gallagher, MD

Introduction

Red cell membrane disorders have historically been classified according to the associated abnormalities of erythrocyte shape observed on peripheral blood smear. These disorders include hereditary spherocytosis, hereditary elliptocytosis, hereditary pyropoikilocytosis, and the hereditary stomatocytosis syndromes. There is significant clinical, laboratory, and genetic heterogeneity in disorders of the erythrocyte membrane.[1] Hereditary spherocytosis is more likely to bring patients to medical attention due to hemolytic anemia and its complications. Hereditary elliptocytosis is the most common primary red cell membrane disorder; however, most patients are asymptomatic and do not require therapy. The red cell membrane and its skeleton provide the strength and flexibility needed to maintain its normal shape and deformability. This allows the erythrocyte to undergo significant shape change without fragmentation or loss of integrity while travelling through the microcirculation and to withstand the high shear stress of the arterial circulation.[1,13,17–19] Perturbation of membrane-associated proteins leads to membrane dysfunction and associated disease pathophysiology.

Hereditary Spherocytosis

Etiology and Epidemiology

The hereditary spherocytosis (HS) syndromes are a heterogeneous group of disorders associated with a primary defect in proteins of the red cell membrane.[2] HS occurs worldwide in all racial and ethnic groups; it is the most common inherited anemia in individuals of northern European ancestry. The incidence of HS is estimated to be ~1:2,000–2,500 individuals, likely an underestimate due to undiagnosed mild HS cases.[3]

HS is inherited in an autosomal dominant manner in ~two-thirds of patients, due to heterozygous mutations in the ankyrin, beta-spectrin, or band 3 genes.[2] In the remaining patients, inheritance is nondominant due to autosomal recessive inheritance or *de novo* mutations.[3,4] Autosomal recessive inheritance is associated with mutations of either the alpha-spectrin or protein 4.2 genes. *De novo* mutations are not uncommon in HS.[5,6]

Pathophysiology

The primary defect in HS red cells is a loss of membrane surface area relative to intracellular volume leading to sphere-shaped erythrocytes with decreased deformability and increased fragility.[7] Surface area loss is due to primary and/or secondary abnormalities of the red cell membrane proteins ankyrin-1, band 3, alpha and beta spectrin, and protein 4.2 (Figure 14.1). Although the primary defects in HS red cells are heterogeneous, a common feature is weakening of the linkages between the lipid bilayer and the underlying membrane skeleton. Impairment of these interactions leads to destabilization of the membrane with vesiculation and membrane loss, which, in turn, results in decreased membrane surface area and formation of poorly deformable spherocytes.

The secondary defect in HS red cells is the selective retention of poorly deformable HS erythrocytes that are selectively retained and further damaged in the hostile environment of the spleen. Low pH, low levels of ATP and glucose, high local concentrations of oxidants, and contact with splenic macrophages condition the red cell for removal.[8,9] Splenic destruction of HS erythrocytes is the primary cause of hemolysis in HS patients.[8,9]

Clinical Presentation

The clinical presentation of HS is variable. HS patients may present at any age from infancy to the elderly. Most patients present in childhood with anemia, pallor, jaundice, and splenomegaly.[3,10] The degree of anemia varies from mild, moderate, to severe depending on the degree of compensation for the associated hemolysis (Table 14.1).[11] In most HS patients, there is mild to moderate anemia with incompletely compensated hemolysis. These patients suffer from complications of chronic anemia and hemolysis. Approximately 25 percent of HS patients are not anemic with well-compensated hemolysis, that is, red cell production and destruction are balanced. These patients are largely asymptomatic.[12] Five to 10 percent of HS patients suffer from moderate to severe anemia, with the most severe patients requiring intermittent or chronic transfusion. The most severely affected patients almost always have recessive HS.[13–15] These patients

Table 14.1 Classification of hereditary spherocytosis (HS)[a]

	HS Carrier	Mild HS	Moderate HS	Severe HS[b]
Hemoglobin (g/dL)	Normal	11–15	8–12	6–8
Reticulocytes (%)	≤3	3–6	≥6	≥10
Bilirubin (mg/dL)	0–1	1–2	≥2	≥2
Spectrin content (% of normal)	100	80–100	50–80	40–60
Peripheral smear	Normal	Mild spherocytosis	Spherocytosis	Spherocytosis
Osmotic fragility fresh blood	Normal	Normal or slightly increased	Distinctly increased	Distinctly increased
Incubated blood	Slightly increased	Distinctly increased	Distinctly increased	Distinctly increased

[a] From Eber SW, Armbrust R, Schroter W. Variable clinical severity of hereditary spherocytosis: relation to erythrocytic spectrin concentration, osmotic fragility, and autohemolysis. *J Pediatr.* 1990; 117:409–416.
[b] Values in untransfused patients.

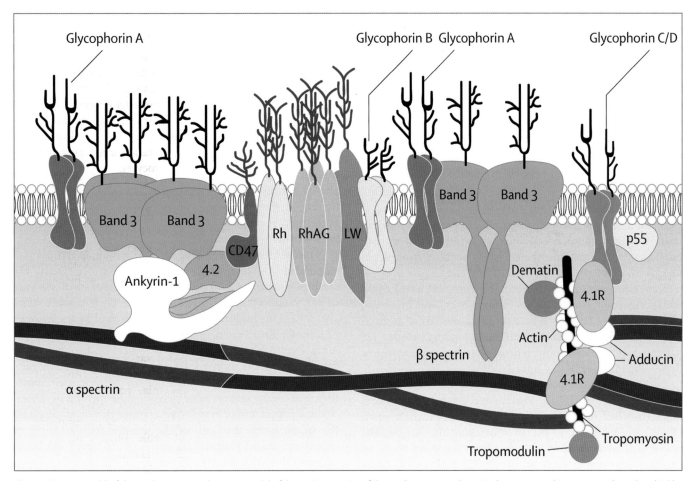

Figure 14.1 A model of the erythrocyte membrane. A model of the major proteins of the erythrocyte membrane is shown: α– and β-spectrin, ankyrin, band 3 (the anion exchanger), 4.1 (protein 4.1) and 4.2 (protein 4.2), actin, and glycophorin.
From Perrotta S, Gallagher PG, Mohandas N. Hereditary spherocytosis. *Lancet* 2008; 372:1411–1426, with permission.

suffer from complications of chronic anemia and hemolysis as well as complications of frequent transfusion.

Jaundice is frequently observed in HS patients, especially during viral illness or other stress. Palpable splenomegaly is found in most HS patients.

Complications

Chronic hemolysis predisposes to the formation of bilirubinate gallstones, the most common complication in HS, which are usually detected in late childhood and young adulthood.

Chronic hemolytic disorders, including HS, may be complicated by aplastic, hemolytic, or megaloblastic crises. Aplastic crises are due to parvovirus B19-mediated marrow suppression after infection and apoptosis of erythroid progenitor cells.[16] Aplastic crises typically last 7–10 days, about half the life span of the typical HS erythrocyte, which is ~20 days. During the aplastic phase, the hemoglobin falls to approximately half of its normal level, thus the degree of anemia and clinical symptomatology observed with parvovirus infection is related to the severity of the HS before infection. "Epidemics" of HS have been reported when multiple affected family members experience parvovirus B19 aplastic crises at the same time.[17] In some patients, parvovirus infection may be the first manifestation of HS.

Hemolytic crises are less severe than aplastic crises. They present with worsening anemia and reticulocytosis, jaundice, and increased splenomegaly, though in rare cases the anemia may be significant enough to require transfusion and hospitalization. They are typically associated with viral infection.

Megaloblastic crises present with worsening anemia caused by exhaustion of folate reserves due to increased folate demands.[18] This typically occurs in during periods of rapid growth in childhood, during pregnancy, and during recovery from an aplastic crisis.

Rare HS-associated complications include chronic leg ulcers, extramedullary masses due to extramedullary hematopoiesis,[19,20] cardiomyopathy, and neuromuscular abnormalities.

Diagnostic Evaluation and Laboratory Findings

Evaluation of a patient with suspected HS includes history of anemia, pallor, jaundice, gallstones ,and splenectomy in both the patient and family members. Pallor, jaundice, and splenomegaly may be found on physical examination.

Laboratory testing should include a complete blood count with peripheral blood smear, reticulocyte count, and incubated osmotic fragility (OF) or flow cytometric analysis of eosin-5-maleimide-labeled erythrocytes (EMA binding). Most HS patients exhibit anemia and reticulocytosis of varying degree depending on severity (Table 14.1).[12,21]

Mean corpuscular hemoglobin concentration (MCHC) is increased ($\geq$34.5 g/dL) due to relative cellular dehydration in more than half of HS patients.[22] Red cell distribution width (RDW) is increased (>14) in most patients. An MCHC >35.4 g/dL and an RDW >14 has been suggested to be an excellent screening strategy to identify HS patients.[23,24] Mean corpuscular volume (MCV) is normal except in severe HS patients, when it is decreased due to membrane loss and cellular dehydration.[23]

Peripheral blood smear usually reveals spherocytes, erythrocytes lacking central pallor, which are distinctive but not diagnostic for HS (Figure 14.2A). In severe cases, numerous small, hyperdense spherocytes and bizarre erythrocyte morphology with anisocytosis and poikilocytosis may be seen (Figure 14.2B).

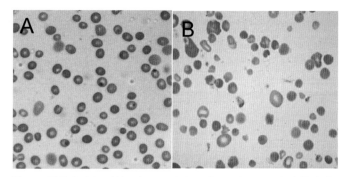

Figure 14.2 Peripheral blood smears in hereditary spherocytosis. A. Typical hereditary spherocytosis. Characteristic spherocytes lacking central pallor are seen. B. Severe, recessively inherited spherocytosis. Numerous small, dense spherocytes and bizarre erythrocyte morphology with anisocytosis and poikilocytosis associated with severe hemolysis are seen.

EMA binding and osmotic fragility testing are the primary laboratory tests utilized in the diagnosis of HS. EMA, a fluorescent dye, is a flow cytometry-based test that quantitates fluorescence intensity as a read out of EMA binding to band 3 and Rh-related proteins in the erythrocyte membrane. In typical HS, a reduction in band 3 and related membrane proteins in the membrane leads to a decrease in fluorescence intensity, to approximately two-thirds of normal (Figure 14.3A). Decreased EMA binding is seen not only in HS cases associated with band 3 deficiency but also in HS cases due to defects in ankyrin or spectrin, presumably due to altered transmission of long-range effects from varying protein defects in the membrane. EMA binding is simple, rapidly performed, it can be performed on stored samples, and it has high sensitivity and specificity.

Osmotic fragility measures the *in vitro* lysis of erythrocytes suspended in saline solutions of decreasing osmolarity. HS erythrocytes cannot tolerate the introduction of small amounts of free water as they are placed in increasingly hypotonic saline solutions. This leads to hemolysis, determined by the amount of hemoglobin released, of HS erythrocytes more readily than normal erythrocytes (Figure 14.3B). After incubation at 37°C for 24 hours, the stressed HS erythrocyte loses membrane surface area more readily than normal because their membranes are leaky and unstable, revealing the membrane defect. A small population of very fragile erythrocytes conditioned by the spleen forms the "tail" of the osmotic fragility curve in unsplenectomized patients (Figure 14.3B). Neither EMA binding nor OF testing detects 100 percent of HS patients.

Both tests struggle in the identification of cases of mild HS. Decreased EMA binding may be seen in other disorders such as Southeast Asian ovalocytosis, hereditary pyropoikilocytosis, and congenital dyserythropoietic anemia type II. OF testing is unreliable in patients who have small numbers of spherocytes, and it is abnormal in other conditions where spherocytes are present, such as autoimmune-mediated anemia, *Clostridial* sepsis, severe hypophosphatemia, transfusion reaction with hemolysis, and after thermal burns.

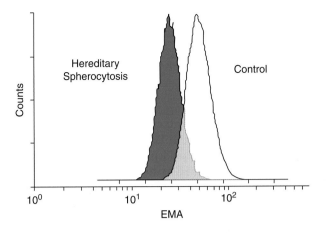

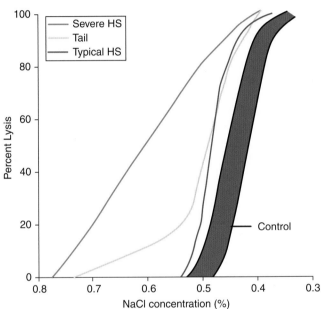

Figure 14.3 Diagnosis of hereditary spherocytosis. A. Eosin-5-maleimide (EMA) binding. Histogram of fluorescence of EMA-labeled erythrocytes from a normal control and a patient with typical hereditary spherocytosis. Decreased fluorescence is observed from HS erythrocytes. B. Osmotic fragility curves in hereditary spherocytosis. The shaded region is the normal range. Results representative of both typical and severe spherocytosis are shown. A tail, representing fragile erythrocytes conditioned by the spleen, is common in spherocytosis patients prior to splenectomy.

Molecular testing, if desired, is available in several commercial laboratories.

Nonspecific markers of ongoing hemolysis, such as increased bilirubin, increased lactate dehydrogenase, increased urinary and fecal urobilinogen, and decreased haptoglobin, are common.

Splenomegaly is typically detected on abdominal ultrasound examination or radionuclide scanning. Cholelithiasis may be detected on abdominal ultrasound. Longitudinal ultrasounds are recommended to provide timely diagnosis and treatment of gallstones, avoiding complications of symptomatic biliary tract disease including biliary obstruction, cholecystitis, and cholangitis.

Treatment and Prognosis

Treatment of HS involves supportive care and, when indicated, splenectomy.[25,26] Longitudinal visits should monitor the degree of anemia, the development of complications, such as gallstones, and in children, to follow growth and development. Folate supplementation is recommended for HS patients with moderate to severe hemolysis. Patient education about HS and its complications and study of other family members when appropriate should be provided. Serial parvovirus B19 antibody titers should be followed until positive to assess risk for parvovirus-associated aplastic crisis.

The sequestration and destruction of HS erythrocytes in the spleen is the primary determinant of erythrocyte survival and disease severity in HS. Splenectomy cures the hemolytic anemia and decreases the incidence of cholelithiasis in most HS patients.[27] Even severely affected patients exhibit improvement in their anemia postsplenectomy.[13] Early splenectomy complications include localized infection or bleeding and pancreatitis due to injury during surgery. The most feared long-term complication of splenectomy is overwhelming postsplenectomy infection (OPSI). An uncommon but potentially fatal complication, OPSI is typically associated with sepsis from encapsulated organisms, particularly in children.[28] Widespread immunization with pneumococcal vaccine, patient education, and early use of antibiotic therapy for the asplenic febrile patient have led to decreases in the incidence of OPSI. An emerging postsplenectomy complication is an increased risk of cardiovascular disease, especially thrombosis and pulmonary hypertension.[29-31]

Splenectomy was once a routine operation in HS patients. Now, the risk of OPSI, increased recognition of postsplenectomy-associated cardiovascular disease, and increased international travel with consideration of the role of the spleen in protection from malaria and other parasitic diseases have contributed to a change in the use of splenectomy in the treatment of HS.[32]

It is now recommended that patients, family members, and health care providers review the risks and benefits of splenectomy before proceeding to operation.[32,33] Most experts agree that it is reasonable to splenectomize severe HS patients and those with growth failure, skeletal changes, extramedullary hematopoietic tumors, and leg ulcers.[25] Patients with moderate HS and compensated, asymptomatic anemia should be evaluated on an individual basis. Mild HS patients with well-compensated hemolysis can be managed expectantly, deferring splenectomy unless indicated.[11] Splenectomy for mild to moderate HS with cholelithiasis is also controversial, as current treatment including laparoscopic cholecystectomy, endoscopic sphincterotomy, and extracorporal choletripsy, lower the risk of treating this complication. Laparoscopic splenectomy is the method of choice, due to decreased postoperative discomfort, shorter length of stay, and decreased costs.[34,35] Partial splenectomy has been utilized for infants with severe HS,[36,37] to ameliorate hemolysis while maintaining residual splenic immune function. Prior to splenectomy, all patients should be immunized against pneumococcus, *Haemophilus influenzae* type b, and meningococcus.[25,38]

Hereditary Elliptocytosis, Hereditary Pyropoikilocytosis, and Related Disorders

Introduction

Hereditary elliptocytosis (HE) is a heterogeneous group of inherited disorders distinguished by the finding of elliptical, cigar-shaped erythrocytes on blood smear.[39,40] A few HE subtypes are associated with symptomatic hemolytic disease, but most are clinically asymptomatic and are discovered incidentally when a blood smear is reviewed. The elliptocytosis syndromes occur worldwide in all racial and ethnic groups. They are much more common in areas of endemic malaria, particularly in people of African and Mediterranean ancestry, and some studies suggest elliptocytes confer some resistance to malaria.[41] The incidence of HE is 1:2000 to 4000, approaching 1:100 in parts of Africa.[40,42]

Pathophysiology

The primary defect in HE and HPP erythrocytes is mechanical weakness of the membrane skeleton due to qualitative or quantitative defects in several membrane proteins,[7] including alpha- and beta-spectrin, protein 4.1, and glycophorin C. Disruption of erythrocyte membrane skeleton protein interactions by mutations that alter protein structure, function, or amount leads to diminished membrane mechanical stability and, in severe cases, to hemolysis. Most cases are due to abnormalities in spectrin, the principal structural protein of the erythrocyte membrane skeleton, in the region of spectrin self-association,[43] disrupting the integrity and mechanical stability of the membrane skeleton critical for erythrocyte shape and function.[44,45]

Inheritance

HE is inherited in an autosomal dominant manner with rare cases of *de novo* mutation.[46,47] In contrast to HS, in which most mutations are private, the HE/HPP syndromes, while also heterogeneous, are associated with specific spectrin mutations in persons of similar genetic backgrounds, suggesting a "founder effect" for these mutations.[48]

Clinical Presentation

Clinical manifestations of the HE syndromes vary widely (Table 14.2). The majority of HE patients have "common" or "typical" HE, discovered incidentally during testing for unrelated conditions. Typical HE patients are asymptomatic. They are not anemic, there is no splenomegaly, and their erythrocyte life span is normal. In one subset of patients, termed hemolytic HE, there is hemolytic anemia of varying severity, the spleen may be enlarged, and the erythrocyte life span is shortened. Complications of chronic hemolysis, including cholelithiasis and crises, may occur.

Hereditary pyropoikilocytosis (HPP), a severe inherited anemia that overlaps severe hemolytic HE, is characterized by erythrocyte morphology on peripheral blood smear that resembles that seen after thermal burns.[49] Affected patients, typically of African ancestry, present in infancy or early childhood with moderate to severe hemolytic anemia. Complications of chronic hemolysis frequently occur.

Southeast Asian ovalocytosis (SAO) is an HE variant found in Malaysia, New Guinea, Indonesia, and the Philippines. SAO patients do not suffer from hemolysis or anemia. SAO erythrocytes, rigid spoon-shaped cells with a longitudinal slit or a transverse ridge, have a normal life span. SAO erythrocytes may confer resistance to cerebral malaria.

Complications

Complications in hemolytic HE and HPP are similar to those in HS.

Table 14.2 Classification of hereditary elliptocytosis

	Common HE	Hemolytic HE	Hereditary Pyropoikilocytosis	Southeast Asian Ovalocytosis
Anemia	None	Moderate-severe	Severe	None
Hemolysis	None-mild	Moderate-severe	Severe	None
Splenomegaly	None	Present	Present	None
Peripheral blood smear	15–90% Elliptocytes	Elliptocytes; poikilocytes; fragments	Poikilocytosis; RBC budding with fragments; elliptocytes; microspherocytes	Rounded elliptocytes, some having a transverse bar dividing cell
Osmotic fragility	Normal	Normal/Increased	Increased	Normal-decreased
Inheritance	Dominant	Recessive	Recessive	Dominant
Other	Poikilocytosis with severe hemolysis, seen transiently in some infants	Normal/low mean corpuscular volume	Low/very low mean corpuscular volume	Rigid erythrocytes

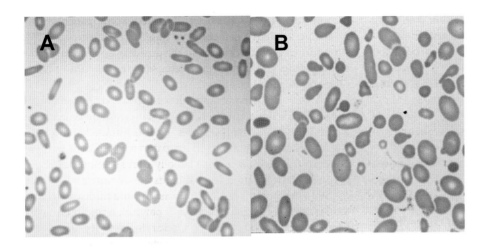

Figure 14.4 Peripheral blood smears in hereditary elliptocytosis. A. Hereditary elliptocytosis. Smooth, cigar-shaped elliptocytes are seen. B. Hereditary pyropoikilocytosis. Pronounced microcytosis, poikilocytosis, and fragmentation of erythrocytes and elliptocytes are seen.

Diagnostic Evaluation and Laboratory Findings

Evaluation of a patient with suspected HE includes history of anemia, pallor, jaundice, gallstones, and splenectomy in both the patient and family members. Pallor, jaundice, and spleno-megaly may be found on physical examination of patients with hemolytic HE and HPP.

Laboratory testing should include a complete blood count with peripheral blood smear and a reticulocyte count. Where indicated, incubated OF or EMA binding may be performed.

Typical HE patients exhibit no anemia. The only laboratory finding is the presence of normochromic, normocytic ellipto-cytes on peripheral blood smear, numbering from 15 to 100 percent (Figure 14.4A). In patients with hemolytic HE and HPP, there is anemia and reticulocytosis. In hemolytic HE, elliptocytes, fragmented cells, and rare ovalocytes, spher-ocytes, and stomatocytes may be seen on peripheral blood smear. In addition to the findings in hemolytic HE, bizarre-shaped cells with fragmentation or budding and microspher-ocytes are seen in HPP (Figure 14.4B).[49] The MCV in HPP is frequently very low, 50–65 fL. OF and EMA binding are normal in typical HE but increased in hemolytic HE and HPP.

Thermal instability of HPP erythrocytes, susceptibility to budding and fragmentation upon heating to 46°C, once thought to be diagnostic of HPP, is not unique, as it is also found in some HE erythrocytes. Unlike HE red cells, HPP erythrocytes are also partially deficient in spectrin.

Splenomegaly is typically detected on abdominal ultra-sound or radionuclide scanning in patients with hemolytic HE and HPP. Cholelithiasis may be detected on abdominal ultrasound.

Treatment

Treatment is rarely necessary for patients with typical HE.[40] In cases of hemolytic HE and HPP, supportive care similar to that in HS, for example, supplemental folic acid, interval examin-ations for cholelithiasis, transfusion during hemolytic or aplas-tic crisis, and so on is indicated. Splenectomy has been curative, with the same indications for splenectomy in HS applied to patients with symptomatic HE or HPP.[26] Ellipto-cytes persist on peripheral smear post splenectomy. No treat-ment is required for patients with SAO.

Disorders of Volume Homeostasis and the Hereditary Stomatocytosis Syndromes

Volume homeostasis in the erythrocyte is primarily deter-mined by the intracellular concentration of monovalent cations. A net increase in sodium and potassium ions causes water to enter, forming stomatocytes or hydrocytes, whereas a net loss of sodium and potassium produces dehydrated red cells, or xerocytes. Many cases of familial hemolytic anemia associated with abnormal cation permeability with perturb-ations in red cell hydration have been reported.[50] These range from severe hydrocytosis to severe xerocytosis.[51] An unusual characteristic of the stomatocytosis syndromes is a predispos-ition to thrombosis after splenectomy.

Overhydrated Stomatocytosis (Hydrocytosis)

The hydrocytoses are a very rare group of disorders character-ized by stomatocytes, erythrocytes with a mouth-shaped (stoma) area of central pallor on peripheral blood smear, hemolysis, marked macrocytosis (110–150 fL), elevated eryth-rocyte sodium concentration, reduced potassium concentra-tion, and increased total Na^+ and K^+ content. Excess cations increase cell water, producing large, osmotically fragile cells with a low MCHC (24–30 percent). Clinical severity in the hydrocytoses is variable from compensated hemolysis to sig-nificant anemia. Missense mutations in the Rh-associated glycoprotein (RhAG) have been identified in a subset of hydro-cytosis patients.[50]

Dehydrated Stomatocytosis (Hereditary Xerocytosis)

Hereditary xerocytosis (HX) is an uncommon disorder of erythrocyte dehydration. Most patients have well-compensated hemolysis, increased MCHC and MCV, decreased osmotic fragility, and decreased potassium concentration and total monovalent cation content. Peripheral blood smear may be unremarkable except for contracted, spiculated red cells, few stomatocytes, and occasional target cells. Dominantly inherited mutations in PIEZO1, encoded by the *FAM38A* gene, have been identified in hereditary xerocytosis patients. PIEZO proteins are the recently identified pore-forming subunits of channels that mediate mechanotransduction in mammalian cells.[52] Association of PIEZO variants with changes in erythrocyte hydration suggest that these proteins play an important role in erythrocyte volume homeostasis. A few HX patients do not have mutations in PIEZO1 but instead have mutations in the Gardos channel, encoded by *KCNN4*.[51]

Intermediate Syndromes and Other Variants

Hydrocytosis and xerocytosis represent the extremes of a spectrum of red cell permeability defects.[50] Patients with features of both conditions have been described. Some patients with severe permeability defects have little or no hemolysis. The proportion of stomatocytes and the degree of sodium influx do not correlate, and neither correlates with the amount of hemolysis or anemia.

Erythrocytes from a subgroup of patients with stomatocytosis, spherocytosis, and sphero-stomatocytosis revealed large cation leaks at low temperatures and membrane band 3 deficiency. Missense mutations in band 3 were discovered in these patients,[53] thought to convert band 3 from an anion exchanger to a nonselective cation leak channel.[54]

Stomatocytosis is also prominent in Rh null disease, sitosterolemia, and familial deficiency of high-density lipoproteins (Tangier disease).

Acquired stomatocytosis has been associated with acute alcoholism and hepatobiliary disease, vinca alkaloid administration, neoplasms, and cardiovascular disease. Stomatocytosis is also sometimes observed as a processing artifact.

References

1. Gallagher PG. Abnormalities of the erythrocyte membrane. *Pediatr Clin North Am.* 2013; 60(6):1349–1362.

2. Perrotta S, Gallagher PG, Mohandas N. Hereditary spherocytosis. *Lancet.* 2008; 372(9647):1411–1426.

3. Eber S, Lux SE. Hereditary spherocytosis – defects in proteins that connect the membrane skeleton to the lipid bilayer. *Semi Hematol.* 2004; 41(2):118–141.

4. Gallagher PG. Update on the clinical spectrum and genetics of red blood cell membrane disorders. *Curr Hematol Rep.* 2004; 3(2):85–91.

5. Miraglia del Giudice E, Francese M, Nobili B, et al. High frequency of de novo mutations in ankyrin gene (ANK1) in children with hereditary spherocytosis. *J Pediatr.* 1998; 132 (1):117–120.

6. Miraglia del Giudice E, Lombardi C, Francese M, et al. Frequent de novo monoallelic expression of beta-spectrin gene (SPTB) in children with hereditary spherocytosis and isolated spectrin deficiency. *Br J Haematol.* 1998; 101 (2):251–254.

7. Mohandas N, Gallagher PG. Red cell membrane: past, present, and future. *Blood.* 2008; 112(10):3939–3948.

8. Lusher JM, Barnhart MI. The role of the spleen in the pathophysiology of hereditary spherocytosis and hereditary elliptocytosis. *Am J Pediatr Hematol Oncol.* 1980; 2:31–39.

9. Safeukui I, Buffet PA, Deplaine G, et al. Quantitative assessment of sensing and sequestration of spherocytic erythrocytes by the human spleen. *Blood.* 2012; 120(2):424–430.

10. Christensen RD, Yaish HM, Gallagher PG. A pediatrician's practical guide to diagnosing and treating hereditary spherocytosis in neonates. *Pediatrics.* 2015; 135(6):1107–1114.

11. Eber SW, Armbrust R, Schroter W. Variable clinical severity of hereditary spherocytosis: relation to erythrocytic spectrin concentration, osmotic fragility, and autohemolysis. *J Pediatr.* 1990; 117(3):409–416.

12. Rocha S, Costa E, Catarino C, et al. Erythropoietin levels in the different clinical forms of hereditary spherocytosis. *Br J Haematol.* 2005; 131 (4):534–542.

13. Agre P, Asimos A, Casella JF, McMillan C. Inheritance pattern and clinical response to splenectomy as a reflection of erythrocyte spectrin deficiency in hereditary spherocytosis. *N Engl J Med.* 1986; 315(25):1579–1583.

14. Agre P, Casella JF, Zinkham WH, McMillan C, Bennett V. Partial deficiency of erythrocyte spectrin in hereditary spherocytosis. *Nature.* 1985; 314(6009):380–383.

15. Agre P, Orringer EP, Bennett V. Deficient red-cell spectrin in severe, recessively inherited spherocytosis. *N Engl J Med.* 1982; 306(19): 1155–1161.

16. Young NS. Hematologic manifestations and diagnosis of parvovirus B19 infections. *Clin Adv Hematol Oncol.* 2006; 4(12):908–910.

17. Lefrere JJ, Courouce AM, Girot R, Bertrand Y, Soulier JP. Six cases of hereditary spherocytosis revealed by human parvovirus infection. *Br J Haematol.* 1986; 62(4): 653–658.

18. Delamore IW, Richmond J, Davies SH. Megaloblastic anaemia in congenital spherocytosis. *Br Med J.* 1961; 1 (5225):543–545.

19. Smith J, Rahilly M, Davidson K. Extramedullary haematopoiesis secondary to hereditary spherocytosis. *Br J Haematol.* 2011; 154(5):543.

20. Rabhi S, Benjelloune H, Meziane M, et al. Hereditary spherocytosis with leg ulcers healing after splenectomy. *South Med J.* 2011; 104(2):150–152.

21. Guarnone R, Centenara E, Zappa M, Zanella A, Barosi G. Erythropoietin production and erythropoiesis in compensated and anaemic states of hereditary spherocytosis. *Br J Haematol.* 1996; 92(1):150–154.

22. Brugnara C, Mohandas N. Red cell indices in classification and treatment of anemias: from M.M. Wintrobes's original 1934 classification to the third millennium. *Curr Opin Hematol.* 2013; 20(3):222–230.

23. Michaels LA, Cohen AR, Zhao H, Raphael RI, Manno CS. Screening for hereditary spherocytosis by use of

automated erythrocyte indexes. *J Pediatr.* 1997; 130(6):957–960.

24. Cynober T, Mohandas N, Tchernia G. Red cell abnormalities in hereditary spherocytosis: relevance to diagnosis and understanding of the variable expression of clinical severity. *J Lab Clin Med.* 1996; 128(3): 259–269.

25. Bolton-Maggs PH, Langer JC, Iolascon A, Tittensor P, King MJ, General Haematology Task Force of the British Committee for Standards in H. Guidelines for the diagnosis and management of hereditary spherocytosis–2011 update. *Br J Haematol.* 2012; 156(1):37–49.

26. Iolascon A, Andolfo I, Barcellini W, et al. Recommendations for splenectomy in hereditary hemolytic anemias. *Haematologica.* 2017; 102 (8):1304–1313.

27. Baird RN, Macpherson AI, Richmond J. Red-blood-cell survival after splenectomy in congenital spherocytosis. *Lancet.* 1971; 2 (7733):1060–1061.

28. Schilling RF. Risks and benefits of splenectomy versus no splenectomy for hereditary spherocytosis – a personal view. *Br J Haematol.* 2009; 145 (6):728–732.

29. Crary SE, Ramaciotti C, Buchanan GR. Prevalence of pulmonary hypertension in hereditary spherocytosis. *Am J Hematol.* 2011; 86(12):E73–76.

30. Hayag-Barin JE, Smith RE, Tucker FC, Jr. Hereditary spherocytosis, thrombocytosis, and chronic pulmonary emboli: a case report and review of the literature. *Am J Hematol.* 1998; 57(1):82–84.

31. Schilling RF, Gangnon RE, Traver MI. Delayed adverse vascular events after splenectomy in hereditary spherocytosis. *J Thromb Haemost.* 2008; 6(8):1289–1295.

32. Casale M, Perrotta S. Splenectomy for hereditary spherocytosis: complete, partial or not at all? *Expert Rev Hematol.* 2011; 4(6):627–635.

33. Schilling RF. Risks and benefits of splenectomy versus no splenectomy for hereditary spherocytosis – a personal view. *Br J Haematol.* 2009; 145 (6):728–732.

34. Wood JH, Partrick DA, Hays T, Sauaia A, Karrer FM, Ziegler MM. Contemporary pediatric splenectomy: continuing controversies. *Pediatr Surg Int.* 2011; 27(11):1165–1171.

35. Rescorla FJ, Engum SA, West KW, Tres Scherer LR, 3rd, Rouse TM, Grosfeld JL. Laparoscopic splenectomy has become the gold standard in children. *Am Surg.* 2002; 68(3):297–301.

36. Buesing KL, Tracy ET, Kiernan C, et al. Partial splenectomy for hereditary spherocytosis: a multi-institutional review. *J Pediatr Surg.* 2011; 46 (1):178–183.

37. Guizzetti L. Total versus partial splenectomy in pediatric hereditary spherocytosis: A systematic review and meta-analysis. *Pediatr Blood Cancer.* 2016; 63(10):1713–1722.

38. Grace RF, Mednick RE, Neufeld EJ. Compliance with immunizations in splenectomized individuals with hereditary spherocytosis. *Pediatr Blood Cancer.* 2009; 52(7):865–867.

39. Dhermy D, Garbarz M, Lecomte MC, et al. Hereditary elliptocytosis: clinical, morphological and biochemical studies of 38 cases. *Nouv Rev Fr Hematol.* 1986; 28(3):129–140.

40. Gallagher PG. Hereditary elliptocytosis: spectrin and protein 4.1R. *Semin Hematol.* 2004; 41(2):142–164.

41. Dhermy D, Schrevel J, Lecomte MC. Spectrin-based skeleton in red blood cells and malaria. *Curr Opin Hematol.* 2007; 14(3):198–202.

42. Glele-Kakai C, Garbarz M, Lecomte MC, et al. Epidemiological studies of spectrin mutations related to hereditary elliptocytosis and spectrin polymorphisms in Benin. *Br J Haematol.* 1996; 95(1):57–66.

43. Morrow JS, Rimm DL, Kennedy SP, Cianci CD, Sinard JH, Weed SA. Of membrane stability and mosaics: the spectrin cytoskeleton. In: Hoffman J, Jamieson J, eds. *Handbook of Physiology.* London: Oxford; 1997:485–540.

44. Gaetani M, Mootien S, Harper S, Gallagher PG, Speicher DW. Structural and functional effects of hereditary hemolytic anemia-associated point mutations in the alpha spectrin tetramer site. *Blood.* 2008; 111 (12):5712–5720.

45. Ipsaro JJ, Harper SL, Messick TE, Marmorstein R, Mondragon A, Speicher DW. Crystal structure and functional interpretation of the erythrocyte spectrin tetramerization domain complex. *Blood.* 2010; 115 (23):4843–4852.

46. Coetzer T, Lawler J, Prchal JT, Palek J. Molecular determinants of clinical expression of hereditary elliptocytosis and pyropoikilocytosis. *Blood.* 1987; 70 (3):766–772.

47. Coetzer T, Palek J, Lawler J, et al. Structural and functional heterogeneity of alpha spectrin mutations involving the spectrin heterodimer self-association site: relationships to hematologic expression of homozygous hereditary elliptocytosis and hereditary pyropoikilocytosis. *Blood.* 1990; 75 (11):2235–2244.

48. Gallagher PG. Red cell membrane disorders. *Hematology Am Soc Hematol Educ Program.* 2005; 2005(1):13–18.

49. Zarkowsky HS, Mohandas N, Speaker CB, Shohet SB. A congenital haemolytic anaemia with thermal sensitivity of the erythrocyte membrane. *Br J Haematol.* 1975; 29(4):537–543.

50. Gallagher PG. Disorders of red cell volume regulation. *Curr Opin Hematol.* 2013; 20(3):201–207.

51. Andolfo I, Russo R, Gambale A, Iolascon A. New insights on hereditary erythrocyte membrane defects. *Haematologica.* 2016; 101 (11):1284–1294.

52. Zarychanski R, Schulz VP, Houston BL, et al. Mutations in the mechanotransduction protein PIEZO1 are associated with hereditary xerocytosis. *Blood.* 2012; 120 (9):1908–1915.

53. Bruce LJ, Robinson HC, Guizouarn H, et al. Monovalent cation leaks in human red cells caused by single amino-acid substitutions in the transport domain of the band 3 chloride-bicarbonate exchanger, AE1. *Nat Genet.* 2005; 37 (11):1258–1263.

54. Guizouarn H, Martial S, Gabillat N, Borgese F. Point mutations involved in red cell stomatocytosis convert the electroneutral anion exchanger 1 to a non-selective cation conductance. *Blood.* 2007; 110(6):2158–2165.

Malaria

Michael A. McDevitt, MD, PhD,[1] and Richard Bucala, MD, PhD[2]

Etiology and Epidemiology

Malaria is a parasitic infection of erythrocytes caused by mosquito-borne protozoa of the genus *Plasmodium*. More than 200 million clinical episodes of infection occur annually, which in 2010 resulted in an estimated global death toll of more than 1.2 million.[1] Malarial disease predominantly affects the poor, pregnant women, and children under the age of 5, with 80% of fatalities occurring in sub-Saharan Africa. Of the five *Plasmodial* strains infecting humans, *Plasmodium falciparum* is both the most prevalent and the most deadly, and death ensues from the inflammatory complications of the infection: severe anemia leading to profound hypoxia and congestive heart failure, cerebral disease producing irreversible coma, and a sepsis-like syndrome with pulmonary and renal failure. Severe malarial anemia has been defined by the World Health Organization as a hemoglobin concentration <5 g/dL or a hematocrit <0.15 in the presence of a *P. falciparum* parasitemia of >10,000 parasites/μL in a normocytic blood film. This characterization is useful for epidemiologic studies and in defining clinical management. In practice, malaria-related anemia is usually defined as a reduction in the hemoglobin or hematocrit below the normal range for the age, sex, and state of pregnancy, in the presence of malarial parasitemia of any density in an endemic area. Severe malarial anemia also occurs most commonly in young children, and there are important distinctions between childhood and adult anemia that impact the clinical pathogenesis of the disease. Baseline hematologic indices, nutritional stores, and coinfections differ in children compared to adults. Moreover, the immunopathogenic mechanisms in children with first infection are distinct from older, surviving individuals with acquired, partial immunity.[2,3]

Anemia results from an imbalance between erythropoiesis and red cell elimination or tissue sequestration. The rupture of parasitized red blood cells is an essential feature of the *Plasmodium* life cycle as intracellular schizonts mature and merozoites are released to infect new red cells. Long-standing clinical observations that anemia is observed in children with low erythrocyte parasitemia and during chronic infection, and persists after antibiotic elimination of *Plasmodium* has given impetus to current notions that mechanisms beyond the parasite-induced destruction of red cells play an important role in malarial anemia.

Pathophysiology

Erythrocytic Destruction and Sequestration. Although the severity of anemia in the early stages of malaria frequently correlates with parasitemia and schizontoemia, uninfected red cells also have a shortened lifespan when compared to that of healthy individuals. Indeed, mathematical modeling of red cell survival kinetics indicates that an average of 8.5 uninfected red cells are destroyed for each parasitized red cell.[4] Nonspecific but immunologically mediated mechanisms contribute to this effect. Serum antibodies recognize malarial antigens and are passively absorbed onto uninfected cells, initiating complement-dependent hemolysis or opsonization.[5] A Coombs-positive hemolytic anemia may develop, and there is evidence for the loss from red cell surfaces of the complement regulatory proteins, CR1 and CD55.[6] Intraerythrocytic parasite metabolism also may produce sufficient reactive oxygen species to damage uninfected bystander cells. The inflammatory sequestration of infected red cells within the liver and spleen together with their adhesion to activated microvasculature and extravasation in different tissues also contributes to the overall reduction in hematocrit.[7]

Dyserythropoiesis. Malaria infection is characterized by a reduction in erythropoietic activity and inappropriately low reticulocyte numbers. Bone marrow cellularity is abnormal, with erythroid hypoplasia and hypoproliferative erythropoiesis most frequently noted during chronic infection, which is surprising for a hemolytic anemia. Detailed hematological studies of patients with severe malaria anemia have established the presence of ineffective erythropoiesis, bone marrow dyserythropoiesis, and lower erythroblast proliferative rates and numbers.[7,8] Erythropoiesis is critically regulated by erythropoietin, which is an obligatory growth factor for erythroid development, and a heme-containing protein within renal peritubular cells senses oxygen need to trigger the release of erythropoietin into the bloodstream. Interaction of erythropoietin with receptor-bearing progenitor cells in the bone marrow rescues them from apoptosis and translates physiologic oxygen demand into increased red cell production. It is not unusual for malaria patients to have a suboptimal reticulocyte count for the degree of anemia, even in the face of elevated erythropoietin levels.[9] These observations are supported by the results of ferrokinetic analysis showing impaired iron utilization consistent with ineffective erythropoiesis.[10] Clinical reports of severe anemia in children with low parasitemia or after successful antibiotic treatment and relocation of patients to non–malarial endemic regions also support a pathogenic role for impaired erythropoiesis.[11] Nevertheless, not all hematologic analyses have been uniform in their support of dyserythropoiesis in particular phases of malaria infection.[4,12]

Host Immunity. Experimental studies suggest several mechanisms by which *Plasmodium* parasites suppress the ability of erythropoietin to stimulate the proliferation and differentiation of hematopoietic progenitors. Chief among these is the impact of hemozoin, or malaria pigment, which results from parasite metabolism of host hemoglobin. The accumulation of malaria pigment in the bone marrow of infected patients is well described and may be directly toxic to erythroid precursors.[13] Circulating hemozoin-containing monocyte numbers correlate negatively with hematocrit and poor reticulocyte responses, which may be expected in the context of high parasite sequestration and disease severity.[14] Histologic examination of bone marrow from children with severe malaria also has revealed dysmorphic erythroid progenitors in proximity to hemozoin-laden macrophages suggestive of abnormal development.

Immune cytokines originating from macrophages, T cells, and natural killer (NK) cells are critical mediators in the host response to malaria. *Plasmodium* products such as hemozoin, glycosylphosphatidylinositol protein anchors, and CpG DNA activate innate immune responses via Toll- and NOD-like receptors to initiate inflammatory cytokine release.[15] Because infected red cells are cleared by activated macrophages, the differentiation of the adaptive immune response into a Th1-type T cell response favoring macrophage cytotoxicity rather than an antibody predominant Th2 response is expected to enhance the initial clearance of infected (and noninfected) red cells. Strong production of the innate cytokine IL-12 by macrophages, dendritic cells, and NK cells drives CD4 T cell IFNγ expression to further activate macrophages and favor clearance mechanisms. Th1 T cell mediated immune effector responses also would augment macrophage production of TNFα and IL-1, which have been correlated with bone marrow suppression, although neither these cytokines nor IFNγ appear to be central culprits in experimental mouse models.[16] Th2 T cell–derived cytokines (i.e., IL-4, IL-10, IL-13), on the other hand, counteract Th1 cytokines to drive B cell antibody production and may exert a protective role in chronic infection or in the recovery period.[15] Of note, a sustained elevation in circulating inflammatory cytokines may continue for weeks after treatment of malaria and may be associated with hypoproliferative erythropoiesis and anemia persistence.[17] Low circulating IL-10 concentrations have been described in African children with severe malarial anemia, and the ratio of TNFα to IL-10 is higher in patients with severe malarial anemia, suggesting that an insufficient IL-10 response may contribute to the pathophysiology of severe malarial anemia.[18] Clinical evidence also indicates that inflammatory cytokines decrease erythrocyte lifespan, but perhaps not via antibody-dependent mechanisms. Looareesuwan et al.[19] studied erythrocyte survival times in Thai subjects following clearance of asexual *P. falciparum* or *P. vivax* parasitemia and reported significant differences in the mean red cell lifespan in infected patients versus controls but without associated increases in cell-bound IgG or C3 complement.

As part of a cytokine-driven acute phase response, the peptide hepcidin is released from hepatocytes, increasing serum ferritin concentrations and reducing bioavailable iron for hemoglobin synthesis.[20] Hepcidin binds to the iron exporter ferroportin, which is expressed on macrophages, resulting in its internalization, degradation, and a reduction of iron recycling for bone marrow erythropoiesis. Serum iron concentrations rapidly decrease during acute malaria infection, and iron is sequestered in the bone marrow. Clinical studies have affirmed the importance of hepcidin in the anemia of chronic inflammation, although to date, there is conflicting data about this mediator in malaria. Uncomplicated malaria infections also may differ from severe malaria anemia with respect to hepcidin expression and its role in iron homeostasis.[21]

Impact of the Immune Response on Erythropoiesis. During malaria infection, inflammatory cells including macrophages appear in the spleen and bone marrow and may act to inhibit the erythroid progenitor response to erythropoietin. There is an inverse log-linear relationship between circulating erythropoietin levels and total hemoglobin: as hemoglobin decreases, erythropoietin levels rise. Serum erythropoietin is markedly elevated in children with severe malarial anemia and is inappropriately low for the degree of anemia.[22,23] As for other inflammation-related anemias, it has been proposed that inflammatory cytokines blunt erythropoietin synthesis or, more likely, inhibit the responsiveness of bone marrow progenitors to its signal transduction effects.[16]

Several studies support a role for predominantly macrophage-derived cytokines in the development of ineffective erythropoiesis or dyserythropoiesis. Inhibition of human erythroid colony formation by TNFα has been demonstrated *in vitro*, and there are corollary observations that BFU-E growth in bone marrow cultured with mononuclear cells from patients with rheumatoid arthritis can be reversed with anti-TNFα antibody. However, while TNFα may act directly on BFU-E, its effect on CFU-E colony formation is indirect and mediated instead by the paracrine release of other cytokines, such as IFNγ or MIF (macrophage migration inhibitory factor; reviewed in.[2] IL-1 shares many systemic inflammatory actions with TNFα, and malarial hemozoin activates the inflammasome to initiate the release of IL-1β.[24] IL-1 decreases erythroid colony counts *in vitro*, but its effects also may be indirect and by the induction of secondary mediators.[16]

IL-12 is produced by activated monocytes/macrophages and is highly inflammatory because it is an early and potent stimulus for T cell production of IFNγ. In human studies, IL-12 is inversely associated with risk of infection and positively associated with circulating concentrations of hemoglobin, IFNγ, and TNFα.[25] Mouse modeling indicates that IL-12 correlates with resistance to infection, protection from anemia, and improved indices of bone marrow erythropoiesis to *Plasmodium* infection. This effect is likely due to enhancement of the host response against the parasite, and hematologic studies show corresponding increases in BFU-E and CFU-E formation in bone marrow and spleen.[26] IFNγ inhibits the growth of CFU-E obtained from the spleens of mice, although this effect also may be indirect and require accessory cells. TNFα, IFNγ, and IL-1 each have been reported to inhibit *in vitro* erythropoiesis in cooperative or synergistic fashions. These mediators do not act in isolation, and feedback loops with sequential patterns of activation also occur.[2,16]

Multiple candidate gene association studies examining relationships between different effector cytokines and malaria susceptibility or clinical severity, including anemia, have been reported. Promoter polymorphisms in the TNFα gene have been associated with malaria susceptibility, with homozygosity at TNF-308A, for instance, associated with increased risk of cerebral malaria. A different polymorphism in the TNFα gene (TNF-238A), however, has been associated with severe anemia in Gambians. In Western Kenya, where severe malarial anemia is more common than cerebral malaria, an analysis of distributions of TNFα, IFNγ, TGFβ, IL-6, and IL-10 alleles showed a marked bias toward genotypes associated with low expression of IFNγ and IL-6.[15,27]

Macrophage migration inhibitory factor (MIF) is released from macrophages and T cells and acts by paracrine and autocrine pathways to augment the activation of numerous cell types. *Mif*-KO mice were observed to sustain similar parasitemias as their wild-type counterparts but were protected from lethal anemia, focusing interest on the primary role of this innate cytokine in the pathogenesis of malarial anemia.[28] MIF inhibits BFU-E differentiation *in vitro* and strongly synergizes with the inhibitory actions of cytokines such as TNFα and IFNγ to reverse the normal pattern of MAPK activation induced by erythropoietic stimuli. MIF is encoded in a functionally polymorphic locus, and variant *MIF* alleles occur commonly in different populations (minor allele frequency >5%). Of note, the highest prevalence of low-expression *MIF* alleles (78%) occurs in sub-Saharan Africa, where HbS occurs infrequently.[29] A protective role for low-expression *MIF* alleles in severe malarial anemia has been reported in a Kenyan population and confirmed recently in an Indian cohort.[30,31] Expression studies also have shown that hemozoin drives macrophage MIF production in an *MIF* allele-dependent fashion.[28] As the persistence of accumulated hemozoin within bone marrow may induce a prolonged state of MIF release, the risk of anemia conferred by high-expression *MIF* alleles is plausible and has prompted the development of MIF-specific biochips for use in resource-poor settings.[29]

Clinical Presentation and Diagnosis

The clinical presentation and manifestations of malaria can vary tremendously relative to the geographical location of the patient, age, immunity parameters, comorbidities, and other variables including pregnancy. Malaria should be considered in any patient with a febrile illness following exposure to mosquitoes in an endemic region. Associated symptoms can be quite nonspecific including chills, sweats, fatigue, myalgias, arthralgias, headache, anorexia, nausea, vomiting, cough, abdominal pain, diarrhea. Clinical signs include tachycardia, tachypnea, scleral icterus, and splenomegaly. Besides anemia, laboratory studies can reveal thrombocytopenia, transaminitis, coagulopathy, and elevated BUN and creatinine. To establish the diagnosis of malaria, blood smears or a rapid diagnostic test is essential.

Blood smears show parasitemia: fewer than 5,000 parasites/μL of blood - less than 0.1% parasitized RBCs for uncomplicated malaria compared to >100,000 parasites/μL of blood (typically) for those with complicated or severe malaria (5–10% of RBCs parasitized). The WHO considers 5% (low-transmission areas) and 10% (high-transmission areas) as cutoffs for the diagnosis of hyperparasitemia. *Plasmodium falciparum, vivax, ovale, malariae,* and *knowlesi* can all cause uncomplicated malaria. As described, most severe and complicated malaria is usually due to *P. falciparum* infection, but serious *P. vivax* infections have been reported. Young children including first-time infection-nonimmune individuals, immunocompromised individuals such as those with lymphoma, HIV, or asplenia are at greatest risk for severe disease. Diagnosed US cases should be reported to the Centers for Disease Control.

The differential diagnosis includes babesiosis, other febrile illnesses that relate to epidemiological and geographical considerations such as dengue or typhoid fever, and less common viral conditions. More common sepsis, meningitis, pneumonia, and less common leptospirosis and tick-borne diseases must be included in the differential. Complicating diagnosis and treatment is the fact that severe malaria anemia is often multifactoral and associated with nutritional deficiencies and certain coinfections; one infection particularly associated with severe anemia is parvovirus B19.

Treatment and Prognosis

The approach to selection of antimalarial therapy is complex, with geographical antibiotic resistance patterns, parasitic subtype, and the severity of disease at presentation among the considerations. Patients with severe malaria treated with artesunate should be evaluated at 4 weeks after treatment, as recent reports emphasize the risk of a delayed and poorly understood hemolytic anemia.[32] Beyond appropriate antibiotic therapy, which will become increasingly problematic with emerging resistance to artemisinins, blood transfusion is a mainstay for treatment of severe malarial anemia.[33] The decision when to transfuse severe malarial anemia is not clear-cut, and guidelines have not been established. A hematocrit cutoff of 20% is typically employed in adults, with clinical consideration for comorbidities. A recently published study from Kenya of 1,200 children with malarial anemia, 65% of whom received transfusion, used a hemoglobin threshold of 4 g/dL, with an increase to 5 g/dL in those with respiratory distress, impaired consciousness, or hyperparasitemia. The overall data appeared supportive, although the time to transfusion and the initial density of parasitemia also appeared important for outcome.[34] There remain concerns over the potential adverse effects of transfusion, such as the management of circulatory overload and transfusion reactions, even with a safe and available blood supply.

Exchange transfusion also is employed, usually in the setting of high parasitemia (>10%) and complications such as cerebral malaria, high-output cardiac failure, respiratory distress, renal insufficiency, older age or pregnancy. Beyond the correction of anemia and acidosis, the therapeutic rationale is parasite removal, reduction of *Plasmodium* toxins, and the improved rheology provided by uninfected red cells.[35] Exchange transfusion has come to be recommended, especially in well-resourced facilities where safe blood is available, for all patients in whom the parasitemia exceeds 30% even in the absence of other clinical manifestations.[33] As in the case of direct transfusion, there are no controlled clinical trials supporting this approach. Recent approaches also have employed erythrocytapheresis, or the removal only of the diseased red blood cell fraction by apheresis. This intervention may offer the advantage over standard exchange transfusion in returning leukocytes, platelet fractions, and other plasma components to the patients. However, its application to resource-poor settings remains limited.[36]

Conclusions

Malarial anemia remains a major global health problem that produces morbidity and death in millions of individuals every year. It also places a significant economic burden on developing societies and their health care facilities. Current paradigms for this common manifestation of malaria emphasize the proximate role of host immunity and an excessive or deleterious inflammatory effector response, which accelerates red cell elimination and inhibits compensatory erythropoiesis. There is increasing evidence for the importance of functional antagonism between erythropoietin signaling and immune cytokines on bone marrow progenitor cells. As severe malaria anemia arises from complex interactions between the parasite and the host, who often suffer comorbidity and coinfection by other pathogens, defining the exact interplay between different molecular and genetic influences remains challenging. It is nevertheless hoped that continued investigation of pathogenic signaling pathways coupled with the identification of genetic predispositions will lead to new and more effective diagnostic, preventative, and therapeutic approaches.

Acknowledgments

We regret the citation limit and our inability to credit numerous primary studies. Malaria studies in the authors' laboratories were supported by funding from the NIH, Yale Downs Fellowships, and Novartis.

References

1. Murray CJ, Rosenfeld LC, Lim SS, Andrews KG, Foreman KJ, Haring D, Fullman N, Naghavi M, Lozano R, Lopez AD. Global malaria mortality between 1980 and 2010: a systematic analysis. *Lancet.* 2012; 379:413–431.

2. McDevitt M, Xie J, Gordeuk V, Bucala R. The anemia of malaria infection: role of inflammatory cytokines. *Curr Hematol Rep.* 2004; 3:97–106.

3. Haldar K, Mohandas N. Malaria, erythrocytic infection, and anemia. *Hematology Am Soc Hematol Educ Program.* 2009:87–93.

4. Jakeman PH, Saul A, Hogarth WL, Collins WE. Anaemia of acute malaria infections in non-immune patients primarily results from destruction of uninfected erythrocytes. *Parasitology.* 2004; 119:127–133.

5. Waitumbi J, Opollo M, Muga R, Misore A, Stoute J. Red cell surface changes and erythrophagocytosis in children with severe *Plasmodium falciparum* anemia. *Blood.* 2000;95:1481–1486.

6. Stoute JA, Odindo AO, Owuor BO, Mibei EK, Opollo MO, Waitumbi JN. Loss of red blood cell-complement regulatory proteins and increased levels of circulating immune complexes are associated with severe malarial anemia. *J Infect Dis.* 2003; 187: 522–525.

7. Weatherall D, Kwiatkowski D, Roberts D. Hematologic manifestations of systemic disease in children of the developing world. In: Orkin SH, Ginsburg D, Nathan DG, Look TA, Fisher DE, Lux SE, editors, *Nathan and Oski's Hematology and Oncology of Infancy and Childhood*, 8th edition, Amsterdam: Elsevier; 2008.

8. Wickramasinghe S, Abdalla S. Blood and bone marrow changes in malaria. *Baillieres Best Pract Res Clin Haematol.* 2003; 13:277–299.

9. Abdalla SH. Hematopoiesis in human malaria. *Blood Cells.* 1990; 16:401–416.

10. Srichaikul T, Wasanasomsithi M, Poshyachinda V, Panikbutr N, Rabieb T. Ferrokinetic studies and erythropoiesis in malaria. *Arch Intern Med.* 1969; 124:623–628.

11. Biemba G, Gordeuk V, Thuma P, Mabeza GF, Weiss G. Prolonged macrophage activation and persistent anemia in children with complicated malaria. *Trop Med Int Health.* 1998; 3:60–65.

12. Das B, Nanda N, Rath P, Satapathy R, Das D. Anaemia in acute *Plasmodium falciparum* malaria in children from the Orissa state, India. *Ann Trop Med Parasitol.* 1999; 93:109–118.

13. Lamikanra AA, Theron M, Kooij TW, Roberts DJ. Hemozoin (malarial pigment) directly promotes apoptosis of erythroid precursors. *PLoS One.* 2009;4: e8446.

14. Kremsner PG, Valim C, Missinou MA, Olola C, Krishna S, Issifou S, Kombila M, Bwanaisa L, Mithwani S, Newton CR, Agbenyega T, Pnder M, Bojang K,

Wypij D, Taylor T. Prognostic value of circulating pigmented cells in African children with malaria. *J Infect Dis.* 2009; 199:142–150.

15. Stevenson MM, Riley EM. Innate Immunity to Malaria. *Nat Revs Immunol.* 2004; 4:169–180.

16. Yap GS, Stevenson MM. Inhibition of *in vitro* erythropoiesis by soluble mediators during *Plasmodium chabaudi AS* malaria: lack of a major role for interleukin-1, tumor necrosis factor-α, and γ-interferon. *Infect Immun.* 1994; 62:357–362.

17. Kwiatkowski D, Cannon JG, Manogue KR, Cerami A, Dinarello CA, Greenwood BM. Tumour necrosis factor production in Falciparum malaria and its association with schizont rupture. *Clin Exp Immunol.* 1989; 77:361–366.

18. Thuma PE, van Dijk J, Bucala R, Debebe Z, Nekhai S, Kuddo T, Nouraie M, Weiss G, Gordeuk VR. Distinct clinical and immunologic profiles in severe malarial anemia and cerebral malaria in Zambia. *J Infect Dis.* 2011; 203:211–219.

19. Looareesuwan S, Merry AH, Phillips RE, Pleehachinda R, Wattanagoon Y, Ho M, Charoenlarp P, Warrell DA, Weatherall DJ. Reduced erythrocyte survival following clearance of malarial parasitaemia in Thai patients. *Br J Haematol.* 1987; 67:473–478.

20. Nicolas G, Chauvet C, Viatte L, Danan JL, Bigard X, Devaux I, Beaumont C, Kahn A, Vaulont S. The gene encoding the iron regulatory peptide hepcidin is regulated by anemia, hypoxia, and inflammation. *J Clin Invest.* 2002; 110:1037–1044.

21. Burté F, Brown BJ, Orimadegun AE, Ajetunmobi WA, Afolabi NK, Akinkunmi F, Kowobari O, Omokhodion S, Osinusi K, Akinbami FO, Shokunbi WA, Sodeinde O, Fernandez-Reyes D. Circulatory hepcidin is associated with the anti-inflammatory response but not with iron or anemic status in childhood malaria. *Blood.* 2013; 121:3016–3022.

22. Burchard G, Radloff P, Philipps J, Nkeyi M, Knobloch J, Kremsner P. Increased erythropoietin production in children with severe malarial anemia. *Am J Trop Med Hyg.* 1995; 53:547–551.

23. Burgmann H, Looareesuwan S, Kapiotis S, Viravan C, Vanijanonta S, Hollenstein U, Wiesinger E, Presterl E, Winkler S, Graninger W. Serum levels of erythropoietin in acute *Plasmodium falciparum* malaria. *Am J Trop Med Hyg.* 1996; 54:280–283.

24. Griffith JW, Sun T, McIntosh MT, Bucala R. Pure hemozoin is inflammatory *in vivo* and activates the NALP3 inflammasome via release of uric acid. *J Immunol.* 2009; 183:5208–5220.

25. Dodoo D, Omer FM, Todd J, Akanmori BD, Koram KA, Riley EM. Absolute levels and ratios of proinflammatory and anti-inflammatory cytokine production in vitro predict clinical immunity to *Plasmodium falciparum* malaria. *J Infect Dis.* 2002; 185:971–979.

26. Mohan K, Stevenson MM. Interleukin-12 corrects severe anemia during blood-stage *Plasmodium chabaudi AS* in susceptible A/J mice. *Exp Hematol.* 1998; 26:45–52.

27. Mcguire W, Knight JC, Hill AVS, Allsopp CEM, Greenwood BM, Kwiatkowski D. Severe malarial anemia and cerebral malaria are associated with different tumor necrosis factor promoter alleles. *J Infect Dis.* 1999; 179:287–290.

28. McDevitt MA, Xie J, Shanmugasundaram G, Griffith J, Liu A, McDonald C, Thuma P, Gordeuk VR, Metz CN, Mitchell R, Keefer J, David J, Leng L, Bucala R. A critical role for the host mediator macrophage migration inhibitory factor in the pathogenesis of malarial anemia. *J Exp Med.* 2006; 203:1185–1196.

29. Zhong XB, Leng L, Beitin A, Chen R, McDonald C, Hsiao B, Jenison RD, Kang I, Park SH, Lee A, Gregersen P, Thuma P, Bray-Ward P, Ward DC, Bucala R. Simultaneous detection of microsatellite repeats and SNPs in the macrophage migration inhibitory factor (MIF) gene by thin-film biosensor chips and application to rural field studies. *Nucleic Acids Res.* 2005;33:121–129.

30. Awandare GA, Martinson JJ, Were T, Ouma C, Davenport GC, Ong'echa JM, Wang WK, Leng L, Ferrell RE, Bucala R, Perkins DJ. *MIF* promoter polymorphisms and susceptibility to severe malarial anemia. *J Infect Dis.* 2009; 15:629–637.

31. Jha AN, Sundaradival P, Pati SS, Patra PK, Thandaraj K. Variations in ncRNA gene LOC284889 and MIF-794CATT repeats are associated with malaria susceptibility in Indian populations. *Malar J.* 2013;12:345–353.

32. Published Reports of Delayed Hemolytic Anemia After Treatment with Artesunate for Severe Malaria – Worldwide, 2010–2012. *Morb Mortal Wkly Rep.* 2013; 62(1):5–8.

33. Akinosoglou KS, Solomou EE, Gogos CA. Malaria: a haematological disease. *Hematology.* 2012; 17:106–114.

34. English M, Ahmed M, Ngando C, Berkley J, Ross A. Blood transfusion for severe anaemia in children in a Kenyan hospital. *Lancet.* 2002; 359:494–495.

35. van Genderen PJ, Hesselink DA, Bezemer JM, Wismans PJ, Overbosch D. efficacy and safety of exchange transfusion as adjunct therapy for severe *Plasmodium falciparum* malaria in nonimmune travelers: a 10 year single-center experience with a standardized treatments protocol. *Transfusion.* 2010; 50:787–794.

36. Nieuwenhuis JA, Meertens JH, Zijlstra JG, Ligtenberg JJ, Tulleken JE, van der Werf TS. Automated erythrocytapheresis in severe falciparum malaria: a critical appraisal. *Acta Trop.* 2006; 98:201–206.

Microangiopathic Hemolytic Anemia

Elaine M. Majerus, MD, PhD, and J. Evan Sadler, MD, PhD

Etiology/Epidemiology

Microangiopathic hemolytic anemia (MAHA) is caused by disruptions of microvascular blood flow that lead to hemolysis and fragmentation of red blood cells into schistocytes[1] (Figure 16.1). The combination of MAHA and thrombocytopenia is referred to as thrombotic microangiopathy, which is a characteristic feature of three main clinical disorders and can occur in several other settings (Table 16.1).

Thrombotic thrombocytopenic purpura (TTP). TTP refers to thrombotic microangiopathy without another apparent cause or disseminated intravascular coagulation and without acute renal failure. The majority of patients with TTP are adults with acquired autoantibodies against the metalloprotease ADAMTS13 that reduce plasma ADAMTS13 activity to <10% of normal. Approximately 20%[2] to 50%[3] of patients with a clinical picture consistent with autoimmune TTP prove to have normal or slightly decreased ADAMTS13 levels. This variability has not been explained but may reflect different referral patterns and case definitions.

The demographics of autoimmune TTP are similar to those of systemic lupus erythematosis, and patients sometimes have serologic findings of autoimmune disorders.[4] The median age of presentation is approximately 40 years, with an interquartile range of 33–50 years of age.[5] Demographic risk factors include female gender, African ancestry, and obesity.[3]

The reported annual incidence of MAHA is 5–6 cases per million in the United States[6] but a lower 2.2 per million in the United Kingdom.[7] Of those in the United States, about 2–3 per million are associated with severe acquired ADAMTS13 deficiency.

Congenital TTP, also known as Upshaw-Schulman syndrome, is caused by homozygous or compound heterozygous mutations in ADAMTS13, which have an estimated prevalence of 1 per million.[8] Congenital TTP accounts for a few% of patients presenting with TTP.

Shiga toxin-producing *Escherichia coli*-hemolytic uremic syndrome (STEC-HUS). Ingestion of food or water contaminated with Shiga toxin-producing *E. coli* (STEC) can cause hemolytic uremic syndrome (STEC-HUS), which is distinguished from TTP by acute renal failure, usually oliguric or anuric, with a prodrome of abdominal pain and diarrhea that becomes bloody. STEC-HUS usually occurs in children less than 5 years old but is rare before 6 months of age. STEC-HUS is a common cause of chronic renal failure in children.[9]

The incidence of STEC-HUS varies with sporadic or epidemic exposure to STEC but is approximately 10–30 per million children per year. Most cases occur in the summer and autumn. In the United States and most of the world, *E. coli* O157:H7 is the most common serotype associated with STEC-HUS. Of children less than 10 years of age with bloody diarrhea and *E. coli* O157:H7 infection, approximately 15% will develop STEC-HUS.[9] Non-O157:H7 *E. coli* serotypes have caused STEC-HUS in Europe and Australia.[10] *Shigella dysenteriae* serotype 1 causes some cases in Africa and South Asia.[9]

Atypical hemolytic uremic syndrome (aHUS). Like STEC-HUS, aHUS is characterized by thrombotic microangiopathy and acute renal failure. Unlike STEC-HUS, aHUS is not classically preceded by bloody diarrhea. Inherited heterozygous mutations in proteins that regulate the alternate complement pathway or acquired autoantibodies against complement factor H have been identified in 60–70% of patients with

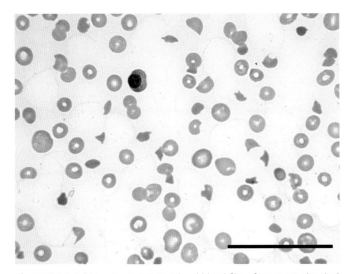

Figure 16.1 Schistocytes in TTP. Peripheral blood film of a patient who died with TTP shows schistocytes, polychromasia, and nucleated red blood cells. Scale bar is 50 μm.

Table 16.1 Classification of Thrombotic Microangiopathies

Thrombotic thrombocytopenic purpura (TTP)

- Autoimmune – Antibodies against ADAMTS13

- Congenital – *ADAMTS13* mutations (Upshaw-Schulman Syndrome)

Shiga toxin-producing *Escherichia coli* hemolytic uremic syndrome (STEC-HUS)

- Shiga toxin-producing *E. coli*

- *Shigella dysenteriae*

Atypical hemolytic uremic syndrome (aHUS)

- Complement alternate pathway regulatory defects

- Diacylglycerol kinase epsilon defects

- Cobalamin metabolic defects

Secondary thrombotic microangiopathy, associated with:

- Malignant hypertension

- Mechanical hemolysis – malfunctioning aortic or mitral valve prostheses

- Pregnancy – preeclampsia/eclampsia, HELLP syndrome

- Infections – viral, bacterial, fungal

- Disseminated intravascular coagulation

- Cancer

- Hematopoietic stem cell or solid organ transplantation

- Antiphospholipid antibody syndrome

- Autoimmune disease

- Vasculitis

- Ionizing radiation

- Drugs – calcineurin inhibitors, mitomycin C, gemcitabine, VEGF inhibitors, ticlopidine, quinine

aHUS (Table 16.2). The disease appears to be familial in approximately 20% of cases, with approximately 50% penetrance.

Children <18 years old comprise approximately one-half of patients. Approximately 70% of affected children have their first episode of aHUS before age 2 years and 25% before age 6 months. In contrast, STEC-HUS is uncommon before age 6 months.

Homozygous or compound heterozygous mutations in diacylglycerol kinase ε (DGKE) cause aHUS with high penetrance that presents before 1 year of age with hypertension, hematuria, and proteinuria. *DGKE* mutations may account for a few% of aHUS.[11]

Atypical HUS affects approximately 5% as many children as develop STEC-HUS, with an estimated incidence of 2 per million per year,[12]

Secondary thrombotic microangiopathy. Many other conditions can cause microangiopathic hemolytic anemia with thrombocytopenia (Table 16.1). In most of these cases, the clinical course is dictated by the underlying disorder rather than the thrombotic microangiopathy.

Pathophysiology

Thrombotic thrombocytopenic purpura (TTP). Severe deficiency of ADAMTS13 allows excessive von Willebrand factor (VWF)–dependent platelet adhesion, microvascular thrombosis and tissue injury (Figure 16.2). Increased shear stress associated with these lesions causes microangiopathic hemolysis and platelet consumption. Plasma ADAMTS13 >10% is sufficient to prevent thrombotic microangiopathy in nearly all patients with acquired or congenital TTP.

Affected tissues have arteriolar occlusions that contain VWF and platelets but minimal fibrin (Figure 16.3). Endothelial cells are usually intact. Lesions occur in kidney, heart, brain, pancreas, adrenals, skin, spleen, bone marrow, liver, and most other tissues. The lungs are spared.

Table 16.2 Complement Defects in Atypical Hemolytic Uremic Syndrome

Gene or subgroup	Prevalence in aHUS	Low C3	Progression to end stage renal disease	Death
CFH	25–30%	50–60%	50–60%	5–20%
CFI	4–10%	20–50%	~60%	0–10%
MCP	7–10%	6–30%	6–35%	0%
CFB	<1.5%	≤100%	~50%	0%
C3	4–8%	70–80%	55–70%	0%
THBD	<5%	~50%	~50%	~30%
Anti-CFH antibody	3–7%	~40%	30–60%	0%
No mutation	30–50%	~20%	~40%	3–7%

Based on outcomes after 5 years from the International Registry of Recurrent and Familial HUS/TTP (18) and after 3 years from the French Study Group for aHUS (37).

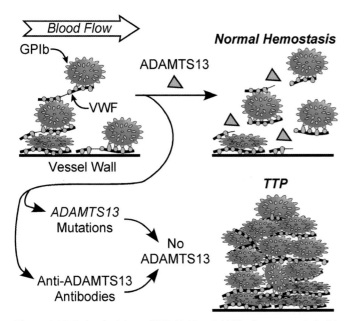

Figure 16.2 Pathophysiology of TTP. Multimeric VWF adheres to endothelial cells or connective tissue in the vessel wall. Platelets adhere to VWF through platelet membrane GPIb. Flowing blood stretches the VWF and exposes a cleavage site (thin lines) for ADAMTS13. Cleavage limits the growth of intravascular thrombi. Congenital or acquired ADAMTS13 deficiency allows excessive platelet deposition, causing microvascular thrombosis and TTP.

Almost all *ADAMTS13* mutations in congenital TTP impair ADAMTS13 secretion. Residual plasma ADAMTS13 activity levels higher than ~2 to 3% have been associated with less frequent recurrences, avoidance of prophylactic plasma therapy, and a tendency to present in adulthood rather than childhood.[13]

Shiga toxin-producing *Escherichia coli*-hemolytic uremic syndrome (STEC-HUS). STEC can make two types of Shiga toxin (Stx), Stx1 and Stx2, both of which have an AB_5 structure: pentamers of B subunits bind globotriaosylceramide (Gb3) on cell surfaces, and the active (A) subunit is responsible for cytotoxicity. Stx1 is identical to the major toxin of *S. dysenteriae* serotype 1. Stx2 is ~50% identical to Stx1 and occurs in several variants. Most STEC isolated in the United States express both Stx1 and Stx2.

STEC colonize the gut and secrete Stx that is transported into the blood, where cells, probably neutrophils, deliver it to tissues that express Gb3 including renal tubular epithelial, mesangial, and glomerular endothelial cells and other organs. Stx is retrotranslocated into the cytoplasm, where the A subunit damages 28S ribosomal RNA, inhibits protein synthesis, and causes apoptosis. This injury promotes thrombotic microangiopathy and renal failure.

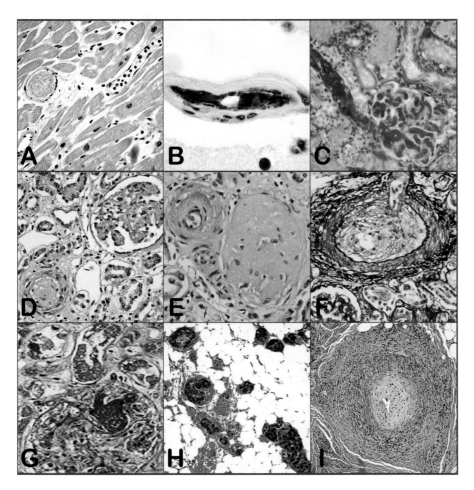

Figure 16.3 Pathology of Thrombotic Microangiopathy. A, (TTP) Arteriolar thrombosis in the heart, with intact endothelium and vessel wall. B, (TTP) Immunochemical stain shows VWF in the arterioles in the brain. C, (STEC-HUS) prominent fibrin deposits (magenta). Platelet and fibrin stain of Carstair. D, (aHUS) A reorganizing renal arteriolar thrombosis with loss of the endothelial cells. The glomerulus is contracted with thickened subendothelial and mesangial matrix. E, (aHUS) Marked subendothelial expansion, arteriolar fibrosis, and stenosis without thrombosis in the kidney. F, (aHUS) renal thrombotic microangiopathy with marked subendothelial expansion and cellular proliferation causing arteriolar stenosis. The interal elastic lamina is intact. Jones silver stain. Stained with hematolylin and eosin unless otherwise stated.
(Reproduced with permission from Tsai H-M. Thrombotic thrombocytopenic purpura, hemolytic-uremic syndrome, and related disorders. In: Greer JP, Arber DA, Glader B, List AF, Means RT Jr., Paraskevas F, Rodgers GM, eds. *Wintrobe's Clinical Hematology*, 13th edition Philadelphia: Lippincott Williams & Wilkins; 2014.)

Renal lesions in STEC-HUS contain fibrin with few platelets in glomerular capillaries, blood vessels, and tubules, in contrast to the platelet-rich and fibrin-poor thrombi that characterize TTP (Figure 16.3). Glomeruli are enlarged, with endothelial swelling, and capillaries are distended by red cells and fibrin. Renal cortical necrosis is common. Lesions occur less frequently in pancreas, adrenal glands, brain, and heart.[14]

Atypical hemolytic uremic syndrome (aHUS). Complement component C3b is deposited on cells in response to activation that depends on antibodies (classical pathway), bacterial glycans (lectin pathway), or spontaneous conversion of C3 to C3b (alternative pathway). Under normal circumstances, C3b production is limited by the serine protease complement factor I (CFI) and the cofactors complement factor H (CFH), MCP, and thrombomodulin (THBD) (Figure 16.4). Defects in CFH, MCP, CFI, or THBD impair the feedback inhibition of C3b activation and promote the production of C5a and membrane attack complexes. Gain-of-function mutations in C3 or CFB can increase complement activation by promoting C3 convertase formation or impairing its inactivation by CFI. These effects cause complement deposition on renal glomerular and arteriolar endothelium and basement membrane, which leads to vascular damage and thrombotic microangiopathy.

As in STEC-HUS, renal lesions in aHUS are rich in fibrin but poor in platelets or VWF. Subendothelial glomerular basement thickening, mesangial cell proliferation, endothelial swelling, fibrinoid necrosis, and thrombosis may be seen (Figure 16.3). Late changes include basement membrane

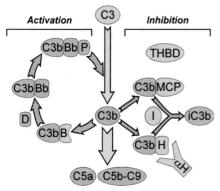

Figure 16.4 The Alternative Complement Pathway and aHUS. Slow spontaneous hydrolysis of the C3 thioester bond creates a C3b-like species that attaches to cell surfaces. When C3b binds to complement factor B (CFB), which is a serine protease zymogen, complement factor D (CFD) cleaves and activates CFB to form the alternative pathway C3 convertase (C3bBb). The C3 convertase generates more C3b in a positive feedback loop (*green arrows*). Binding of a second C3b changes C3 convertase (C3bBb) into a C5 convertase (C3bC3bBb), which cleaves C5 into C5a (anaphylatoxin) and C5b. C5b initiates the formation of membrane attack complexes (C5b-9). Amplification of the initial C3b response is limited (*red arrows*) by complement factor I (CFI), which cleaves and inactivates C3b in a reaction that is accelerated by complement factor H (CFH), which is recruited from the blood, or MCP, which is present in membranes of all cells except erythrocytes. Thrombomodulin (THBD) also can bind C3b and CFH to accelerate the inactivation of C3b. Mutations in certain factors (*orange*) or antibodies against CFH increase the activity of the alternative complement pathway and predispose to aHUS.

duplication and mesangial expansion, with regression of thrombosis and endocapillary swelling.[15] Arterial lesions, mesangial proliferation, and basement membrane duplication are not described in STEC-HUS.

How DGKE mutations cause aHUS is not established.

Secondary thrombotic microangiopathy. For many disorders the cause of secondary thrombotic microangiopathy is not understood, with some exceptions. Quinine-induced thrombotic microangiopathy is caused by quinine-dependent autoantibodies against platelet proteins that activate platelets. Disease can be triggered within hours by a single dose of quinine or quinine-containing beverage taken months after a sensitizing exposure.

Ticlopidine-associated TTP is caused by autoantibodies against ADAMTS13 that do not depend on continued presence of the drug, and ticlopidine-associated TTP responds to plasma exchange. Other thienopyridines such as clopidogrel and prasugrel do not appear to induce TTP by this mechanism.

Hemolytic uremic syndrome can occur with invasive *Streptococcus pneumoniae* infections, particularly pneumonia complicated by empyema or pleural effusion, with an incidence of approximately 0.6 per million children (0–18 years of age). Few cases occur in adults. The mechanism of thrombotic microangiopathy appears to involve the action of bacterial neuraminidase on erythrocytes, platelets, and endothelial cells, which exposes Thomsen-Friedenreich (T) antigen to attack by endogenous anti-T antibodies.

Clinical Presentation

The clinical features that are characteristic of TTP, STEC-HUS, and aHUS are helpful but do not distinguish perfectly among these diagnoses.

Thrombotic thrombocytopenic purpura (TTP). Patients with acquired TTP may present acutely or subacutely with symptoms of anemia and thrombocytopenia, including fatigue, dyspnea, weakness, headache, petechiae, bruising, and mucosal bleeding. Many patients describe a prior upper respiratory tract infection or flu-like symptoms. Patients with severe deficiency of ADAMTS13 can remain asymptomatic for varying lengths of time but develop active TTP in response to an inflammatory stress or other trigger such as pregnancy, surgery, infection, or thyrotoxicosis. Recognizing TTP in such settings can be a challenge because many of them can cause thrombotic microangiopathy by other mechanisms.

Symptoms may reflect widespread microvascular thrombosis in almost any tissue. Fever occurs in a minority of patients with TTP. Neurological complaints are common, occurring in approximately one-half of patients, and vary from headache, confusion, or paresthesias to focal deficits, blindness, seizures, or coma. Some patients have neurological events before developing overt thrombotic microangiopathy. Patients can rarely have apparent occlusion of the middle cerebral artery or other large arteries on admission or during the course of illness.

Cardiac involvement is common and may cause symptomatic or fatal arrhythmias, myocardial infarction, or congestive heart failure.

Abdominal pain and tenderness are relatively common. Nausea, vomiting, and diarrhea occur in a few patients. Bloody diarrhea is uncommon.

Patients with congenital TTP often have neonatal jaundice and thrombocytopenia that cannot be explained by ABO or Rh incompatibility. Approximately half of patients have repeated episodes of thrombocytopenia during childhood that may be misdiagnosed as ITP or Evans syndrome. The rest have their first experience with thrombotic microangiopathy as adults. For women, TTP occurs predictably during the second or third trimester of pregnancy. Rare patients, usually men, never become symptomatic. Renal insufficiency is not a common feature of congenital TTP, but renal failure that may require dialysis can develop after repeated episodes of inadequately treated disease.[16]

Shiga toxin-producing *Escherichia coli*-hemolytic uremic syndrome (STEC-HUS). Diarrhea and abdominal pain begin between 2 and 12 days after ingestion of STEC, with a mean incubation period of 3–7 days and a median of 3 days. After 1–3 days of nonbloody diarrhea, often with nausea and vomiting, the diarrhea becomes bloody in 90% of cases. However, STEC has been isolated from the stool of patients with STEC-HUS who never have diarrhea. Fever is characteristically absent in the hospital. The abdominal pain is greater than is typical for other forms of gastroenteritis, with tenderness on examination, and defecation is often painful.[9]

Atypical hemolytic uremic syndrome (aHUS). Approximately 20% of patients with aHUS have a subacute or chronic course with anemia, variable thrombocytopenia, and relatively preserved renal function. However, patients usually present acutely with symptoms of anemia such as pallor, fatigue, and weakness. Children may have poor feeding, vomiting, drowsiness, and edema.[17,18] Most patients have a potential triggering event such as an upper respiratory infection, influenza, varicella, diarrhea, or gastroenteritis. Approximately 20% of women with aHUS have disease in association with a pregnancy; 80% develop aHUS postpartum, and most of the rest develop symptoms during the third trimester.

Extrarenal involvement is evident in approximately 20% of patients. Neurological symptoms are the most common. Myocardial infarction can occur. Necrosis of peripheral digits or skin is present in a few% of patients. Gastrointestinal symptoms may include pancreatitis or diarrhea in approximately 25% of patients. Painful, bloody diarrhea is very uncommon. Multiorgan failure has been described in up to 10% of patients.

Diagnostic Evaluation and Laboratory Findings

A diagnosis of thrombotic microangiopathy is established by finding anemia, thrombocytopenia, and increased schistocytes on examination of a peripheral blood film. The frequency of schistocytes is variable but usually greater than 1%, compared to 0.05% in healthy controls.

Table 16.3 Laboratory Testing in Thrombotic Microangiopathy

Diagnosis and planning therapy:

- CBC and platelet count
- Reticulocyte count
- Peripheral blood film
- Bilirubin
- Haptoglobin
- LDH
- Direct antiglobulin test
- PT, aPTT, fibrinogen
- BUN, creatinine
- Urinalysis
- AST, ALT, alkaline phosphatase
- Hepatitis B and C

TTP:

- ADAMTS13 activity, inhibitor, antibodies

STEC-HUS:

- Stool culture for STEC, *C. difficile*, other pathogens
- Shiga toxin immunoassay or PCR assay

aHUS:

- Plasma C3, C4, CFH, CFI
- Anti-CFH antibodies
- MCP by flow cytometry on peripheral blood mononuclear cells
- Mutation screening for *CFH, CFI, MCP, C3, CFB, THBD, DGKE*

Depending on clinical context:

- Pregnancy test
- Lupus anticoagulant
- Anticardiolipin antibodies
- Anti-PF4 antibodies, serotonin release assay
- Anti-DsDNA, ANA, anti-centromere antibodies, anti-ACL-70
- Plasma B12, methylmalonic acid, homocysteine, methionine
- Urine methylmalonic acid, homocysteine
- Viral testing for HIV, influenza, CMV, EBV
- Bacterial cultures (e.g., *S. pneumoniae*)

Specific diagnosis depends on additional laboratory testing (Table 16.3). Hemolysis can cause increased indirect bilirubin, absent haptoglobin, and increased LDH. Some of the increase in LDH may be due to release from injured tissues. Direct antiglobulin testing (Coombs test) is characteristically negative. Fibrinogen is typically normal or elevated. The prothrombin time and partial thromboplastin time are normal or minimally prolonged.

Most secondary causes (Table 16.1) can be excluded by history and laboratory testing. Depending on the setting, tests should be considered for pregnancy, cobalamin deficiency, systemic lupus erythematosis, scleroderma, antiphospholipid antibody syndrome, HIV, and various other pathogens (Table 16.3).

Thrombotic thrombocytopenic purpura. At presentation, patients with TTP have median platelet counts of 10,000–17,000 platelets/μL. Urinalysis usually shows microhematuria, granular or red cell casts, and proteinuria. The serum creatinine is usually within the normal range or slightly elevated: values are seldom >2 mg/dL and almost never >4 mg/dL unless the patient has had several previous episodes of MAHA or a long delay before the initiation of treatment.

ADAMTS13 activity is characteristically <10% in congenital or acquired TTP during active disease. The normal range (±2 SD) of ADAMTS13 activity in human plasma is approximately 60–140%, but a level of >10% appears sufficient to prevent thrombotic microangiopathy. ADAMTS13 is synthesized in the liver, and severe ADAMTS13 deficiency has been observed rarely in acute or chronic liver failure.

Polyclonal autoantibody inhibitors of ADAMTS13, usually IgG but occasionally IgA or IgM, can be demonstrated in at least 65% of patients with acquired TTP. Nearly 100% of patients with acquired TTP have anti-ADAMTS13 autoantibodies that can be detected by ELISA or western blotting, some of which promote ADAMTS13 clearance. Detection of anti-ADAMTS13 autoantibodies by ELISA or western blotting supports the diagnosis of acquired TTP, with the caveat that anti-ADAMTS13 autoantibodies occur in approximately 4% of healthy controls and up to 13% of patients with systemic lupus erythematosis who have normal plasma ADAMTS13 activity.[19] Conversely, severe ADAMTS13 deficiency with no anti-ADAMTS13 antibodies is consistent with congenital TTP, but the diagnosis may require confirmation based on genetic studies or a complete response to simple plasma infusion.

VWF multimer patterns should not be relied upon to identify TTP or distinguish it from other causes of thrombotic microangiopathy.

STEC-HUS. The platelet count and serum creatinine may be normal upon presentation. When HUS develops, the average platelet count is approximately 40,000/μL and the serum creatinine is elevated. ADAMTS13 activity is characteristically normal.

Stool samples should be cultured for *E. coli* O157:H7 on selective media and tested for Shiga toxins to detect non-O157 STEC. STEC are detected in at least 90% of patients during the first 6 days but in <30% at later times. Fecal leukocytes may or may not be present. *Clostridium difficile* can cause acute bloody diarrhea, and coinfection with both STEC and *C. difficile* has been reported.

Serum obtained at diagnosis and at 2 weeks can be assayed for antibodies to lipopolysaccharide antigens of major STEC serogroups, which rise after infection and persist for 8–12 weeks.

aHUS. The mean platelet count in aHUS is approximately 40,000/μL. The serum creatinine is usually markedly elevated and associated with proteinuria if patients are not anuric. ADAMTS13 activity is normal.

Values for complement component C4 are usually normal. The likelihood of observing a low C3 value depends on the underlying mutation (Table 16.2). Approximately 3–7% of aHUS patients have autoantibodies against CFH that can be detected by ELISA.

Measuring levels of C3, C4, CFH, and CFI and cell surface MCP may be useful for prognosis and considering transplantation options.[12] However, patients with mutations are usually heterozygous, and factor levels may not be clearly decreased.

DNA sequencing should be considered to detect *CFH, CFI, MCP, C3, CFB,* and *THBD* mutations before renal transplantation. Sequencing of *DGKE* should be considered for infants with aHUS.

Treatment/Prognosis

Prompt diagnosis and treatment is critical to preserve renal function and prevent extrarenal tissue injury. The possibility of misdiagnosis or multiple diagnoses should be considered for patients with unusual clinical features or an inadequate response to treatment.

TTP. Plasma exchange should be started as soon as feasible in patients who may have acquired TTP, because delay is associated with inferior outcomes. If plasma exchange must be delayed more than a few hours, patients can be treated by infusion of plasma 7.5 ml/kg every 6 hours, if tolerated, until plasma exchange is possible.[16,20]

The volume exchanged is generally 1–1.5 plasma volumes (40–60 ml/kg) daily with fresh frozen plasma (FFP) as the replacement fluid. Solvent-/detergent-treated plasma, methylene blue–treated plasma, and psoralen-treated plasma are used in some localities. Cryosupernatant (cryopoor) plasma is theoretically attractive because it contains a similar concentration of ADAMTS13 but much less von Willebrand factor. However, limited comparisons have not demonstrated an advantage for cryosupernatant plasma.

For acquired TTP, glucocorticoids such as prednisone or methylprednisolone 1–2 mg/kg/day are given routinely for immunosuppression. Alternatively, methylprednisolone 1 g/day intravenously for 3 days has been used.[16]

Laboratory monitoring should include daily CBC, electrolytes, calcium, and LDH (Table 16.3). As patients respond to treatment, the platelet count rises, LDH falls, the hemoglobin stabilizes, and signs of tissue injury improve.

Plasma exchange should continue daily until the patient has a treatment response, which is defined as normalization of the platelet count for at least 2 days.[16] The median number of plasma exchanges to treatment response is approximately 11, with a wide range of 4–55 sessions.[21] Normalization of serum LDH lags behind the platelet count by approximately

9 days, and persistent elevation of LDH appears not to correlate with the risk of exacerbation or relapse.[22]

Exacerbations are defined as TTP recurring within 30 days after a treatment response and are common during the first week after stopping plasma exchange. A durable treatment response, lasting more than 30 days, is achieved eventually in approximately 80% of patients. Relapses occur within 2 years after a durable treatment response in approximately 40% of patients after therapy with plasma exchange and glucocorticoids alone.

Refractory and relapsing TTP have been treated effectively with rituximab, usually 375 mg/m^2 weekly for 4 weeks. Almost all patients have a durable treatment response within 2–3 weeks after the first dose of rituximab associated with normalization of plasma ADAMTS13 activity. Relapses are uncommon during the subsequent 2 years and usually respond to retreatment with rituximab.

Rituximab has been combined with plasma exchange and glucocorticoids for the initial treatment of TTP. The use of rituximab at diagnosis appears to shorten the time to treatment response and reduce the incidence of relapse.[16]

Some patients achieve a treatment response despite ongoing severe ADAMTS13 deficiency, but the duration of such responses is unpredictable. Relapses are always associated with persistent or recurrent severe ADAMTS13 deficiency. Limited experience suggests that almost all of these relapses can be prevented by monitoring ADAMTS13 levels and giving rituximab preemptively when severe ADAMTS13 deficiency recurs.[23,24]

Benefits of rituximab must be balanced against potentially increased susceptibility to infection and other risks. For example, some patients with malignancy or HIV infection treated with rituximab have developed progressive multifocal leukoencephalopathy due to JC virus reactivation or fulminant hepatitis and hepatic failure due to hepatitis B reactivation. However, these complications are very rare after the use of rituximab in autoimmune diseases.[25,26]

Patients who may receive rituximab should be screened for hepatitis B. Ideally, naïve patients should be vaccinated for hepatitis B well before receiving rituximab, and those with evidence of prior infection should receive antiviral prophylaxis. Patients should be monitored for signs of hepatic injury and hepatitis B reactivation for 6–12 months after treatment with rituximab.

Other treatments that have been used for refractory TTP include splenectomy, cyclophosphamide, cyclosporine, vincristine,[16] bortezomib,[27] mycophenolate,[28] and N-acetylcysteine.[29] Agents under development can block the binding of platelets to VWF and have the potential to arrest microvascular thrombosis despite persistent ADAMTS13 deficiency.[30,31]

Congenital TTP can be treated with plasma infusion alone, typically 15–20 ml/kg for 1–3 days. Some patients have prolonged symptom-free intervals and can be treated on demand. Others require prophylactic plasma infusions of 5–20 mg/kg every 2–3 weeks to maintain a plasma ADAMTS13 level >5%. Inadequately treated patients are at risk for developing chronic renal failure and stroke.[16].

Patients with severe allergic reactions to plasma have been treated successfully with plasma-derived factor VIII/VWF concentrates that contain significant amounts of ADAMTS13 (16).

Pregnancy is a frequent trigger of congenital TTP. If untreated, pregnancies usually end in spontaneous abortion, stillbirth, or premature delivery. Fetal loss and premature birth can be prevented by plasma infusions 10 ml/kg every 2 weeks beginning at 8 weeks' gestation, increasing to weekly in the second trimester. Any sign of thrombotic microangiopathy is an indication to increase the volume or frequency of plasma infusion. Plasma exchange may be necessary to avoid fluid overload.[16,32]

STEC-HUS. Patients with acute bloody diarrhea should be presumed to have STEC infection and admitted to the hospital for management and infection control. If the patient does have STEC infection, intravenous hydration protects against the development of renal failure. Edema is common, and patients should be monitored closely for fluid overload.[9]

Diarrhea improves with a few days, and most patients recover spontaneously, but approximately 15% develop HUS an average of 7 days (range 5–13 days) after the start of diarrhea. Thrombocytopenia and hemolysis develop after bloody diarrhea and generally before renal failure. Most patients require red cell transfusions and hemolysis can persist as HUS resolves. A rising platelet count signals the end of the risk period for HUS.[9]

Extrarenal involvement can be serious. The incidence of neurological symptoms varies from 10% to 65% among outbreaks and is increased for older patients. Cardiac dysfunction occurs in 10% of children and a higher%age of adults. Gastrointestinal complications can include peritonitis, pancreatitis, rectal prolapse, hemorrhagic colitis, necrosis and perforation.[9,33,34]

The risks and benefits of antibiotic use in STEC-HUS may depend on the stage of illness. Case-control studies indicate that antibiotics early in the course of acute diarrheal illness caused mainly by *E. coli* O157:H7 increase the risk of developing HUS.[35] However, retrospective analysis of a 2011 outbreak of *E. coli* O104:H4 infection suggests that treatment with multiple antibiotics *after* the development of HUS reduced the incidence of seizures and death.[33] Better data would be useful.

Antimotility agents and narcotics are associated with an increased risk of HUS and neurological complications. No convincing evidence supports the efficacy of antiplatelet agents, anticoagulants, plasma exchange, glucocorticoids, rituximab, or eculizumab.[9,20,33]

Mortality associated with STEC-HUS is approximately 1–5%. Long-term sequelae include proteinuria, hypertension, and chronic kidney disease in 9–18%. End-stage renal disease occurs in 3%.

aHUS. In the absence of a prior diagnosis of aHUS, empiric plasma exchange 1–2 volumes daily for adults, or 50–100 ml/kg for children, is appropriate[12,20] and can be effective at least transiently except for patients with MCP mutations. The duration and intensity of plasma exchange can be guided by the clinical response of hemolysis and thrombocytopenia.

After excluding STEC, severe ADAMTS13 deficiency, and other causes of thrombotic microangiopathy, plasma exchange should be stopped and eculizumab started at 900 mg intravenously every week for 4 weeks, followed by 1200 mg in week 5 and every other week thereafter.[36] For patients less than 18 years of age, doses are adjusted based on body weight. Supplementary doses are recommended during concomitant plasma exchange or infusion. Additional treatment with glucocorticoids and rituximab should be considered for patients with autoantibodies to FH.[12]

Early use of eculizumab is important because treatment with plasma exchange alone is associated with up to 8% mortality during the first episode of disease and rapid progression to end-stage renal failure in most survivors. Other common sequelae include hypertension, neurological deficits, and cardiac damage.[18,37] In contrast, treatment with eculizumab is associated with normalization of the platelet count, improvement in renal function, and prevention of relapses. In one study, half of patients had a normal platelet count by day 7, and all had a normal platelet count by week 26. Renal injury responded more slowly, but most patients lowered their serum creatinine at least 25% by week 26, and 4 of 5 patients who required hemodialysis were able to discontinue it.[36] These benefits appear to be sustained for the duration of therapy.

For aHUS caused by autoantibodies to FH, eradication of autoantibodies by immunosuppression should permit discontinuation of eculizumab.

The severity of aHUS varies considerably. Some patients have infrequent relapses that respond to plasma exchange alone and normal renal function. However, many patients require treatment with eculizumab indefinitely to prevent recurrence and renal failure.

Patients should be vaccinated against *Neisseria meningitides* if possible at least 2 weeks before receiving eculizumab, but because treatment for aHUS cannot be delayed, patients typically receive prophylactic antibiotics for 2 weeks after vaccination at the time eculizumab is started. Children should also be vaccinated for *S. pneumoniae* and *H. influenza* type b.

Renal transplantation is associated with a high rate of aHUS recurrence that can be treated or prevented with eculizumab. Living related donors are seldom used because the donated kidney may be at risk for aHUS, and some donors have subsequently developed aHUS. Mutations in *MCP* have a relatively favorable prognosis because the grafted kidney typically expresses enough MCP to prevent recurrence. HUS has not recurred after renal transplantation in children with *DGKE* mutations.[12,38]

Secondary thrombotic microangiopathy. The control of secondary thrombotic microangiopathy depends on the successful treatment of the underlying disorder. With the exception of ticlopidine-induced TTP, which responds to plasma exchange, treatment of secondary thrombotic microangiopathy from any cause with plasma exchange, rituximab, or eculizumab is not known to be beneficial.

References

1. Zini G, d'Onofrio G, Briggs C, Erber W, Jou JM, Lee SH, et al. ICSH recommendations for identification, diagnostic value, and quantitation of schistocytes. *Int J Labor Hematol.* 2012; 34(2):107–116.

2. Furlan M, Robles R, Galbusera M, Remuzzi G, Kyrle PA, Brenner B, et al. von Willebrand factor-cleaving protease in thrombotic thrombocytopenic purpura and the hemolytic-uremic syndrome. *N Engl J Med.* 1998; 339 (22):1578–1584.

3. Kremer Hovinga JA, Vesely SK, Terrell DR, Lammle B, George JN. Survival and relapse in patients with thrombotic thrombocytopenic purpura. *Blood.* 2010; 115(8):1500–1511.

4. Coppo P, Bengoufa D, Veyradier A, Wolf M, Bussel A, Millot GA, et al. Severe ADAMTS13 deficiency in adult idiopathic thrombotic microangiopathies defines a subset of patients characterized by various autoimmune manifestations, lower platelet count, and mild renal involvement. *Medicine (Baltimore).* 2004; 83(4):233–244.

5. Terrell DR, Vesely SK, Kremer Hovinga JA, Lammle B, George JN. Different disparities of gender and race among the thrombotic thrombocytopenic purpura and hemolytic-uremic syndromes. *Am J Hematol.* 2010; 85 (11):844–847.

6. Terrell DR, Williams LA, Vesely SK, Lammle B, Hovinga JA, George JN. The incidence of thrombotic thrombocytopenic purpura-hemolytic uremic syndrome: all patients, idiopathic patients, and patients with severe ADAMTS-13 deficiency. *J Thromb Haemost.* 2005; 3 (7):1432–1436.

7. Miller DP, Kaye JA, Shea K, Ziyadeh N, Cali C, Black C, et al. Incidence of thrombotic thrombocytopenic purpura/hemolytic uremic syndrome. *Epidemiology.* 2004; 15(2):208–215.

8. Miyata T, Kokame K, Matsumoto M, Fujimura Y. ADAMTS13 activity and genetic mutations in Japan. *Hamostaseologie.* 2013; 33(2):131–137.

9. Tarr PI, Gordon CA, Chandler WL. Shiga-toxin-producing *Escherichia coli* and haemolytic uraemic syndrome. *Lancet.* 2005; 365(9464):1073–1086.

10. Frank C, Werber D, Cramer JP, Askar M, Faber M, an der Heiden M, et al. Epidemic profile of Shiga-toxin-producing *Escherichia coli* O104:H4 outbreak in Germany. *N Engl J Med.* 2011; 365(19):1771–1780.

11. Lemaire M, Fremeaux-Bacchi V, Schaefer F, Choi M, Tang WH, Le Quintrec M, et al. Recessive mutations in DGKE cause atypical hemolytic-uremic syndrome. *Nat Genet.* 2013; 45(5):531–536.

12. Taylor CM, Machin S, Wigmore SJ, Goodship TH, working party from the Renal Association tBCfSiH, the British

Transplantation S. Clinical practice guidelines for the management of atypical haemolytic uraemic syndrome in the United Kingdom. *Br J Haematol.* 2010; 148(1):37–47.

13. Lotta LA, Garagiola I, Palla R, Cairo A, Peyvandi F. ADAMTS13 mutations and polymorphisms in congenital thrombotic thrombocytopenic purpura. *Hum Mutat.* 2010; 31(1):11–19.

14. Inward CD, Howie AJ, Fitzpatrick MM, Rafaat F, Milford DV, Taylor CM. Renal histopathology in fatal cases of diarrhoea-associated haemolytic uraemic syndrome. British Association for Paediatric Nephrology. *Pediatr Nephrol.* 1997; 11(5):556–559.

15. Taylor CM, Chua C, Howie AJ, Risdon RA, British Association for Paediatric N. Clinico-pathological findings in diarrhoea-negative haemolytic uraemic syndrome. *Pediatr Nephrol.* 2004; 19 (4):419–425.

16. Scully M, Hunt BJ, Benjamin S, Liesner R, Rose P, Peyvandi F, et al. Guidelines on the diagnosis and management of thrombotic thrombocytopenic purpura and other thrombotic microangiopathies. *Br J Haematol.* 2012; 158(3):323–335.

17. Loirat C, Fremeaux-Bacchi V. Atypical hemolytic uremic syndrome. *Orphanet J Rare Dis.* 2011; 6:60.

18. Noris M, Caprioli J, Bresin E, Mossali C, Pianetti G, Gamba S, et al. Relative role of genetic complement abnormalities in sporadic and familial aHUS and their impact on clinical phenotype. *Clin J Am Soc Nephrol.* 2010; 5(10):1844–1859.

19. Rieger M, Mannucci PM, Kremer Hovinga JA, Herzog A, Gerstenbauer G, Konetschny C, et al. ADAMTS13 autoantibodies in patients with thrombotic microangiopathies and other immunomediated diseases. *Blood.* 2005; 106(4):1262–1267.

20. Schwartz J, Winters JL, Padmanabhan A, Balogun RA, Delaney M, Linenberger ML, et al. Guidelines on the use of therapeutic apheresis in clinical practice-evidence-based approach from the Writing Committee of the American Society for Apheresis: the sixth special issue. *J Clin Apher.* 2013; 28(3):145–284.

21. O'Brien KL, Price TH, Howell C, Delaney M. The use of 50% albumin/ plasma replacement fluid in therapeutic plasma exchange for thrombotic thrombocytopenic purpura. *J Clin Apher.* 2013; 28(6):416–421.

22. Zhan H, Streiff MB, King KE, Segal JB. Thrombotic thrombocytopenic purpura at the Johns Hopkins Hospital from 1992 to 2008: clinical outcomes and risk factors for relapse. *Transfusion.* 2010; 50(4):868–874.

23. Westwood JP, Webster H, McGuckin S, McDonald V, Machin SJ, Scully M. Rituximab for thrombotic thrombocytopenic purpura: benefit of early administration during acute episodes and use of prophylaxis to prevent relapse. *J Thromb Haemost.* 2013; 11(3):481–490.

24. Hie M, Gay J, Galicier L, Provot F, Presne C, Poullin P, et al. Preemptive rituximab infusions after remission efficiently prevent relapses in acquired thrombotic thrombocytopenic purpura: experience of the French Thrombotic Microangiopathies Reference Center. *Blood.* 2014; 124(2):204–210.

25. Bharat A, Xie F, Baddley JW, Beukelman T, Chen L, Calabrese L, et al. Incidence and risk factors for progressive multifocal leukoencephalopathy among patients with selected rheumatic diseases. *Arthr Care Res.* 2012; 64(4):612–615.

26. Lunel-Fabiani F, Masson C, Ducancelle A. Systemic diseases and biotherapies: understanding, evaluating, and preventing the risk of hepatitis B reactivation. Joint, bone, spine: revue du rhumatisme. *Joint Bone Spine.* 2014; 81(6):478–484.

27. Shortt J, Oh DH, Opat SS. ADAMTS13 antibody depletion by bortezomib in thrombotic thrombocytopenic purpura. *N Engl J Med.* 2013; 368(1):90–92.

28. Ahmad HN, Thomas-Dewing RR, Hunt BJ. Mycophenolate mofetil in a case of relapsed, refractory thrombotic thrombocytopenic purpura. *Eur J Haematol.* 2007; 78(5):449–452.

29. Li GW, Rambally S, Kamboj J, Reilly S, Moake JL, Udden MM, et al. Treatment of refractory thrombotic thrombocytopenic purpura with N-acetylcysteine: a case report. *Transfusion.* 2014; 54(5):1221–1224.

30. Cataland SR, Peyvandi F, Mannucci PM, Lammle B, Kremer Hovinga JA, Machin SJ, et al. Initial experience from a double-blind, placebo-controlled, clinical outcome study of ARC1779 in patients with thrombotic thrombocytopenic purpura. *Am J Hematol.* 2012; 87(4):430–432.

31. Callewaert F, Roodt J, Ulrichts H, Stohr T, van Rensburg WJ, Lamprecht S, et al. Evaluation of efficacy and safety of the anti-VWF Nanobody ALX-0681 in a preclinical baboon model of acquired thrombotic thrombocytopenic purpura. *Blood.* 2012; 120(17):3603–3610.

32. Scully M, Thomas M, Underwood M, Watson H, Langley K, Camilleri RS, et al. Congenital and acquired thrombotic thrombocytopenic purpura and pregnancy: presentation, management and outcome of subsequent pregnancies. *Blood.* 2014; 124(2):211–219.

33. Menne J, Nitschke M, Stingele R, Abu-Tair M, Beneke J, Bramstedt J, et al. Validation of treatment strategies for enterohaemorrhagic *Escherichia coli* O104:H4 induced haemolytic uraemic syndrome: case-control study. *BMJ.* 2012; 345:e4565.

34. Braune SA, Wichmann D, von Heinz MC, Nierhaus A, Becker H, Meyer TN, et al. Clinical features of critically ill patients with Shiga toxin-induced hemolytic uremic syndrome. *Crit Care Med.* 2013; 41(7):1702–1710.

35. Wong CS, Mooney JC, Brandt JR, Staples AO, Jelacic S, Boster DR, et al. Risk factors for the hemolytic uremic syndrome in children infected with Escherichia coli O157:H7: a multivariable analysis. *Clin Infect Dis.* 2012; 55(1):33–41.

36. Legendre CM, Licht C, Muus P, Greenbaum LA, Babu S, Bedrosian C, et al. Terminal complement inhibitor eculizumab in atypical hemolytic-uremic syndrome. *N Engl J Med.* 2013; 368(23):2169–2181.

37. Fremeaux-Bacchi V, Fakhouri F, Garnier A, Bienaime F, Dragon-Durey MA, Ngo S, et al. Genetics and outcome of atypical hemolytic uremic syndrome: a nationwide French series comparing children and adults. *Clin J Am Soc Nephrol.* 2013; 8(4):554–562.

38. Noris M, Remuzzi G. Managing and preventing atypical hemolytic uremic syndrome recurrence after kidney transplantation. *Curr Opin Nephrol Hypertens.* 2013; 22(6):704–712.

Chapter

17

Extrinsic Nonimmune Hemolytic Anemias

Pavan K. Bendapudi, MD, and Ronald P. McCaffrey, MD

Introduction

Normal red blood cells circulate for 120 days. During that period of time, they are subject to a variety of stresses that can result in a shortened life span. When the life-span of a significant fraction of the circulating red cell mass is shortened, anemia, termed hemolytic anemia, is the outcome.

In this chapter, we will discuss hemolytic destruction of red cells by mechanisms other that immune-mediated damage. Immune-mediated destruction of red cells is covered in a separate chapter. Causes of nonimmune red cell destruction include trauma to the red cell membrane (mechanical red cell fragmentation), exposure to a variety of endogenous and exogenous metabolic and toxic insults, and membrane and metabolic damage from parasitic invasion and bacterial toxins.

A multitude of conditions are associated with extrinsic, nonimmune hemolysis. The recognition of these hemolytic disorders in the spectrum of acquired anemias, the most common of which are discussed here, allows for the rational selection of specific therapy.

Hemolysis Associated with Prosthetic Cardiac Valves

History and Epidemiology

Intravascular hemolysis in the context of prosthetic cardiac valve replacement is a well-described phenomenon. Reports in the 1960s attributed this finding to mechanical intravascular hemolysis resulting from turbulent blood flow around the implanted valve prosthesis.[1,2] In general, replacement of left-sided valves (i.e., mitral and aortic) is associated with higher rates of hemolysis than replacement of right-sided valves. For left-sided valve replacement, no consensus exists as to which position is associated with more hemolysis. At least one study has shown that mitral valve and double-valve prostheses are associated with a greater degree of hemolysis than single-valve and aortic valve prostheses, despite the higher pressures experienced by the aortic valve.[3] Mechanical prosthetic valves carry a higher risk of hemolysis than bioprosthetic valves, in particular ball-and-cage valves and bileaflet valves.[4,5] The reported rates of clinically significant hemolysis have fallen from 5 to 15% in the 1960s–1970s to less than 1% in the

1990s due to improved prosthetic valve design.[6,7] However, subclinical hemolysis continues to occur more commonly.

Pathophysiology

Hemolysis in the setting of cardiac valve replacement is thought to occur as a result of turbulent blood flow through and around the prosthesis, large pressure gradients across the valve, and fragmentation of red blood cells by contact with prosthetic surfaces. The most common mechanism for hemolysis in current prosthesis models is paravalvular leak from a poorly seated valve, which can be minimized with the use of intraoperative transesophageal echocardiography (TEE).[8,9] Late paravalvular leak can be caused by suture dehiscence. In prosthetic valves that have undergone restenosis, a high transvalvular pressure gradient can generate shear forces in excess of the 3000 dynes/cm^2 necessary to cause red cell destruction.[10] One *in vitro* study has also suggested that red cell fragmentation may be more common in patients with a less compliant aortic root, indicating that factors beyond the prosthesis itself may contribute to hemolysis.[11]

Clinical and Laboratory Features

Patients may be asymptomatic or present with pallor, weakness, and signs of congestive heart failure. One report showed higher levels of hemoglobinuria associated with periods of activity, likely due to higher cardiac output during that time.[12] Patients may also have a new or changing murmur. Accompanying laboratory findings include an elevated lactate dehydrogenase (LDH), total and indirect bilirubin and reticulocyte count, a decreased haptoglobin, and hemoglobinuria. Schistocytes are seen on the peripheral blood smear.[13–15]

Treatment

Treatment of hemolytic anemia arising from cardiac valve prosthesis is based on improving erythropoiesis and correcting the underlying valvular structural problem if possible. Reoperation, though usually of higher risk than the primary surgery, is considered the definitive therapy for poorly seated valves or those with paravalvular leak. Percutaneous closure has also been used in this context.[16] From a medical standpoint, iron and folate supplementation has long been employed in this setting to encourage hematopoiesis.[17,18] Erythropoietin has also been reported to defer or obviate the need for additional reoperation in patients who have already undergone repeated heart valve surgeries.[19] Pentoxifylline, a nonselective phosphodiesterase inhibitor used in the management of claudication and alcoholic liver disease, was shown in a small randomized controlled trial to reduce markers of valve-related hemolysis in 60% of patients, compared to 5% in the placebo arm. Patients receiving pentoxifylline at a dose of 400 mg orally three times daily had higher hemoglobin and haptoglobin levels and lower levels of LDH and bilirubin as well as reduced reticulocyte counts. Six patients with severe hemolysis experienced complete remission of their disorder while on pentoxifylline.[20] It is thought that in this setting, pentoxifylline exerts its therapeutic effect by enhancing erythrocyte deformability.

March Hemoglobinuria

March hemoglobinuria refers to mechanical hemolysis resulting from repetitive foot strike or other physical activity. It was first described in 1881 in a German soldier who complained of passing red urine after demanding field marches.[21] Approximately 80 years later, Davidson showed that the pathophysiologic mechanism was mechanical hemolysis due to trauma in the vasculature of the soles of the feet. He encouraged affected athletes to make changes to their strides and wear shoes with padded insoles, which led to resolution of hemolysis with exercise.[22] March hemoglobinuria occurs more commonly in men than in women.[23] Although seen most often with vigorous running or walking, cases have been described following activities as diverse as karate exercises, basketball, and conga drum playing.[24,25] Because it is usually associated with only a small quantity of hemolysis that resolves with the cessation of physical activity, march hemoglobinuria is not usually associated with anemia or morphologic signs of red cell fragmentation and is rarely of clinical significance.

Thermal Injury–Induced Hemolysis

It was initially shown in the 19th century that heating blood above a temperature of approximately 50 degrees centigrade results in the deformation and fragmentation of erythrocytes, eventually leading to the development of spherocytes and other abnormal red cell morphologies.[26] In animal models of thermal injury, plasma-free hemoglobin is significantly increased 1 hour after injury, likely due to direct destruction of red blood cells by heat, and is associated with hemoglobinuria over the first 12–24 hours. Paradoxically, these findings are associated with an increased hematocrit in the early stages of injury due to hemoconcentration.[27,28] Corresponding morphological examination demonstrates marked anisopoikilocytosis, including the formation of acanthocytes, schistocytes, and spherocytes. These cells demonstrate both reduced membrane deformity and increased osmotic fragility, which are thought to lead to hemolysis and clearance of red cells.[29]

Although direct damage from heat is the main cause of hemolysis during the first phase of thermal injury, ongoing red cell destruction in burn patients has been demonstrated. Red cells from normal donors that are transfused into burn victims experience more rapid clearance than expected; this phenomenon is thought to be due to erythrocyte destruction resulting from free radicals elaborated by activated neutrophils in the setting of complement activation and systemic inflammation.[30,31]

Hemolysis Associated with Infectious Parasites

Hemolytic anemia can occur as a result of infection with protozoan parasites of the genera *Plasmodium* (malaria) and *Babesia* (babesiosis) and gram-negative bacilli of the genus *Bartonella*. The complex life cycles of these arthropod-borne organisms are beyond the scope of this chapter, but each involves a direct interaction with host erythrocytes. In the case of malaria, *P. vivax* preferentially parasitizes younger red cells, while *P. falciparum* targets both young and old cells, meaning that patients with *P. falciparum* often have higher burdens of parasitemia and hemolytic anemia.[32,33] Parasitized red cells incur surface membrane defects, including abnormalities in structure and phosphorylation that lead to the clearance of these cells by the spleen.[34] For unclear reasons, unparasitized red blood cells also display a number of internal and membrane abnormalities, including increased osmotic fragility and cation permeability, which likely contribute to their reduced lifespans.[35,36] Together with the red cell fragmentation that occurs when parasite progeny burst from infected erythrocytes, these factors contribute to the hemolytic anemia observed in malaria.

Babesiosis is endemic to the West Coast, the Upper Midwest, and the Northeast. The organism directly invades and destroys red blood cells, causing hemolytic anemia. Individuals at highest risk for poor outcome include those who are elderly, immunocompromised, or asplenic. Agents active against babesiosis include atovaquone, azithromycin, clindamycin, and quinine.[37] In bartonellosis (Oroya fever or Carrión disease), it is thought that the organism does not invade the red cell but rather adheres to the outside of erythrocytes, leading to clearance by the spleen.[38] Additionally, the 130-kD *Bartonella* protein *deformin* causes red cell structural abnormalities, which may also contribute to splenic clearance.[39] Hemolysis is usually of rapid onset and is usually mild to moderate, although cases with profound anemia have also been reported.[40]

Hemolysis Due to Clostridial Sepsis
Clinical Features and Pathophysiology

Massive intravascular hemolysis due to *Clostridium perfringens* or *Clostridium septicum* bacteremia is a rare but well-documented complication of these infections that is associated with a mortality rate of 80% or more.[41] Patients are usually those at risk for anaerobic infection due to abdominal pathology, an immunocompromised state, or the presence of necrotic tissue. Cases present suddenly with a rapid intravascular hemolysis that can lead to death within hours; most patients experience a decline in hematocrit of at least 50%, and at least one case with an undetectable hematocrit has been reported.[42] Traditional markers of intravascular hemolysis tend to be markedly elevated except for the reticulocyte count, which remains normal due to an insufficient time for bone marrow response in most cases; the direct and indirect antiglobin tests are invariably negative.[43,44]

There are two competing pathophysiologic explanations for the hemolysis seen in these cases. First, it has been shown that clostridial species synthesize a neuroaminidase that is capable of removing portions of the glycophorin A and B chains on the surface of erythrocytes, thereby exposing the Thomsen-Friedenreich (T) cryptantigen (a process known as "T antigen activation").[45] It is thought that the uncovered T antigen, normally hidden from the humoral immune system, then provides a target on the erythrocyte surface for naturally occurring anti-T IgM, which subsequently fixes complement and destroys the cell.[46] In support of this concept is the observation that infants who are too young to have generated anti-T isoagglutinins and are infected with *C. perfringens* only develop hemolysis after the infusion of plasma-containing blood products that carry exogenous anti-T.[47]

Alternatively, it has been shown that *C. perfringens* alpha toxin possesses a phospholipiase activity (lysolecithins) and can bind and destroy red cell membranes.[48,49] It has been pointed out in at least two case reports that while serum phospholipase C activity increased significantly during the hemolytic phase of infection, titers of anti-T isoagglutinin and levels of detected T antigen remain low, suggesting that clostridial phospholipase is primarily responsible for hemolysis.[50,51] However, the clinical significance of T antigen or anti-T antibody levels in the setting of rapid hemolysis is not clear, and levels of neuroaminidase activity have never been recorded in this condition.

Treatment

The vast majority of published primary literature concerning the treatment of hemolysis secondary to clostridial infection is derived from case reports. Clinicians should have a low threshold to initiate treatment with high-dose intravenous penicillin and clindamycin if clostridial infection is suspected. Source control should be achieved via surgical intervention if indicated. Whole-blood exchange transfusion and hyperbaric oxygen therapy have been proposed but are of unclear benefit.[52] Supportive treatments for DIC, shock, renal failure, and anemia have proven key in the rare documented cases of survival.[53]

Hemolysis Due to Heavy Metal Exposure

Copper

Exposure to high levels of both copper and lead has been associated with hemolysis. In the case of copper, patients usually have Wilson's disease or present after accidental or intentional ingestion. Patients who have ingested copper-containing solutions experience symptoms of gastrointestinal distress followed approximately 1–2 days later by hemoglobinuria and other signs of intravascular hemolysis.[54] Patients with Wilson's disease may have hepatosplenomegaly, Kayser-Fleischer rings, and other stigmata of this condition.[55] Hemolysis is usually moderate (i.e., 25–50% of red cell mass) but can be more severe. While the mechanism is not completely understood, it has been proposed that copper sulfate leads to enhanced oxidation of NADPH, increasing overall oxidative stress on erythrocytes; patients with underlying G6PD deficiency may therefore be at higher risk for copper-induced hemolysis.[56,57] Copper also inhibits steps in other red cell metabolic pathways, which likely plays a role as well.[58] The copper chelator penicillamine has been used to halt hemolysis by reducing serum copper levels via increased urinary excretion.[59] Plasmapheresis is another maneuver that has been reported to successfully decrease serum copper levels and reduce the pace of hemolysis.[60–62]

Lead

Lead poisoning ("plumbism") was first described in antiquity and in the past was commonplace due to the broad use of lead in the implements of industry and daily life. Today, most cases of lead poisoning are due to occupational exposure or the ingestion of lead-containing paint or other articles. Lead acts broadly to inhibit a range of enzymes by binding sulfhydryl groups and interfering with enzyme function.[63] The inhibition of ALA dehydratase and ferrochelatase, two enzymes in the heme synthesis pathway, leads to the macrocytic anemia commonly associated with plumbism.[64]

Hemolysis is a less frequent but well-described cause of anemia in lead poisoning. It is thought to occur due to obstruction of the pentose phosphate pathway (PPP) in erythrocytes and resultant oxidative stress.[65] Lead has been shown to impair the PPP enzyme pyrimidine 5'-nucleotidase, which leads to accumulation of pyrimidine nucleotides and inhibition of G6PD in both a competitive and noncompetitive fashion.[66] This process in turn leads to increased red cell oxidative stress and hemolysis. In further support of this concept, *in vitro* studies have shown that erythrocytes taken from patients with G6PD deficiency are significantly more sensitive to lead exposure than those from normal controls.[67] Of note, hereditary pyrimidine 5'-nucleotidase deficiency also presents with basophilic stippling of erythrocytes similar to that seen in lead poisoning, leading some to suggest the same mechanism for this characteristic finding in plumbism. Evidence for the treatment of lead-induced hemolytic anemia is limited to level of case reports; however, in at least one instance, treatment with the lead chelator 2,3-dimercaptosuccinic acid (Succimer) was associated with resolution of hemolysis in a patient who experienced lead poisoning from retained shotgun pellets.[68]

Hemolysis Due to Intravenous Immunoglobulin

Intravenous immune globulin (IVIG) is a blood product derived from the fraction of pooled donor plasma that contains high levels of immunoglobulins.[69] Greater than 90% of these products are composed of IgG, with IgM and IgA present in much smaller amounts.[70] Because blood group O is the most common blood type in the general population, IVIG preparations can contain high titers of anti-A, anti-B, or anti-A,B, which are naturally occurring isohemagglutinins generated by group O individuals.[71] Hemolysis occurs when administration of IVIG leads to passive transfer of these isohemagglutinins to a non–group O patient; anti-blood group antibodies from the IVIG then bind recipient red cells, leading to complement-mediated red cell destruction. A common scenario is for a recipient with blood type A1 to encounter anti-A,B IgG in the transfused product, resulting in intravascular hemolysis.[72,73]

Hemolysis in this setting is usually self-limited. An eluate prepared from the recipient's red cells should demonstrate the presence of bound isohemagglutinin. It is thought that performing a "minor crossmatch" between the IVIG product and the recipient's red cells could help prevent this reaction, although the efficacy of this approach is not proven. Likewise, measuring the isohemagglutinin titer of an IVIG product prior to transfusion is of unclear utility.[74] Management of IVIG-induced hemolysis usually involves transfusion of type O blood, which lacks cognate antigens for the offending antibodies.[75]

Hemolysis Due to Hypersplenism or Liver Disease

Liver disease and hypersplenism, two conditions that are often related, can each cause hemolysis. In the spleen, red blood cells must traverse at a relatively slow rate the cords of Billroth, where they are exposed to lymphocytes and macrophages of the reticuloendothelial system. Under normal conditions, aging red cells are detected and removed by splenic macrophages as part of the spleen's so-called "culling function." Discrete abnormalities (i.e., Howell-Jolly bodies or membrane-bound immunoglobulins) may be removed by splenic macrophages without destroying the red cell itself as part of the spleen's "pitting function."[76] This mechanism results in a reduction in red cell surface area-to-volume ratio and the formation of spherocytes.

In the setting of an enlarged spleen, these normal functions can become accentuated and lead to clinical findings of hemolysis. Hemolysis is usually mild to moderate with signs of compensatory bone marrow erythropoiesis and variable severity of anemia. Spherocytes are often detectable. Because an enlarged spleen will sequester leukocytes and platelets from the peripheral circulation, cytopenias in these two lineages may be seen as well. Treatment of hemolysis associated with hypersplenism should be supportive and directed at the underlying cause of the disorder.

Liver disease can lead to hemolysis for a number of reasons, including hypersplenism, metabolic changes, and acquired red cell membrane defects that lead to the formation of spur cells, which are a form of acanthocytes. Spur cells are so named because of their bizarre, spiculated morphology and contain abnormally high levels of free cholesterol.[77] The exact mechanism by which liver disease leads to the accumulation of cholesterol in red cell membranes is not completely understood, but it is thought that impaired cholesterol esterification due to a deficiency of liver-produced lecithin cholesterol acyl transferase (LCAT) is responsible; interestingly, when applied to red cells from healthy donors in vitro, the serum of patients with spur cells can convert normal erythrocytes into spur cells.[78,79] These acanthocytes have impaired red cell deformability and consequently undergo destruction by reticuloendothelial macrophages in the spleen, leading to hemolysis.[80] Metabolic changes involving lipid peroxidation and impairment of pyruvate kinase have also been implicated as a cause of hemolysis in liver disease.[81] More recently, it has been postulated that asialoglycoprotein receptor (ASGP-R) released from damaged hepatocytes in the setting of alcoholic liver disease is capable of binding blood group A1 residues on erythrocytes; this interaction, in conjunction with the binding of anti-ASGP-R autoantibodies that also present in these patients, can lead to red cell agglutination and immune-mediated hemolysis.[82]

For patients with cirrhosis, the presence of acanthocytosis is felt to be a poor prognostic indicator.[83] As is the case in hypersplenism, management of hemolysis associated with liver failure is directed at the underlying cause.

References

1. Rodgers, et al. Hemolytic anemia following prosthetic valve replacement. *Circulation.* 1969; 39:155–161.

2. Eyster E, et al. Chronic intravascular hemolysis after aortic valve replacement. *Circulation.* 1971; 44:657–665.

3. Skoularigis J, et al. Frequency and severity of intravascular hemolysis after left-sided cardiac valve replacement with Medtronic Hall and St. Jude Medical prostheses, and influence of prosthetic type, position, size and number. *Am J Cardiol.* 1993; 71:587–591.

4. Skoularigis J, et al. Frequency and severity of intravascular hemolysis after left-sided cardiac valve replacement with Medtronic Hall and St. Jude Medical prostheses, and influence of prosthetic type, position, size and number. *Am J Cardiol.* 1993; 71:587–591.

5. Chang H, et al. Chronic intravascular hemolysis after valvular surgery. *J. Formos Med Assoc.* 1990; 89:880.

6. Shapira Y, et al. Hemolysis associated with prosthetic heart valves. *Cardiology in Review.* 2009; 17:121–124.

7. Mecozzi G, et al. Intravascular hemolysis in patients with new-generation prosthetic heart valves: a prospective study. *J Thorac Cardiovasc Surg.* 2002; 123:550–556.

8. Shapira Y, et al. Hemolysis associated with prosthetic heart valves. *Cardiol Rev.* 2009; 17:121–124.

9. Demirsoy E, et al. Hemolysis after mitral valve repair: a report of five cases and literature review. *J Heart Valve Dis.* 2008; 17:24–30.

10. Nevaril CG, et al. Erythrocyte damage and destruction induced by shearing stress. *J Lab Clin Med.* 1968; 71:784.

11. Linde T, et al. Aortic root compliance influences hemolysis in mechanical heart valve prostheses: an in-vitro study. *Int J Artif Organs.* 2012; 35: 495–502.

12. Sears DA, et al. Intravascular hemolysis due to intracardiac prosthetic devices: diurnal variations related to activity. *Am J Med.* 1965; 39:341–354.

13. Mecozzi G, et al. Intravascular hemolysis in patients with new-generation prosthetic heart valves: a prospective study. *J Thorac Cardiovasc Surg.* 2002; 123:550–556.

14. Shapira Y, et al. Hemolysis associated with prosthetic heart valves. *Cardiol Rev.* 2009; 17:121–124 .

15. Maraj R, et al. Evaluation of hemolysis in patients with prosthetic heart valves. *Clin Cardiol* 1998; 21:387–392.

16. Shapira Y, et al. Hemolysis associated with prosthetic heart valves. *Cardiol Rev.* 2009; 17:121–124.

17. Rodgers, et al. Hemolytic anemia following prosthetic valve replacement. *Circulation.* 1969; 39:155–161.

18. Shapira Y, et al. Hemolysis associated with prosthetic heart valves. *Cardiol Rev.* 2009; 17:121–124.

19. Shapira Y, et al. Erythropoietin can obviate the need for repeated heart valve replacement in high-risk patients with severe mechanical hemolytic anemia: case reports and literature review. *J Heart Valve Dis.* 2001; 10:431–435.

20. Golbasi I, et al. The effect of pentoxifylline on haemolysis in patients with double cardiac prosthetic valves. *Acta Cardiol.* 2003; 58:379–383.

21. Fleischer R. Uber eine neue Form von Hämoglobinurie beim Menschen. *Klin Wochenschr.* 1881; 18:691.

22. Davidson RJL. Exertional hemoglobinuria: a report on three cases with studies on the haemolytic mechanism. *J Clin Pathol.* 1964; 17:536–540.

23. Gilligan DR, et al. March hemoglobinuria in a woman. *N Engl J Med.* 1950; 243:944–948.

24. Streeton JA. Traumatic haemoglobinuria caused by karate exercises. *Lancet.* 1967; 2(7508): 191–192.

25. Schwartz KA. March hemoglobinuria: report of a case after basketball and congo drum playing. *Ohio State Med J.* 1973; 69:448–49.

26. Ham TH, et al. Studies on the destruction of red blood cells. *Blood.* 1948; 3:373–403.

27. Endoh Y, et al. Causes and time course of acute hemolysis after burn injury in the rat. *J Burn Care Rehab.* 1992; 13:203–209.

28. Ham TH, et al. Studies on the destruction of red blood cells. *Blood.* 1948; 3:373–403.

29. Endoh Y, et al. Causes and time course of acute hemolysis after burn injury in the rat. *J Burn Care Rehab.* 1992; 13:203–209.

30. Loebl EC, et al. The mechanism of erythrocyte destruction in the early post-burn period. *Ann Surg.* 1973; 178:681–686.

31. Hatherill JR, et al. Thermal injury, intravascular hemolysis and toxic oxygen products. *J Clin Invest.* 1986; 78:629–636.

32. Wilson RJM, et al. Invasion and growth of *Plasmodium falciparum* in different types of human erythrocyte. *Bull WHO.* 1977; 55:179–185.

33. Weatherall DJ, et al. Malaria and the red cell. *Hematology(ASH Education Program).* 2002; 35:35–57.

34. Yuthavong Y, et al. The relationship of phosphorylation of membrane proteins with osmotic fragility and filterability of *Plasmodium berghei*-infected mouse erythrocytes. *Biochim Biophys Acta.* 1987; 929:278–287.

35. George JN, et al. Erythrocytic abnormalities in experimental malaria. 1967; 124:1086–1090.

36. Overman RR. Reversible cellular permeability alterations in disease. In vivo studies on sodium, potassium, and chloride concentrations in erythrocytes

of the malarious monkey. 1948; 152:113–121.

37. www.cdc.gov/parasites/babesiosis/ health_professionals/index.html#tx.

38. Ricketts WE. Bartonella bacilliformis anemia (Oroya fever). A study of thirty cases. *Blood.* 1948; 3:1025–1049.

39. Xu YH, et al. Purification of deformin, an extracellular protein synthesized by Bartonella bacilliformis which causes deformation of erythrocyte membranes. *Biochim Biophys Acta.* 1995; 1234:173–183.

40. Reynafarje C, et al. The hemolytic anemia of human bartonellosis. *Blood.* 1961; 17:562–578.

41. Van Bunderen CC, et al. *Clostridium perfringens* septicaemia with massive intravascular haemolysis: a case report and review of the literature. *Neth J Med.* 2010; 68:343–346.

42. Terebelo H, et al. Implication of plasma free hemoglobin in massive clostridial hemolysis. *JAMA.* 1982248:2028–2029.

43. Bätge B, et al. Clostridial sepsis with massive intravascular hemolysis: rapid diagnosis and successful treatment. *Intensive Care Med.* 1992; 18:488–490.

44. Paulino C, et al. *Clostridium perfringens* sepsis with massive intravascular haemolysis: a rare presentation. *J Med Cases.* 2012; 3:207–210.

45. Bätge B, et al. Clostridial sepsis with massive intravascular hemolysis: rapid diagnosis and successful treatment. *Intensive Care Med.* 1992; 18:488–490.

46. Klein RL, et al. T-cryptantigen exposure in neonatal necrotizing enterocolitis. *J. Pediatric Surg.* 1986; 21:1155–1158.

47. Placzek MM, et al. T activation haemolysis and death after blood transfusion. *Arch Dis Child.* 1987; 62:743–744.

48. McPharlane RG, et al. Hemolysis and production of opalescence in serum and lecitho-vitillin by a toxin of *Clostridium welchii. J Pathol Bacteriol.* 1941; 522:99–103.

49. Bennett JM, et al. Spherocytic hemolytic anemia and acute cholecystitis caused by *Clostridium welchii. N Engl J Med.* 1968; 268:1070–1072.

50. Hübel W, et al. Investigation of the pathogenesis of massive hemolysis in a case of *Clostridium perfringens* septicemia. *Ann Hematol.* 1993; 67:145–147.

51. Bätge B, et al. Clostridial sepsis with massive intravascular hemolysis: rapid diagnosis and successful treatment. *Intensive Care Med.* 1992; 18:488–490.

52. Paulino C, et al. *Clostridium Perfringens* sepsis with massive intravascular haemolysis: a rare presentation. *J Med Cases.* 2012; 3:207–210.

53. Bätge B, et al. Clostridial sepsis with massive intravascular hemolysis: rapid diagnosis and successful treatment. *Intensive Care Med.* 1992; 18:488–490.

54. Fairbanks VF, et al. Copper sulfate-induced hemolytic anemia. *Arch Intern Med.* 1967; 120:428–432.

55. Robitaille GA, et al. Hemolytic anemia in Wilson's Disease. *JAMA.* 1977; 237:2402–2403.

56. Valsami S, et al. Acute copper sulphate poisoning: a forgotten cause of severe intravascular haemolysis. *BJH.* 2011; 156:294.

57. Fairbanks VF, et al. Copper sulfate-induced hemolytic anemia. *Arch Intern Med.* 1967; 120:428–432.

58. Boulard M, et al. The effect of copper on red cell enzyme activities. *J Clin Invest.* 1972; 51:459–461.

59. Robitaille GA, et al. Hemolytic anemia in Wilson's Disease. *JAMA.* 1977; 237:2402–2403.

60. Kiss JE, et al. Effective removal of copper by plasma exchange in fulminant Wilson's disease. *Transfusion.* 1998; 38:327–331.

61. Asfaha S, et al. Plasmapheresis for hemolytic crisis and impending acute liver failure in Wilson disease. *J Clin Apher.* 2007; 22:295–298.

62. Matsumura K, et al. Plasma exchange for hemolytic crisis in Wilson disease. *Ann of Int Med.* 1999; 131:866.

63. Vallee BL, et al. Biochemical effects of mercury, cadmium, and lead. *Ann Rev Biochem.* 1972; 41:91–128.

64. Champe PC, Harvey RA, eds. *Biochemistry*, 4th ed. Baltimore: Lippincott Williams and Wilkins; 2008:279.

65. Lachant NA, et al. Inhibition of the pentose phosphate shunt by lead: a potential mechanism of hemolysis in lead poisoning. *Blood.* 1984; 63:518–524.

66. Lachant NA, et al. Inhibition of the pentose phosphate shunt by lead: a potential mechanism of hemolysis in lead poisoning. *Blood.* 1984; 63:518–524.

67. Osband M, et al. The hemolytic effect of lead on glucose-6-phosphate dehydrogenase deficient erythrocytes. *Ped Res.* 1981; 15:583.

68. Aly MH, et al. Hemolytic anemia associated with lead poisoning from shotgun pellets and the response to Succimer treatment. *Am J Hematol.* 1993; 44:280–283.

69. Gelfand EW, et al. Intravenous immune globulin in autoimmune and inflammatory diseases. *NEJM.* 2012; 367:2015–2025.

70. Simon TL, et al. eds. *Rossi's Principles of Transfusion Medicine.* Oxford: Blackwell Publishing, Ltd; 2009:262.

71. Kahwaji J, et al. Acute hemolysis after high-dose intravenous immunoglobulin therapy in highly HLA sensitized patients. *Clin J Am Soc Nephrol.* 2009; 4:1993–1997.

72. Pintova S, et al. IVIG—A hemolytic culprit. *NEJM.* 2012; 367:974–976.

73. Thomas MJ, et al. Hemolysis after high-dose intravenous Ig. *Blood.* 1993; 82:3789.

74. Pintova S, et al. IVIG—A hemolytic culprit. *NEJM.* 2012; 367:974–976.

75. Pintova S, et al. IVIG—A hemolytic culprit. *NEJM.* 2012; 367:974–976.

76. Crosby WH. Normal functions of the spleen relative to red blood cells: a review. *Blood.* 1959; 14:399–408.

77. Cooper RA, et al. An analysis of lipoproteins, bile acids, and red cell membranes associated with target cells and spur cells in patients with liver disease. *J Clin Invest.* 1972; 51:3182.

78. Morse EE. Mechanisms of hemolysis in liver disease. *Ann Clin Lab Sci.* 1990; 20:169–174.

79. Cooper RA. Anemia with spur cells: a red cell defect acquired in serum and modified in the circulation. *J Clin Invest.* 1969; 48:1820–1831.

80. Cooper RA, et al. Role of the spleen in membrane conditioning and hemolysis of spur cells in liver disease. *NEJM.* 1974; 290:1279–1284.

81. Morse EE. Mechanisms of hemolysis in liver disease. *Ann Clin Lab Sci.* 1990; 20:169–174.

82. Hilgard P, et al. Asialoglycoprotein receptor facilitates hemolysis in patients with alcoholic liver cirrhosis. *Hepatology.* 2004; 39:1398–1407.

83. Ricard MP. Spur cell hemolytic anemia of severe liver disease. *Haematologica.* 84:654 1999.

Acquired Aplastic Anemia and Pure Red Cell Aplasia

Daria Babushok, MD, PhD, and Monica Bessler, MD, PhD

Acquired Aplastic Anemia

Acquired aplastic anemia (aAA) is a rare, life-threatening blood disorder, characterized by a failure of the bone marrow to produce sufficient cells to sustain normal blood production. While a variety of inherited defects can impair hematopoiesis and cause congenital bone marrow failure (BMF), aAA is a prototypical syndrome of acquired BMF. Here, we focus on the pathophysiology, diagnosis, and treatment of aAA. Congenital syndromes are discussed in Chapter 20 of this book.

Epidemiology and Etiology

aAA has an incidence of 2.0 per million in the Western countries and a two- to threefold higher incidence in Asia.[1] No consistent gender bias has been identified, with a male-to-female ratio of approximately 1:1. There is a bimodal age distribution, with a peak incidence in patients under 25 years and in the elderly.

Several environmental, infectious, and genetic factors have been linked to aAA (Table 18.1), including toxins such as benzene and pesticides, medications such as chloramphenicol, as well as several geographically restricted risk factors such as exposure to waterfowl in Thailand.[1] A small fraction of patients (2–5% in Western countries and up to 10% in Asia) develop aAA within 6 months after an episode of seronegative hepatitis. Genetically, aAA has been linked to certain human leukocyte antigen (HLA) subtypes (particularly HLA-DR2 and HLA-B*40:02 and HLA-B*14:02),[2–4] polymorphisms in cytokine genes (e.g., interferon-γ), and detoxifying enzymes (e.g., GSTT1).[5]

Pathophysiology

From the original description of aAA by Paul Ehrlich in 1888[6] through the later part of the 20th century, the etiology of aAA remained largely enigmatic, historically attributed to marrow toxicity from environmental exposures. In the late 1960s, reports of failed syngeneic bone marrow engraftment in patients who received marrow infusion without conditioning[7] and, conversely, of recovery of autologous hematopoiesis after failed allografts, attributed to the immunosuppressive conditioning,[8] suggested a possible immune-mediated etiology of aAA (Figure 18.1). Bone marrow of aAA patients produced fewer hematopoietic colonies *in vitro*, which improved with pretreatment of patients' cells with antithymocyte globulin (ATG). Bone marrow of aAA patients suppressed the colony-forming ability of cells from normal donors,[9] and this inhibitory ability was traced to patients' lymphocytes. Cytokine profiling and T cell receptor studies revealed frequent oligoclonal T lymphocyte expansion and increased T-helper 1 response cytokines in aAA patients; regulatory T cells were frequently decreased.[5] Depletion of lymphocytes in aAA patients allowed for hematopoietic recovery.[5] To date, the immunogenic targets in aAA remain unknown.

Table 18.1 Etiologic Factors Associated with Acquired Aplastic Anemia

Etiologic Factors Associated with Acquired Aplastic Anemia
Idiopathic
Environmental Exposures   Benzene, pesticides, solvents, fertilizers
Radiation

Drugs
   Cytotoxic chemotherapy agents (e.g., alkylating agents, antimetabolites)
   Anticonvulsants (e.g., carbamazepine)
   Antibiotics (e.g., chloramphenicol, sulfonamides)
   Antimalarials (e.g., quinacrine)
   Antithyroid drugs (e.g., methimazole)
   Nonsteroidal anti-inflammatory agents
   Metals (e.g., gold)

Infectious and Inflammatory Conditions
   Viral: Epstein-Barr virus (EBV), Human Immunodeficiency Virus (HIV), Parvovirus B19
   Seronegative Hepatitis
   Eosinophilic Fasciitis

Graft-versus-host disease
Pregnancy

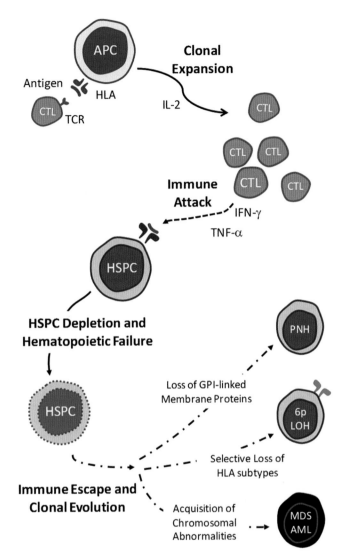

Figure 18.1 Pathophysiology of acquired aplastic anemia.

Clonal hematopoiesis is a frequent finding in aAA and is a product of clonal depletion, immune escape and, less commonly, malignant transformation (Figure 18.1). More than 20% of aAA patients have an expansion of cells lacking glycosylphosphatidylinositol- (GPI-) anchored membrane proteins due to an acquired mutation in the *PIG-A* gene; this phenomenon is called Paroxysmal Nocturnal Hemoglobinuria (PNH).[10] The clonal expansion and long-term persistence of PNH cells is hypothesized to represent "immune escape".[5] More than 10% of aAA patients have clonal expansion of cells with an acquired copy-number neutral loss of heterozygosity (LOH) at chromosome arm 6p, leading to the loss of specific HLA alleles, which may lead to loss of immune recognition.[11] An estimated 10% of aAA patients treated with immunosuppression will develop myelodysplastic syndrome (MDS), and 7% will evolve to acute leukemia; up to 12% of patients without overt transformation may carry cytogenetic abnormalities.[12]

Clinical Presentation

Most aAA patients come to medical attention due to manifestations of cytopenias – easy bruising and bleeding due to thrombocytopenia and fatigue and dyspnea due to anemia. Fevers and infections may be present at diagnosis, although this is less common. Generally, there is no long-standing history of illness. A history of hepatitis is seen in up to 10% of cases. Medication or toxin exposure history may be present, but a causal link is often difficult to establish.

Diagnostic Evaluation and Laboratory Findings

For a patient presenting with new cytopenias, the aim of the diagnostic evaluation is to rapidly screen for a number of treatable and life-threatening diagnoses that can present with low blood counts (Table 18.2). A comprehensive history, physical exam, complete blood count with a differential, peripheral blood smear, reticulocyte count, and a bone marrow aspirate and biopsy will quickly narrow down the possibilities. In patients with pancytopenia and hypoplastic bone marrow concerning for aAA, the evaluation should exclude its common mimickers – inherited BMF, hypoplastic MDS, and transient myelosuppression from an illness or medication. The distinction between inherited BMF and aAA is particularly difficult in young adults, who may have no or only subtle extrahematopoietic manifestations. Routine testing for chromosomal fragility and telomere lengths should be done in younger adults (under 40–50 years) to exclude Fanconi anemia (FA) and dyskeratosis congenita (DC). In the elderly, common mimickers of aAA are hypoplastic myelodysplastic syndrome (MDS) and cytopenias related to medications and comorbidities.

Treatment and Prognosis

For life-threatening cytopenias and infections, supportive measures should be started immediately. Fever in a neutropenic patient should be managed emergently with broad spectrum intravenous antibiotics and a comprehensive evaluation for an underlying etiology, including fungal and opportunistic infections. To limit alloimmunization, overuse of transfusions should be avoided; all blood products should be irradiated and leukoreduced to prevent alloimmunization and transfusion-related graft-versus-host disease (GVHD).

Once the diagnosis of aAA is established, decision to institute definitive therapy is guided by severity of cytopenias (Table 18.3). While active observation may be appropriate for patients with moderate aAA, patients with severe aAA require rapid institution of definitive treatment; referral to a tertiary care center with expertise in aAA is strongly advised. Definitive therapy for aAA aims to restore normal hematopoiesis; current first-line approaches are bone marrow transplantation (BMT) and immunosuppressive therapy (IST) (Figure 18.2).

Table 18.2 Differential Diagnosis and Diagnostic Evaluation of Pancytopenia

	Differential Diagnosis of Pancytopenia	Diagnostic Evaluation

Pancytopenia with Cellular Bone Marrow	Malignancy
	  Myelodysplastic syndrome
	  Lymphomas
	  Acute myeloid leukemia
	  Acute lymphoblastic leukemia
	  Multiple myeloma
	  Metastatic cancer
	  Myeloproliferative neoplasms
	  (myelofibrosis, systemic mastocytosis)
	  Large granular lymphocytic leukemia
		Bone marrow aspirate and biopsy
		Flow cytometry
		Cytogenetics and fluorescence in situ hybridization (FISH)
		Disease-specific testing as needed

	Systemic Inflammatory and Autoimmune Disorders
	  Systemic lupus erythematosus, Still's disease, Sjögren's disease
	  Hemophagocytic lymphohistiocytosis (HLH)
	  Sarcoidosis
		History and physical exam
		Complete metabolic panel
		Inflammatory markers (ESR, CRP) autoimmune serologies
		HLH evaluation incl. liver function tests, ferritin, triglycerides, sIL2-R, NK cell function

	Infections
	  Viral infections (e.g., HIV, CMV, EBV, parvovirus B19)
	  Mycobacterial infections
	  Sepsis
		History and physical exam
		Viral serologies and polymerase chain reaction (PCR)
		Blood and bone marrow cultures
		Acid-fast bacilli (AFB) staining

	Nutritional and Metabolic
	  Vitamin B12, folate, or copper deficiency
	  Alcoholism
		Vitamin B12, folate, copper and ceruloplasmin

Pancytopenia with Hypoplastic Marrow	Acquired Aplastic Anemia Hypoplastic Myelodysplastic Syndrome Graft-versus-Host Disease Hemophagocytic Lymphohistiocytosis	Bone marrow morphology and cytogenetics History, physical exam, chimerism analysis HLH evaluation including liver function tests, ferritin, triglycerides, sIL2-R, NK cell function
	Viral Infections (HIV, CMV, EBV) Large Granular Lymphocytic Leukemia Inherited Bone Marrow Failure Syndromes	Viral serologies and PCR Flow cytometry History, physical exam, family history, and syndrome-specific testing
	Fanconi anemia Dyskeratosis congenita Shwachman-Diamond syndrome Amegakaryocytic thrombocytopenia	Chromosomal breakage studies Peripheral blood lymphocyte telomere lengths Stool fat analysis, *SBDS* gene testing *cMPL* gene testing

Bone Marrow Transplantation (BMT)

In younger aAA patients, matched related donor BMT (MRD-BMT) has excellent outcomes with a 5-year overall survival (OS) of 82% in patients under 20 years and 72% in patients aged 20–40 years.[13] Five-year OS after MRD-BMT in children under 16 years exceeds 90%,[14] making MRD-BMT the preferred first-line approach for children and adults under 40 years old who have a MRD. In older patients, outcomes of BMT are less good, with an estimated 5-year OS of 53% in aAA patients over 40 years of age;[13] thus, in older adults, IST remains the preferred first-line therapy.

The standard BMT conditioning regimen for MRD-BMT for aAA uses cyclophosphamide combined with ATG.[15] Newer regimens incorporating fludarabine have shown promise and may reduce cyclophosphamide-related toxicity.[16] Bone marrow remains the recommended graft source, with superior outcomes compared to peripheral blood stem cells.[17] Rabbit ATG results in lower rates of GVHD than horse ATG, when used as a part of transplant conditioning regimen.[18] Historically, outcomes with matched unrelated donor (MUD)-BMT have been suboptimal; however, with improvements in HLA typing and conditioning regimens, MUD-BMT has become a viable option, particularly in the pediatric setting.[18] Although largely used as second-line therapy for patients refractory to IST, MUD-BMT is increasingly being considered upfront, especially in countries where horse ATG is no longer available. Experience with alternative donor BMT is also growing, with a number of studies showing excellent engraftment with low GVHD rates using haploidentical donor BMT with post-transplant cyclophosphamide (19, 20).

Immunosuppressive Therapy (IST)

IST with horse ATG and cyclosporine A (CsA) remains the standard first-line treatment for adult patients over 40 and in

Table 18.3 Severity Grading of Aplastic Anemia

Moderate (Nonsevere) Aplastic Anemia

Bone marrow cellularity <25% or 25–50% with <30% hematopoietic cells
AND at least TWO of the following:

Neutrophil count	<1.5 ×10⁹/L
Hemoglobin	<10 g/dL
Platelet count	<50×10⁹/L

Severe Aplastic Anemia

Bone marrow cellularity <25% or 25–50% with <30% hematopoietic cells
AND at least TWO of the following:

Neutrophil count	<0.5 ×10⁹/L
Reticulocyte count	<60×10⁹/L
Platelet count	<20×10⁹/L

Very Severe Aplastic Anemia

Bone marrow cellularity <25% or 25–50% with <30% hematopoietic cells
AND Neutrophil count <0.2×10⁹/L
AND at least ONE of the following:

Reticulocyte count	<60×10⁹/L
Platelet count	<20×10⁹/L

younger patients without a MRD. Estimated hematologic response is 65% at 3 months and 70% at 6 months.[21] In a randomized controlled trial, a more lymphodepleting ATG preparation, rabbit ATG (ATGAM) produced inferior hematologic response at 6 months and inferior 3-year overall survival compared to horse ATG (37% versus 68% and 76% versus 96%, respectively).[22] Thus, horse ATG and CsA remain the preferred IST regimen. A brief course of corticosteroids to prevent serum sickness and prophylaxis for *Pneumocystis jiroveci* and invasive fungal infections are advised.[23] Adjunctive granulocyte colony-stimulating factor (G-CSF) does not improve OS or event-free survival; the debate on long-term safety of G-CSF is unresolved.[24] A third of patients relapse if CsA is discontinued at 6 months; prolonged CsA therapy followed by a slow taper can lower relapse rates to 8–16%.[24,25] A promising phase 1–2 study of 92 patients with aplastic anemia used synthetic thrombopoietin-receptor agonist eltrombopag along with the standard IST as an upfront therapy, showing excellent outcomes with complete and overall response rates of up to 58% and 94%, respectively.[26] A large, randomized placebo-controlled trial is underway in Europe, which will help validate these data and will better assess long-term complications, including rates of malignant transformation and relapse.

Second-Line Therapies

Younger patients with refractory disease after the initial IST therapy should be considered for a MUD-BMT. If no MUD is available or if patient is ineligible for transplant, historically, a second course of IST with ATG/CsA or alemtuzumab was attempted with an expected response rate of 30–65%.[24]

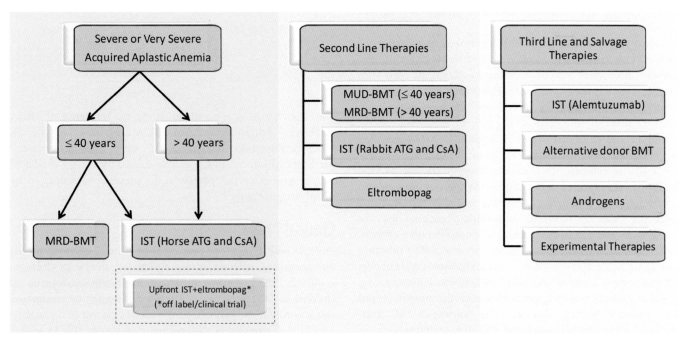

Figure 18.2 Therapeutic approach to acquired aplastic anemia.

Although cyclophosphamide has shown promising activity in aAA, its use has been limited by a significant risk of infectious complications.[5,24] While androgens have ceded way to IST and BMT as the front-line and second-line therapy of aAA in all but the most resource-poor settings, danazol and other androgens can be used as a salvage therapy to achieve a partial response in patients with relapsed or refractory aAA; the improvement is seen primarily in the erythroid lineage (reviewed in [27,28]). More recently, eltrombopag has been added to the standard armamentarium for refractory disease. Hematologic response was achieved in 11 of 25 patients, with 6 patients responding in all three blood lineages and 3 patients recovering bone marrow cellularity after 8 months.[29] A follow-up study of 43 patients with refractory aAA showed a 40% overall response rate at 3–4 months of eltrombopag therapy; however, 8 of the 43 patients developed new chromosomal abnormalities during the study follow-up.[30]

Pure Red Cell Aplasia

Pure red cell aplasia (PRCA) is a rare, heterogeneous group of disorders characterized by severe normochromic and normocytic hypoproliferative anemia, reticulocytopenia, and an absence of erythroblasts in an otherwise normal bone marrow. PRCA can be congenital and acquired. Here, we focus on the pathophysiology, diagnosis, and treatment of acquired PRCA. The congenital form, Diamond Blackfan anemia, is one of the inherited BMF syndromes described in Chapter 20.

Epidemiology, Etiology, and Pathogenesis

Acquired PRCA can be primary or idiopathic or can be caused by several processes that disrupt erythropoiesis, such as infectious, autoimmune, or malignant processes (Table 18.4). PRCA can present at any age and both genders are affected equally.

Most frequently, acquired PRCA is linked to an abnormal expansion of lymphocytes that are cytotoxic to erythroid precursors. Abnormal lymphocytes can be clonal, as seen with large granular lymphocyte (LGL) leukemia and other lymphoproliferative disorders, or polyclonal, as seen with autoimmune diseases, infections, or thymoma.[31]

Other classic causes of PRCA include a parvovirus B19 infection, antibody-mediated PRCA, and medications. Parvovirus B19 is cytotoxic to erythroid progenitors due to viral binding to the erythrocyte P antigen.[32] While an immunocompetent host can mount a neutralizing antibody response and clear the infection, immunocompromised patients may be persistently viremic with a chronic hypoproliferative anemia. In patients with hemolytic anemias, parvovirus B19 infection can cause acute aplastic crises. Anti-erythropoietin antibody, another classic cause of secondary PRCA, was initially recognized in patients receiving recombinant erythropoietin (rEpo) for chronic kidney disease. The incidence of anti-erythropoietin antibody-mediated PRCA rose dramatically in 2001 and 2002 due to the use of a specific formulation of rEpo;

Table 18.4 Etiology and Diagnostic Evaluation of Acquired Pure Red Cell Aplasia

Etiologic Factors Associated with Acquired PRCA	Diagnostic Evaluation
Primary PRCA	
Autoimmune, Idiopathic	Bone marrow aspirate and biopsy
Secondary PRCA	
Infectious	Viral serologies and PCR
Parvovirus B19	
Other (viral hepatitis, EBV, CMV, HTLV-1, HIV)	
Drug-associated	History
Thymoma	History, chest computed tomography (CT) or magnetic resonance imaging (MRI)
Autoimmune	History, physical exam, autoimmune serologies
Collagen vascular disorders	
Other autoimmune	
Antibody-mediated	History, antibody testing (anti-ABO or anti-erythropoietin)
Post ABO-incompatible BMT	
Anti-erythropoietin antibodies	
Malignancy-Associated	Bone marrow aspirate and biopsy, cytogenetics, flow cytometry, T-cell receptor rearrangement. Additional disease-specific studies as necessary.
Lymphoproliferative disorders	
Myelodysplastic syndrome	
Myeloproliferative disorders	
Plasma cell dyscrasias	
Solid tumors	
Severe nutritional deficiencies	Vitamin B12, folate, copper, and ceruloplasmin
Severe renal failure	History, kidney function tests
Pregnancy	History, urine pregnancy test

after the change in rEpo formulation, the incidence of PRCA declined.[33] Antibody-mediated PRCA can also occur after an ABO-incompatible hematopoietic stem cell transplant.[34] Medication-induced PRCA can be caused by an IgG-mediated suppression of erythropoiesis in the presence of a drug or by direct drug toxicity.[31]

Clinical Presentation

Patients with PRCA can present with either a chronic, insidious anemia or with an acute, self-limited illness. In children, acquired PRCA, known as transient erythroblastopenia of childhood, is frequently self-limited. Congenital anomalies and a family history of cytopenias are suggestive of a congenital PRCA (Diamond Blackfan anemia, Chapter 20). In adults, PRCA presents predominantly as a chronic anemia, with symptoms of pallor, fatigue, and dyspnea on exertion; transient PRCA may escape diagnosis due to the long lifespan of red blood cells. In patients with secondary PRCA, clinical features of the associated disease can be present.

Diagnostic Evaluation and Laboratory Findings

In a patient with a hypoproliferative anemia, the diagnosis of PRCA is established by a bone marrow biopsy showing an absence of erythroblasts in an otherwise normal marrow. Further evaluation with a history, physical exam, and laboratory studies should be targeted at possible secondary causes, including medication exposures, infections, malignancies, and autoimmune disorders (Table 18.3). In addition to a comprehensive metabolic panel with liver and renal function tests, specialized laboratory testing may include viral serologies or polymerase chain reaction (PCR), peripheral blood flow cytometry, and T cell receptor rearrangement to look for clonal lymphoproliferative disorders, bone marrow cytogenetics, autoimmune serologies, and imaging to look for thymoma and lymphoproliferative disorders. Careful morphologic and immunophenotypic assessment for large granular lymphocytes is essential, as the diagnosis of large granulocytic leukemia (LGL) can be difficult, especially in patients without an overt lymphocytosis.[31]

Treatment and Prognosis

Therapeutic approach to PRCA includes treatment of the underlying cause in patients with secondary PRCA and immunosuppression for patients with primary PRCA (Figure 18.3). Supportive transfusions are frequently needed, and patients with chronic transfusion requirements and

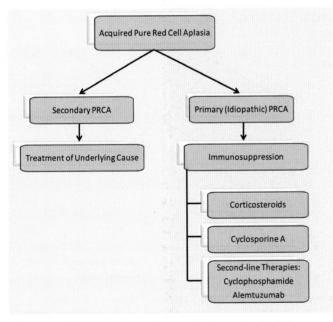

Figure 18.3 Therapeutic approach to acquired pure red cell aplasia

adequate renal function should be considered for iron chelation.

Secondary PRCA

The therapeutic approach in secondary PRCA is aimed at the underlying etiology. All potentially offending medications should be discontinued, nutritional deficiencies corrected, and infections treated. Malignancies should be treated with appropriate therapy. In immunocompromised patients with a persistent parvovirus B19 viremia, intravenous immunoglobulin can be effective at clearing the infection and restoring erythropoiesis.[35] In patients with thymoma-associated PRCA, thymectomy was historically recommended as a first-line therapy, with an expected recovery in 25–30% of patients.[36] More recent data bring into question the role of thymectomy, as PRCA can develop after a thymectomy, and thymectomy alone is frequently insufficient to restore hematopoiesis.[36] In patients with anti-erythropoietin antibodies due to the rEpo administration, further rEpo should be discontinued; peptide-based erythropoietin receptor agonist has shown promise at achieving transfusion independence, but further studies are needed to confirm efficacy and long-term safety.[37]

Primary PRCA

Because 10–12% of cases of primary or idiopathic PRCA run a self-limited course, primary PRCA should be managed supportively for at least 1 month after the diagnosis.[36] Patients with persistent idiopathic PRCA, as well as patients with secondary PRCA who fail to recover despite appropriate treatment of the underlying cause, should be started on immunosuppression, with antimicrobial prophylaxis as appropriate.

In the absence of randomized trials comparing immunosuppressive regimens, corticosteroids have been historically favored in the first-line setting. In the largest published series, 10 of 27 patients treated with corticosteroids achieved a remission with a median time to response of 2.5 weeks (range 1–4 weeks).[38] The majority relapsed upon a corticosteroid taper, and only 11% remained in remission at 5 years.[38] Standard therapy is prednisone at 1mg/kg/day with weekly monitoring of reticulocyte count and hematocrit, followed by a slow taper once hematocrit reaches 35%. Because most remissions occur within 4 weeks of therapy, prolonged corticosteroid treatment in the absence of response is not recommended.

CsA is an alternative to corticosteroids in the first-line setting. In a retrospective analysis from the Japan PRCA Collaborative Study Group,[39] 10 of 31 (32%) patients treated with CsA achieved a complete response and 13 of 31 (42%) a partial response. The initial dose of CsA was 4.8 mg/kg. Relapse-free survival was significantly better with CsA than with corticosteroids (82 months versus 9 months) and was related to the timing of CsA discontinuation. Patients who remained on CsA maintenance relapsed less frequently: 11% versus 86% in patients who discontinued CsA.[39]

Cyclophosphamide was evaluated in multiple small case series[36] and has an estimated overall response rate of 40–60%, with a median time to respond of 12 weeks; higher response and longer response duration can be achieved by combining cyclophosphamide with corticosteroids. In practice, cyclophosphamide has often been reserved for second-line therapy because of the long-term risks of malignancy and gonadal toxicity.

Several other immunosuppressive agents have been used for PRCA including alemtuzumab and ATG; however, published experience with these agents is limited to small case series.[36] In the largest study using alemtuzumab for PRCA, 13 patients were treated with alemtuzumab and CsA with an overall response rate of 84% at 1–4 months, and the majority of patients relapsed; additional studies are needed to confirm the long-term efficacy and safety of this regimen.[40]

Acknowledgments

We thank all patients for participating in studies of bone marrow failure at the Children's Hospital of Philadelphia and the Hospital of the University of Pennsylvania. We thank Dr. Michele E. Paessler for providing the photomicrograph in Figure 18.4A. This work is supported by NHLBI K08 HL132101 to D.B. and the NCI NIH R01 CA105312 and NIDDK DK084188 to M.B.

A 40-year-old previously healthy male presented with petechiae, ecchymoses, and gum bleeding. A complete blood count revealed pancytopenia, with a white blood cell count of 2.1 thousand/μL, neutrophil count of 320 cells/μL, hemoglobin of 11.5 g/dL with 0.2% reticulocytes, and platelets of 3 thousand/μL. A peripheral blood smear confirmed rare neutrophils and severe thrombocytopenia but was otherwise unremarkable. There was no history of recent illnesses. He was not on any medications. Family history was unrevealing. His physical exam was remarkable for scattered petechiae and ecchymoses. A bone marrow biopsy revealed a markedly hypocellular marrow (<5%), with virtual absence of normal trilineage hematopoiesis, consistent with aplastic anemia (Figure 18.4A; photomicrograph of a patient with AA courtesy of Dr. Michele Paessler). Viral serologies and nutritional markers were unremarkable. A presumed diagnosis of acquired aplastic anemia was made. Due to his young age, telomere lengths were sent on peripheral blood lymphocytes and were within normal distribution, thus not suggestive of dyskeratosis congenita. Chromosome breakage studies were normal. At the age of 40, both a MSD-BMT and IST would be an acceptable first-line treatment option, but the patient did not have a matched sibling donor. Immunosuppressive therapy with horse ATG and CsA was started within 3 weeks of initial diagnosis. His treatment course (Figure 18.4B) was complicated by multiple life-threatening infections. He became transfusion independent 6 months after IST, and at 12 months after IST had a complete hematologic response. At 21 months after therapy, he is well and remains on a slow taper of CsA.

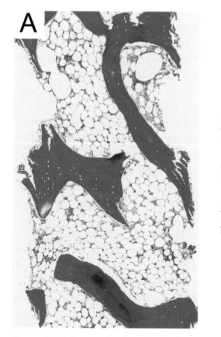

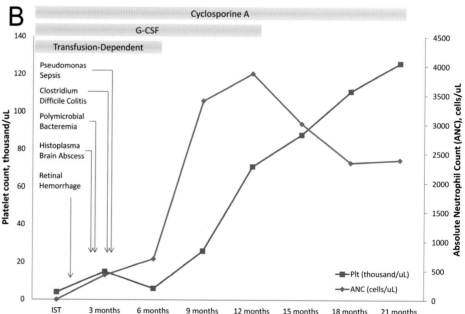

Figure 18.4 Case study of acquired aplastic anemia

References

1. Young NS, Kaufman DW. The epidemiology of acquired aplastic anemia. *Haematologica*. 2008; 93 (4):489–492.

2. Zaimoku Y, Takamatsu H, Hosomichi K, Ozawa T, Nakagawa N, Imi T, et al. Identification of an HLA class I allele closely involved in the autoantigen presentation in acquired aplastic anemia. *Blood*. 2017; 129 (21):2908–2916.

3. Babushok DV, Duke JL, Xie HM, Stanley N, Atienza J, Perdigones N, et al. Somatic HLA mutations expose the role of class I-mediated autoimmunity in aplastic anemia and its clonal complications. *Blood Adv*. 2017; 1:1900–1910.

4. Nakao S, Takamatsu H, Chuhjo T, Ueda M, Shiobara S, Matsuda T, et al. Identification of a specific HLA class II haplotype strongly associated with susceptibility to cyclosporine-dependent aplastic anemia. *Blood*. 1994; 84(12):4257–4261.

5. Young NS, Calado RT, Scheinberg P. Current concepts in the pathophysiology and treatment of aplastic anemia. *Blood*. 2006; 108 (8):2509–2519.

6. Ehrlich P. Uber einen Fall von Anamie mit Bemerkungen uber regenerative Veranderungen des Knochenmarks. *Charite-Annalen*. 1888; 13:300.

7. Pegg DE, Fleming WJ, Compston N. A case of aplastic anaemia treated by isologous bone marrow infusion. *Postgrad Med J*. 1964; 40:213–216.

8. Thomas ED, Storb R, Giblett ER, Longpre B, Weiden PL, Fefer A, et al. Recovery from aplastic anemia following attempted marrow transplantation. *Exp Hematol*. 1976; 4 (2):97–102.

9. Ascensao J, Pahwa R, Kagan W, Hansen J, Moore M, Good R. Aplastic anaemia: evidence for an immunological mechanism. *Lancet*. 1976; 1 (7961):669–671.

10. Dunn DE, Tanawattanacharoen P, Boccuni P, Nagakura S, Green SW, Kirby MR, et al. Paroxysmal nocturnal hemoglobinuria cells in patients with bone marrow failure syndromes. *Ann Intern Med*. 1999; 131(6):401–408.

11. Katagiri T, Sato-Otsubo A, Kashiwase K, Morishima S, Sato Y, Mori Y, et al. Frequent loss of HLA alleles associated with copy number-neutral 6pLOH in acquired aplastic anemia. *Blood*. 2011; 118(25):6601–9660.

12. Socie G, Rosenfeld S, Frickhofen N, Gluckman E, Tichelli A. Late clonal diseases of treated aplastic anemia. *Semin Hematol*. 2000; 37(1):91–101.

13. Gupta V, Eapen M, Brazauskas R, Carreras J, Aljurf M, Gale RP, et al. Impact of age on outcomes after bone marrow transplantation for acquired aplastic anemia using HLA-matched sibling donors. *Haematologica*. 2010; 95 (12):2119–2125.

14. Locasciulli A, Oneto R, Bacigalupo A, Socie G, Korthof E, Bekassy A, et al. Outcome of patients with acquired aplastic anemia given first line bone marrow transplantation or immunosuppressive treatment in the last decade: a report from the European Group for Blood and Marrow Transplantation (EBMT). *Haematologica*. 2007; 92(1):11–18.

15. Storb R, Etzioni R, Anasetti C, Appelbaum FR, Buckner CD, Bensinger W, et al. Cyclophosphamide combined with antithymocyte globulin in preparation for allogeneic marrow transplants in patients with aplastic anemia. *Blood*. 1994; 84 (3):941–949.

16. Maury S, Bacigalupo A, Anderlini P, Aljurf M, Marsh J, Socie G, et al. Improved outcome of patients older than 30 years receiving HLA-identical sibling hematopoietic stem cell transplantation for severe acquired aplastic anemia using fludarabine-based conditioning: a comparison with conventional conditioning regimen. *Haematologica*. 2009; 94 (9):1312–1315.

17. Bacigalupo A, Socie G, Schrezenmeier H, Tichelli A, Locasciulli A, Fuehrer M, et al. Bone marrow versus peripheral blood as the stem cell source for sibling transplants in acquired aplastic anemia: survival advantage for bone marrow in all age groups. *Haematologica*. 2012; 97 (8):1142–1148.

18. Bacigalupo A, Marsh JC. Unrelated donor search and unrelated donor transplantation in the adult aplastic anaemia patient aged 18–40 years without an HLA-identical sibling and failing immunosuppression. *Bone Marrow Transplant*. 2013; 48 (2):198–200.

19. DeZern AE, Zahurak M, Symons H, Cooke K, Jones RJ, Brodsky RA. Alternative donor transplantation with high-dose post-transplantation cyclophosphamide for refractory severe aplastic anemia. *Biol Blood Marrow Transplant*. 2017; 23(3):498–504.

20. Esteves I, Bonfim C, Pasquini R, Funke V, Pereira NF, Rocha V, et al. Haploidentical BMT and post-transplant Cy for severe aplastic anemia: a multicenter retrospective study. *Bone Marrow Transplant*. 2015; 50(5):685–689.

21. Frickhofen N, Kaltwasser JP, Schrezenmeier H, Raghavachar A, Vogt HG, Herrmann F, et al. Treatment of aplastic anemia with antilymphocyte globulin and methylprednisolone with or without cyclosporine. The German Aplastic Anemia Study Group. *N Engl J Med*. 1991; 324(19):1297–1304.

22. Scheinberg P, Nunez O, Weinstein B, Biancotto A, Wu CO, Young NS. Horse versus rabbit antithymocyte globulin in acquired aplastic anemia. *N Engl J Med*. 2011; 365(5):430–438.

23. Hochsmann B, Moicean A, Risitano A, Ljungman P, Schrezenmeier H. Supportive care in severe and very severe aplastic anemia. *Bone Marrow Transplant*. 2013; 48(2):168–73.

24. Young NS, Bacigalupo A, Marsh JC. Aplastic anemia: pathophysiology and treatment. *Biol Blood Marrow Transplant*. 2010; 16(1 Suppl): S119–125.

25. Saracco P, Quarello P, Iori AP, Zecca M, Longoni D, Svahn J, et al. Cyclosporin A response and dependence in children with acquired aplastic anaemia: a multicentre retrospective study with long-term observation follow-up. *Br J Haematol*. 2008; 140(2):197–205.

26. Townsley DM, Scheinberg P, Winkler T, Desmond R, Dumitriu B, Rios O, et al. Eltrombopag added to standard immunosuppression for aplastic anemia. *N Engl J Med*. 2017; 376 (16):1540–1550.

27. Fureder W, Valent P. Treatment of refractory or relapsed acquired aplastic anemia: review of established and experimental approaches. *Leuk Lymphoma*. 2011; 52(8):1435–1445.

28. Shahani S, Braga-Basaria M, Maggio M, Basaria S. Androgens and erythropoiesis: past and present.

J Endocrinol Invest. 2009; 32 (8):704–716.

29. Olnes MJ, Scheinberg P, Calvo KR, Desmond R, Tang Y, Dumitriu B, et al. Eltrombopag and improved hematopoiesis in refractory aplastic anemia. *N Engl J Med.* 2012; 367 (1):11–19.

30. Desmond R, Townsley DM, Dumitriu B, Olnes MJ, Scheinberg P, Bevans M, et al. Eltrombopag restores trilineage hematopoiesis in refractory severe aplastic anemia that can be sustained on discontinuation of drug. *Blood.* 2014; 123(12):1818–1825.

31. Sawada K, Hirokawa M, Fujishima N. Diagnosis and management of acquired pure red cell aplasia. *Hematol Oncol Clin North Am.* 2009; 23(2):249–259.

32. Brown KE, Anderson SM, Young NS. Erythrocyte P antigen: cellular receptor for B19 parvovirus. *Science.* 1993; 262 (5130):114–117.

33. Macdougall IC. Antibody-mediated pure red cell aplasia (PRCA): epidemiology, immunogenicity and risks. *Nephrol Dial Transplant.* 2005; 20 Suppl 4:iv9–15.

34. Bolan CD, Leitman SF, Griffith LM, Wesley RA, Procter JL, Stroncek DF, et al. Delayed donor red cell chimerism and pure red cell aplasia following major ABO-incompatible nonmyeloablative hematopoietic stem cell transplantation. *Blood.* 2001; 98 (6):1687–1694.

35. Kurtzman G, Frickhofen N, Kimball J, Jenkins DW, Nienhuis AW, Young NS. Pure red-cell aplasia of 10 years' duration due to persistent parvovirus B19 infection and its cure with immunoglobulin therapy. *N Engl J Med.* 1989; 321(8):519–523.

36. Sawada K, Fujishima N, Hirokawa M. Acquired pure red cell aplasia: updated review of treatment. *Br J Haematol.* 2008; 142(4):505–514.

37. Macdougall IC, Rossert J, Casadevall N, Stead RB, Duliege AM, Froissart M, et al. A peptide-based erythropoietin-receptor agonist for pure red-cell aplasia. *N Engl J Med.* 2009; 361 (19):1848–1855.

38. Clark DA, Dessypris EN, Krantz SB. Studies on pure red cell aplasia. XI. Results of immunosuppressive treatment of 37 patients. *Blood.* 1984; 63 (2):277–286.

39. Sawada K, Hirokawa M, Fujishima N, Teramura M, Bessho M, Dan K, et al. Long-term outcome of patients with acquired primary idiopathic pure red cell aplasia receiving cyclosporine A. A nationwide cohort study in Japan for the PRCA Collaborative Study Group. *Haematologica.* 2007; 92 (8):1021–1028.

40. Risitano AM, Selleri C, Serio B, Torelli GF, Kulagin A, Maury S, et al. Alemtuzumab is safe and effective as immunosuppressive treatment for aplastic anaemia and single-lineage marrow failure: a pilot study and a survey from the EBMT WPSAA. *Br J Haematol.* 2010; 148(5):791–796.

Paroxysmal Nocturnal Hemoglobinuria

Robert A. Brodsky, MD

Etiology/Epidemiology

Paroxysmal nocturnal hemoglobinuria (PNH) is a rare hematopoietic stem cell disorder that manifests with hemolytic anemia, bone marrow failure, and thrombophilia.[1–4] The median age of onset is roughly 40 years; onset before age 18 years may occur but is very rare. The disease is caused by clonal expansion of a multipotent hematopoietic stem cell that harbors a somatic mutation on the X-chromosome phosphatidylinositol glycan complementation class A gene (*PIGA*)(5, 6). The *PIGA* gene product is one of more than 20 genes involved in the synthesis of glycosylphosphatidylinositol (GPI) anchors. Theoretically, any gene defect in this pathway could lead to PNH, but since all the genes in this pathway except *PIGA* reside on autosomes, virtually all cases of PNH are due to *PIGA* mutations. Varying degrees of immune-mediated bone marrow failure may underlie PNH. Indeed, many PNH patients evolve out of acquired aplastic anemia.[7] Up to 70% of patients with acquired aplastic anemia have evidence of small PNH clones at diagnosis, which serves as further evidence of the pathophysiologic link between aplastic anemia and PNH.[8] These data suggest that autoimmune attack that is associated with acquired forms of aplastic anemia leads to a conditional survival advantage to the PNH stem cell over normal stems and accounts for the clonal expansion in PNH.[9]

Pathophysiology

GPI is a glycolipid moiety that anchors scores or different proteins to the cell surface (Figure 19.1). There are more than a dozen GPI anchored proteins (GPI-AP) on human blood cells. CD59 and CD55 are GPI-APs that serve as important regulators of the complement cascade. Their absence on the surface of PNH cells explains most of the clinical manifestations of PNH. Hemolytic anemia in PNH results from the increased susceptibility of PNH erythrocytes to complement. CD59 and CD55 act at different levels of the complement cascade. CD55 blocks C3 convertases, and CD59 blocks the addition of C9 into the terminal membrane attack complex.[10,11] Thus, the absence of CD55 and CD59 on PNH red cells allows C3 and C5 convertases to proceed unchecked and ultimately leads to increased deposition of membrane attack complexes on the red cell membrane. This results in lysis of the red cell and release of free hemoglobin and other cell contents (e.g., lactate dehydrogenase [LDH]) into the intravascular space.[12]

Thrombosis is the leading cause of mortality from PNH and leads to more than a 60-fold increase in risk for thromboembolism, making PNH more of a thrombophilic risk factor than other known hypercoagulable states such as factor V Leiden deficiency or deficiencies of antithrombin, protein C, or protein S. The mechanisms for thrombophilia in PNH are multifactorial, but increased elaboration of C5a through unchecked complement activation, nitric oxide scavenging from the elaboration of free hemoglobin, and an increase in platelet-derived microparticles all seem to contribute.

Diagnostic Evaluation/Laboratory Findings

Patients with a Coombs negative hemolytic anemia, aplastic anemia, unexplained pancytopenia, and unexplained thrombosis in conjunction with cytopenias or hemolysis should be screened for PNH. Peripheral blood flow cytometry is the most sensitive and specific method to diagnose PNH.[13,14] Flow cytometry should be performed using a panel of monoclonal antibodies directed against GPI-AP and FLAER (a fluorescent proaerolysin variant that binds the GPI anchor).[15,16] A good flow cytometry report should determine the percentage of GPI-AP–deficient (PNH) granulocytes, monocytes, and red

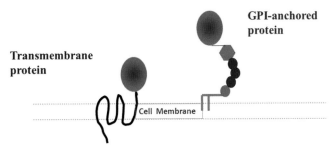

Figure 19.1 Schematic Structure of the GPI Anchor. In contrast to transmembrane proteins (left), GPI-anchored proteins do not traverse the lipid bilayer. The GPI anchor, comprised of phosphatidylinositol (grey), N-glucosamine (green), 3 mannoses (blue), and phosphoethanolamine (red), anchors the protein (light blue) to the cell membrane.

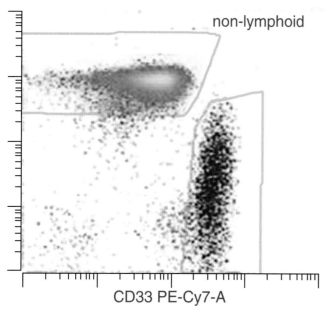

Figure 19.2 Multiparameter Flow Cytometry Analysis of Peripheral Blood in PNH. (A–D) Aplastic anemia patient with small (2%) PNH clone; (E–H) classic PNH patient. (A, E) Forward scatter (FSC)/side scatter (SSC) display showing initial gate to exclude lymphocytes and debris. (B, F) Granulocytes (green) are identified as bright CD15 and low CD33, whereas monocytes (blue) are bright CD33 and low CD15. (C, G) Population of GPI anchor protein–deficient granulocytes showing lack of staining with both anti-CD24 and FLAER. (D, H) Population of GPI anchor protein–deficient monocytes showing lack of staining with both anti-CD14 and FLAER. (Reproduced with permission from Brodsky, *Blood*, 2009; 113.)

cells (Figure 19.2). In addition, red cell phenotyping should report on the percentage of type III cells (absent GPI-APs), type II cells (decreased GPI-APs), and type I cells (normal GPI-APs). Solely screening red cells for PNH can lead to falsely negative tests, especially in the setting of a recent hemolytic episode or a recent blood transfusion. Since granulocytes and monocytes have a short half-life and are not affected by blood transfusions, the percentage of PNH cells in these lineages best reflects the size of the PNH clone.

What Percentage of PNH Cells Is Relevant?

PIG-A mutant blood cells are readily detected in the blood and bone marrow of healthy control subjects at a frequency of roughly 1 in 50,000 (0.002%);[17,18] thus, a PNH clone of <0.01% should be viewed as negative. Meticulous molecular and statistical analysis reveals that unlike *PIG-A* mutations in PNH, *PIG-A* mutations in healthy controls arise from colony-forming cells and not multipotent hematopoietic stem cells.[18] However, expanded populations of PNH cells can be detected in most patients with acquired aplastic anemia, and some patients with myelodysplastic syndromes. Similar to PNH patients the GPI-AP deficient cells in aplastic anemia are clonal and arise from multipotent hematopoietic stem cells; in contrast, the PNH-like cells in MDS patients are usually not relevant in that they are often transient and appear to

arise from colony-forming cells.[19] This explains why PNH so often arises from aplastic anemia but seldom arises from MDS.

PNH patients may be classified as either "classical" or "hypoplastic." This can usually be accomplished by ordering a complete blood count, reticulocyte count, LDH, peripheral blood flow cytometry for PNH, and a bone marrow aspirate, biopsy, and cytogenetics. Patients with classical PNH tend to have mild to moderate cytopenias, a normocellular to hypercellular bone marrow, an elevated reticulocyte count, a markedly elevated LDH, and a relatively large PNH granulocyte population (>30%). Hypoplastic PNH patients, also referred to as "subclinical PNH" or "PNH with underlying bone marrow failure," present with manifestations similar to that of aplastic anemia. These patients typically present with moderate to severe cytopenias, a hypocellular bone marrow (<25% cellularity), a decreased corrected reticulocyte count, a normal or mildly elevated LDH, and a relatively small (<20%) PNH granulocyte population. Most but not all patients can be readily subdivided into classical versus hypoplastic PNH, a distinction that aids with therapeutic decisions; however, patients may evolve over time from hypoplastic to classical PNH.[20]

Clinical Presentation

Hemolysis is often the most conspicuous feature in patients with classical PNH. Many patients, particularly those with coexisting bone marrow failure ("hypoplastic"), exhibit mild to barely detectable hemolysis. The hemoglobin concentration may be normal to severely depressed. The reticulocyte count is often elevated but usually lower than expected for the degree of anemia. Patients with PNH manifest all the usual clinical and laboratory signs of chronic hemolytic anemia: weakness, fatigue, pallor, and dyspnea on exertion. In patients with prominent hemolysis, the magnitude of fatigue may be out of proportion to the degree of anemia. Morphology of the red cells is usually normal, with slight macrocytosis. The haptoglobin levels are usually low, and the LDH is frequently elevated, sometimes greater than 3,000 IU/L, depending on the degree of intravascular hemolysis.

Multiple factors influence the degree of hemolysis in PNH, including the size and type of the PNH clone and the degree of complement activation. In general, the percentage of PNH erythrocytes correlates with the degree of hemolysis. However, the type of PNH erythrocytes may also influence the degree of hemolysis. Type III erythrocytes are more readily lysed than type II erythrocytes and almost always constitute a larger percentage of the PNH red cells. Thus, patients with a large percentage of type III erythrocytes tend to have more hemolysis than patients with a large percentage of type I or type II cells. Finally, hemolysis is frequently exacerbated by viral or bacterial infections, surgery, strenuous exercise, excessive alcohol intake, blood transfusions, and anything else that initiates complement activation.

Smooth Muscle Dystonia and Nitric Oxide

Many clinical manifestations of PNH are readily explained by hemoglobin-mediated nitric oxide scavenging. Brisk intravascular hemolysis releases free hemoglobin into the plasma. Free hemoglobin scavenges nitric oxide, resulting in fatigue, abdominal pain, esophageal spasm, erectile dysfunction, and possibly thrombosis. Indeed, hemoglobinuria, thrombosis, erectile dysfunction, and esophageal spasm are more common in patients with large PNH populations (>60% of granulocytes) than in patients with relatively small PNH populations.[3]

Thrombophilia and PNH

Thrombosis is the leading cause of death from PNH. Before the era of complement inhibition, it occurred in up to 40% of PNH patients and predominantly involved the venous system. The most common sites of venous thrombosis in PNH are the abdominal veins (i.e., hepatic vein, portal vein, mesenteric vein); other common sites include veins of the central nervous system and dermal veins. Abdominal pain, ascites, splenomegaly, intractable headaches, or a painful skin rash should prompt a work-up to document thrombosis. It is important to recognize that patients can have small-vessel thrombosis in the skin, intestines, or liver that may not be visible with imaging. In these circumstances, biopsy demonstrating fibrin deposition may be required to establish the diagnosis. Patients with greater than 50% PNH granulocytes and classical symptoms (hemolytic anemia and hemoglobinuria) have a greater propensity for thrombosis than do patients with small PNH clones.

The mechanism of thrombosis in PNH is not entirely understood and appears to be multifactorial. Indeed, nitric oxide depletion has been associated with increased platelet aggregation, increased platelet adhesion, and accelerated clot formation.[12] In an attempt to repair damage, PNH platelets undergo exocytosis of the complement attack complex.[21] This results in the formation of microvesicles with phosphatidylserine externalization, a potent *in vitro* procoagulant. These prothrombotic microvesicles have been detected in the blood of PNH patients.[22] Fibrinolysis may also be perturbed in PNH given that PNH blood cells lack the GPI-anchored urokinase receptor.[23] Lastly, tissue factor pathway inhibitor (TFPI), a major inhibitor of tissue factor, has been shown to require a GPI-anchored chaperone protein for trafficking to the endothelial cell surface.[24]

Renal Manifestations

Renal damage in PNH is associated with chronic hemosiderosis and microvascular thrombosis. Renal insufficiency is present in up to 65% of patients but is usually mild (stage I or II); only rare patients progress to stage IV or V renal disease.[25] Therapeutic complement inhibition can stabilize or reverse renal function in patients with PNH.

Treatment and Prognosis

Classical PNH

For patients with classical PNH, allogeneic bone marrow transplantation (BMT) and complement inhibition with eculizumab are the only proven effective therapies. Corticosteroids can improve hemoglobin levels and reduce hemolysis in some PNH patients, but the long term toxicity for minimal clinical benefit dampens enthusiasm for these agents. Before the availability of effective drug therapy the median survival for PNH patients was 15–20 years, and thrombosis was the leading cause of death. Complement inhibition has markedly decreased the risk of thrombosis and appears to have improved survival.

Eculizumab

Eculizumab, a humanized monoclonal antibody against C5, is the only FDA-approved drug for the treatment of PNH. The drug is highly effective in controlling the alternative pathway of complement by blocking the formation of the membrane attach complex (Figure 19.3). All patients should be vaccinated against *Neisseria meningitides*, because inhibition of complement at C5 increases the risk for developing infections with encapsulated organisms, particularly *Neisseria meningitides* and *Neisseria gonorrhoeae*. Eculizumab is administered intravenously at a dose of 900 mg weekly for the first 4 weeks. On week five, the dose can be reduced to 600 mg IV, and thereafter the drug is dosed at 600 mg IV every 14 days. Eculizumab is safe and well tolerated but must be continued indefinitely since it does not decrease the size of the PNH clone. The most common side effect, headache, occurs in roughly 50% of patients, predominantly with the initial dose. *Neisserial* sepsis is the most serious complication of terminal complement inhibition. Patients with terminal complement blockade have a 0.5% yearly risk of acquiring *Neisserial* sepsis even after vaccination. Therefore, patients should be revaccinated against *Neisseria meningitidis* every 3–5 years after starting eculizumab. Additional drawbacks of eculizumab include cost (~$400,000/year), the requirement for lifelong treatment, and the requirement for intravenous dosing.

Not all PNH patients require treatment with eculizumab. Watchful waiting is appropriate for asymptomatic patients or those with mild symptoms. Strong indications for initiating treatment include disabling fatigue, thrombosis due to PNH, transfusion dependence due to intravascular hemolysis, and frequent pain paroxysms. Eculizumab was granted FDA approval for the treatment of PNH in 2007 based on efficacy in two pivotal phase III clinical trials. Since C5 is common to all pathways of complement activation, blockade at this point aborts progression of the cascade regardless of the stimuli. Moreover, prevention of C5 cleavage blocks the generation of the potent proinflammatory and cell lytic molecules C5a and C5b-9, respectively. C5 blockade preserves the critical immunoprotective and immunoregulatory functions of upstream

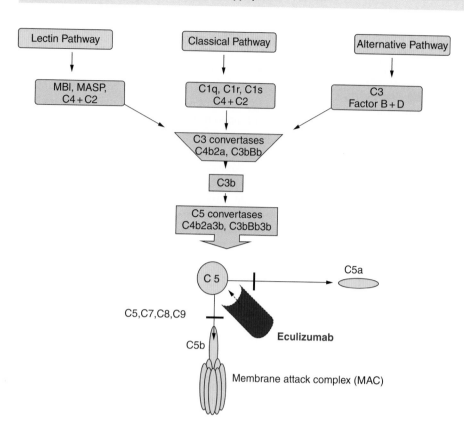

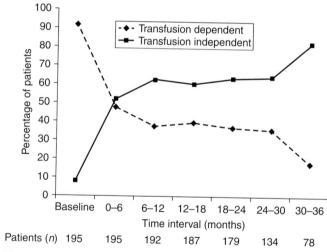

Figure 19.3 Overview of the Complement Cascade. Classic, alternative, and lectin pathways converge at the point of C3 activation. The lytic pathway is initiated with the formation of C5 convertase and leads to the assembly of the C5, C6, C7, C8, (n) C9 membrane attack complex. Eculizumab is a monoclonal antibody that binds to C5, thereby preventing the formation of C5a and C5b. C5b is the initiating component of the MAC. (Reproduced with permission from Brodsky, *Blood*, 2009; 113.)

components that culminate in C3b-mediated opsonization and immune complex clearance. Eculizumab is highly effective in reducing intravascular hemolysis in PNH; it does not stop extravascular hemolysis, and it does not treat bone marrow failure. Thus, eculizumab is most effective in patients with classical PNH. Treatment with eculizumab decreases or eliminates the need for blood transfusions, improves quality of life, and reduces the risk of thrombosis.[26–28]

Most patients managed with complement blockade will have significant medical improvement, but up to 30% will still need occasional blood transfusions (Figure 19.4). Even patients who become transfusion independent will often continue to have a mild to moderate anemia and an elevated reticulocyte count. This is due to C3b deposition on the PNH erythrocytes and subsequent extravascular hemolysis in the spleen. While eculizumab is quite effective at mitigating the CD59 deficit that leads to intravascular hemolysis, it does not reduce C3b deposition that is a direct consequence of the CD55 deficiency.

Other mechanisms of anemia to be considered in PNH patients on eculizumab are bone marrow failure due to concomitant aplastic anemia and insufficient complement blockade from the eculizumab. Most of these etiologies can be distinguished by ordering the following laboratory tests: complete blood count, reticulocyte count, and LDH 2–7 days after the last dose of eculizumab and immediately before the next scheduled dose.

In classical PNH patients who are transfusion dependent, a marked decrease in red cell transfusions is observed in

Figure 19.4 Percentage of Transfusion-Independent and Transfusion-Dependent Patients Over Time. Transfusion-independent patients were those who did not require a blood transfusion during the previous 6 months; transfusion-dependent patients had received at least one blood transfusion in the previous 6 months. (Reproduced with permission from Hilmen et al., *Br J of Haematol*, 2013; 162).

most patients, with more than 60% achieving transfusion independence. Breakthrough intravascular hemolysis and a return of PNH symptoms occurs in less than 5% of PNH patients treated with eculizumab. This typically occurs 1 or 2 days before the next scheduled dose and is accompanied by a spike in the LDH level. If this occurs on a regular basis, the interval between dosing can be shortened to 12 or 13 days, or the dose of eculizumab can be increased to 1,200 mg every 14 days.

It is also important to recognize that increased complement activation that accompanies infections (for example, influenza or viral gastroenteritis) or trauma can also result in transient breakthrough hemolysis. These single episodes of break-through hemolysis do not require a change in dosing.

Bone Marrow Transplantation

BMT is the only curative therapy for PNH, but it is associated with significant morbidity and mortality. The International Bone Marrow Transplant Registry (IBMTR) reported a 2-year survival probability of 56% in 48 recipients of HLA-identical sibling transplants between 1978 and 1995.[29] The median age was 28 years. The majority of the deaths in this study occurred within 1 year of transplantation. The European Blood and Marrow Transplant group reported a 5-year survival rate of 70% following allogeneic BMT for PNH; however, only 54% met criteria for classical PNH. The median age in the study was 30 years. Graft failure occurred in 6% of patients, and acute and chronic graft-versus-host disease occurred in 15% and 20% of patients, respectively. Most bone marrow transplants for PNH have used myeloablative conditioning. More recently, it has been demonstrated that reduced-intensity stem cell transplants from HLA-matched or HLA-haploidentical donors can cure PNH patients (30, 31). Thus, while BMT should not be used as front-line therapy for most PNH patients, it should still be considered as a treatment option in patients with life-threatening cytopenias or suboptimal responders to eculizumab therapy.

References

(1) Hillmen P, Lewis SM, Bessler M, Luzzatto L, Dacie JV. Natural history of paroxysmal nocturnal hemoglobinuria. *N Engl J Med*. 1995; 333:1253–1258.

(2) Socie G, Mary JY, de Gramont A, Rio B, Leporrier M, Rose C, et al. Paroxysmal nocturnal haemoglobinuria: long-term follow-up and prognostic factors. *Lancet*. 1996 Aug 31; 348 (9027):573–577.

(3) Moyo VM, Mukhina GL, Garrett ES, Brodsky RA. Natural history of paroxysmal nocturnal hemoglobinuria using modern diagnostic assays. *Brit J Haematol*. 2004; 126:133–138.

(4) Brodsky RA. Narrative review: paroxysmal nocturnal hemoglobinuria: the physiology of complement-related hemolytic anemia. *Ann Intern Med*. 2008 Apr 15; 148(8):587–595.

(5) Miyata T, Takeda J, Iida Y, Yamada N, Inoue N, Takahashi M, et al. The cloning of PIG-A, a component in the early step of GPI-anchor biosynthesis. *Science*. 1993; 259:1318–1320.

(6) Miyata T, Yamada N, Iida Y, Nishimura J, Takeda J, Kitani T, et al. Abnormalities of PIG-A transcripts in granulocytes from patients with paroxysmal nocturnal hemoglobinuria. *N Engl J Med*. 1994; 330:249–255.

(7) Nagarajan S, Brodsky R, Young NS, Medof ME. Genetic defects underlying paroxysmal nocturnal hemoglobinuria that arises out of aplastic anemia. *Blood*. 1995; 86:4656–4661.

(8) Mukhina GL, Buckley JT, Barber JP, Jones RJ, Brodsky RA. Multilineage glycosylphosphatidylinositol anchor deficient hematopoiesis in untreated aplastic anemia. *Br J Haematol*. 2001; 115:476–482.

(9) Luzzatto L, Bessler M, Rotoli B. Somatic mutations in paroxysmal nocturnal hemoglobinuria: A blessing in disguise? *Cell*. 1997; 88(January 10):1–4.

(10) Medof ME, Kinoshita T, Nussenzweig V. Inhibition of complement activation on the surface of cells after incorporation of decay-accelerating factor (DAF) into their membranes. *J Exp Med*. 1984; 160:1558–1578.

(11) Rollins SA, Sims PJ. The complement-inhibitory activity of CD59 resides in its capacity to block incorporation of C9 into membrane C5b-9. *J Immunol*. 1990 May 1; 144(9):3478–3483.

(12) Rother RP, Bell L, Hillmen P, Gladwin MT. The clinical sequelae of intravascular hemolysis and extracellular plasma hemoglobin: a novel mechanism of human disease. *JAMA*. 2005 Apr 6; 293(13):1653–1662.

(13) Hall SE, Rosse WF. The use of monoclonal antibodies and flow cytometry in the diagnosis of paroxysmal nocturnal hemoglobinuria. *Blood*. 1996; 87:5332–5340.

(14) Borowitz MJ, Craig FE, DiGiuseppe JA, Illingworth AJ, Rosse W, Sutherland DR, et al. Guidelines for the diagnosis and monitoring of paroxysmal nocturnal hemoglobinuria and related disorders by flow cytometry. *Cytometry B Clin Cytom*. 2010;78(4):211–230.

(15) Brodsky RA, Mukhina GL, Nelson KL, Lawrence TS, Jones RJ, Buckley JT. Resistance of paroxysmal nocturnal hemoglobinuria cells to the glycosylphosphatidylinositol-binding toxin aerolysin. *Blood*. 1999; 93(5): 1749–1756.

(16) Brodsky RA, Mukhina GL, Li S, Nelson KL, Chiurazzi PL, Buckley JT, et al. Improved detection and characterization of paroxysmal nocturnal hemoglobinuria using fluorescent aerolysin. *Am J Clin Pathol*. 2000 Sep;114(3):459–466.

(17) Araten DJ, Nafa K, Pakdeesuwan K, Luzzatto L. Clonal populations of hematopoietic cells with paroxysmal nocturnal hemoglobinuria genotype and phenotype are present in normal individuals. *Proc Natl Acad Sci USA*. 1999 Apr 27; 96(9): 5209–5214.

(18) Hu R, Mukhina GL, Piantadosi S, Barber JP, Jones RJ, Brodsky RA. PIG-A mutations in normal hematopoiesis. *Blood*. 2005 May 15; 105(10): 3848–3854.

(19) Pu JJ, Hu R, Mukhina GL, Carraway HE, McDevitt MA, Brodsky RA. The small population of PIG-A mutant cells in myelodysplastic syndromes do not arise from multipotent hematopoietic stem cells. *Haematologica*. 2012; 97(8): 1225–1233.

(20) Pu JJ, Mukhina G, Wang H, Savage WJ, Brodsky RA. Natural history of paroxysmal nocturnal hemoglobinuria clones in patients presenting as aplastic anemia. *Eur J Haematol*. 2011 Jul;87(1): 37–45.

(21) Wiedmer T, Hall SE, Ortel TL, Kane WH, Rosse WF, Sims PJ. Complement-induced vesiculation and exposure of membrane prothrombinase sites in platelets of paroxysmal nocturnal hemoglobinuria. *Blood*. 1993; 82(4): 1192–1196.

(22) Hugel B, Socie G, Vu T, Toti F, Gluckman E, Freyssinet JM, et al. Elevated levels of circulating procoagulant microparticles in patients with paroxysmal nocturnal hemoglobinuria and aplastic anemia. *Blood*. 1999 May 15; 93(10): 3451–3456.

(23) Ploug M, Plesner T, Ronne E, Ellis V, Hoyer-Hansen G, Hansen NE, et al. The receptor for urokinase-type plasminogen activator is deficient on peripheral blood leukocytes in patients with paroxysmal nocturnal hemoglobinuria. *Blood*. 1992 Mar 15; 79(6):1447–1455.

(24) Maroney SA, Cunningham AC, Ferrel J, Hu R, Haberichter S, Mansbach CM, et al. A GPI-anchored co-receptor for tissue factor pathway inhibitor controls its intracellular trafficking and cell surface expression. *J Thromb Haemost*. 2006 May;4(5):1114–1124.

(25) Hillmen P, Elebute M, Kelly R, Urbano-Ispizua A, Hill A, Rother RP, et al. Long-term effect of the complement inhibitor eculizumab on kidney function in patients with paroxysmal nocturnal hemoglobinuria. *Am J Hematol*. 2010 Aug;85(8): 553–559.

(26) Hillmen P, Young NS, Schubert J, Brodsky RA, Socie G, Muus P, et al. The complement inhibitor eculizumab in paroxysmal nocturnal hemoglobinuria. *N Engl J Med*. 2006 Sep 21; 355(12): 1233–1243.

(27) Brodsky RA, Young NS, Antonioli E, Risitano AM, Schrezenmeier H, Schubert J, et al. Multicenter phase 3 study of the complement inhibitor eculizumab for the treatment of patients with paroxysmal nocturnal hemoglobinuria. *Blood*. 2008 Feb 15; 111(4):1840–1847.

(28) Hillmen P, Muus P, Duhrsen U, Risitano AM, Schubert J, Young NS, et al. The terminal complement inhibitor eculizumab reduces thrombosis in patients with paroxysmal nocturnal hemoglobinuria (abstract). *Blood*. 2006; 106:40a–41a.

(29) Saso R, Marsh J, Cevreska L, Szer J, Gale RP, Rowlings PA, et al. Bone marrow transplants for paroxysmal nocturnal haemoglobinuria. *Br J Haematol*. 1999 Feb;104(2):392–396.

(30) Suenaga K, Kanda Y, Niiya H, Nakai K, Saito T, Saito A, et al. Successful application of nonmyeloablative transplantation for paroxysmal nocturnal hemoglobinuria. *Exp Hematol*. 2001 May;29(5):639–642.

(31) Brodsky RA, Luznik L, Bolanos-Meade J, Leffell MS, Jones RJ, Fuchs EJ. Reduced intensity HLA-haploidentical BMT with post transplantation cyclophosphamide in nonmalignant hematologic diseases. *Bone Marrow Transplant*. 2008 Oct;42(8):523–527.

Congenital Marrow Failure Syndromes

Anupama Narla, MD, and Benjamin L. Ebert, MD, PhD

Introduction

The congenital marrow failure syndromes are uncommon but important causes of anemia in pediatrics. With increased understanding of the clinical genetics of these disorders, it has become clear that there is a wide phenotypic spectrum, and these diseases must be considered in the differential diagnosis of both children and adults with unexplained defects in hematopoiesis. Moreover, these conditions are not as rare as previously believed and may present as aplastic anemia or malignancy. Correct diagnosis is essential, as it has implications for treatment, medical management, cancer screening, and family planning. In this chapter, we will review the inherited bone marrow failure syndromes (IBMFs), which

may present in adult populations (Diamond Blackfan anemia, dyskeratosis congenita, Fanconi anemia, and Schwachman-Diamond Syndrome). These diseases are summarized in Table 20.1 later in the chapter. We will also briefly discuss other IBMFs, which present almost exclusively in the pediatric population (amegakaryocytic thrombocytopenia, Pearson syndrome, severe congenital neutropenia, and thrombocytopenia absent radii syndrome). While a comprehensive review of each disorder is beyond the scope of this textbook, our goal is to highlight insights into normal and disordered hematopoiesis, review cryptic presentations of these genetic syndromes, and provide useful references for the practicing hematologist.

Table 20.1. Summary of the IBMFs That May Present in Adults

Disease	Presentation in Adults	Initial Work-Up	Useful Clinical References
Diamond Blackfan anemia	- Macrocytic anemia with reticulocytopenia - History of congenital anomalies/short stature - Family history	- Elevated ADA - Elevated Hgb F - If high suspicion, send testing for RP mutations	- How I treat DBA (Vlachos A and Muir E). Blood 2010 - Diagnosing and treating DBA: results of an international consensus conference (Vlachos A et al.). *Br J Haematology* 2008 - DBA Registry: www.dbar.org
Dyskeratosis congenita	- Classic: triad + bone marrow failure - Cryptic: aplastic anemia, MDS, pulmonary fibrosis, or AML - Family history (pulmonary fibrosis, BMF, cancer in young people, especially head/neck or anogenital)	- Telomere length testing - If short telomeres identified, genetic testing	- Dyskeratosis Congenita (Savage and Alter) 2009. Heme Onc Clinics of North America - www.marrowfailure.cancer.gov (etiologic investigation of cancer susceptibilities in inherited bone marrow failure syndromes)
Fanconi anemia	- Young adults with hypoplastic or aplastic anemia or cytopenias - Young adults with MDS or AML and congenital malformations - Patients presenting with cancers at an unusually young age - Sensitivity to toxic effects of chemotherapy or radiation - Family history (cancer susceptibility, inherited marrow failure)	- Chromosomal breakage blood test	- Fanconi anemia: guidelines for diagnosis and management www.fanconi.org/index.php/publications/guidelines_for_diagnosis_and_management - International Fanconi Anemia Registry (IFAR): http://lab.rockefeller.edu/smogorzewska/ifar/
Schwachman-Diamond syndrome	- Pancreatic exocrine insufficiency and neutropenia	- Pancreatic enzymes - SBDS gene testing	- Draft consensus guidelines for diagnosis and treatment of Schwachman-Diamond syndrome (Dror Y et al.). *Ann NY Acad Sci* 2011 - SDS registry: http://sdsregistry.org/

IBMFs That May Present in Adults

Diamond Blackfan Anemia

Diamond Blackfan anemia (DBA) was originally described by Josephs in 1936 and further characterized by Diamond and Blackfan in 1938 as a congenital hypoplastic anemia.[1] In addition to the hypoplastic anemia, the disorder is characterized by macrocytosis, reticulocytopenia, elevated levels of erythrocyte adenosine deaminase, presence of fetal membrane antigen "i," and a selective decrease or absence of erythroid precursors in an otherwise normocellular bone marrow (Figure 20.1). Additionally, half of patients with DBA also present with physical abnormalities including short stature, thumb abnormalities (classically a triphalangeal thumb), craniofacial defects, and cleft lip/palate. DBA typically presents in infancy, most commonly with pallor and lethargy, at an estimated incidence of four or five cases per million live births, and there is often a family history of the disease.[2]

DBA was the first disease to be linked to impaired ribosome function and is the founding member of a group of disorders now known as ribosomopathies.[3] Several other inherited bone marrow failure syndromes (including Schwachman-Diamond Syndrome and dyskeratosis congenita) and the 5q syndrome have subsequently been linked to mutations in genes encoding for ribosomal proteins (RPs) or for proteins required for normal ribosome function (Figure 20.2). Up to 70% of patients with DBA have been identified as having mutations in ribosomal proteins, most frequently in RPS19. Recently, mutations in GATA-1 have been identified in several patients with DBA, suggesting that, in some cases, the disease may arise from causes other than defects in ribosomal protein genes.[4] The disease is also known to have incomplete penetrance, as demonstrated both by the observation of siblings who carry the same mutation discordant for the presence of anemia and by the occurrence of spontaneous remissions in affected patients.

The fundamental question of how a mutation in a ribosomal protein, which would be expected to have widespread and diverse effects throughout an organism, can lead to selective defects remains a focus of investigation. It has been established, in both *in vivo* and *in vitro* models, that when ribosome biogenesis is perturbed, the p53 protein accumulates and activates downstream cell cycle inhibition and apoptotic pathways. A proposed mechanism for the activation of p53 in the setting of ribosome dysfunction reflects the role of MDM2 (HDM2 in humans) in binding and thereby decreasing the activity of p53. It is postulated that accumulation of free ribosomal proteins and subsequent aberrant ribosome assembly decrease MDM2/HDM2, allowing p53 protein to accumulate.[5] The erythroid lineage appears to be more sensitive to activation of this RP-MDM2-p53 pathway, but further work is needed to understand modifying and alternative pathways that contribute to the DBA phenotype.

The current standard of care for DBA includes corticosteroids and/or chronic transfusions, with the only definitive treatment being bone marrow transplantation. With existing treatments, the overall survival of patients, as reported by the Diamond Blackfan Anemia Registry, is 75.1% at 40 years of age; median overall survival is 58 years.[6] As our understanding of the pathophysiology of the ribosomopathies increases, the goal will be to translate these findings into novel therapeutic options for patients with DBA.

Dyskeratosis Congenita

In 1910, the first case report defined a syndrome, ultimately named dyskeratosis congenita (DC), characterized by a triad of abnormal skin pigmentation, oral leukoplakia, and nail dystrophy (Figure 20.3).[7] The spectrum of DC has expanded considerably since then to include effects on every organ system, particularly the bone marrow (BM). Almost 90% of patients with DC will eventually develop a cytopenia of one or more peripheral blood lineages, and bone marrow failure is the major cause of death. Often bone marrow failure develops in the second or third decade of life, but it can occur at birth or as late as the seventh decade of life. The BM abnormalities can evolve into MDS or AML.[8] The diagnostic triad is still important for identifying dyskeratosis congenita, but the disease is now known to affect a variety of organs, so clinical suspicion must remain high when presented with a patient with bone marrow failure and unusual clinical findings. These findings may include early graying of hair or hair loss, short stature, developmental delay, blepharitis, periodontal disease, pulmonary fibrosis, esophageal stenosis, urethral stenosis, liver disease, and avascular necrosis of the hips or shoulders.

The clinical diagnosis of DC can be challenging given its phenotypic heterogeneity, different modes of inheritance (X-linked, autosomal recessive, and autosomal dominant) and

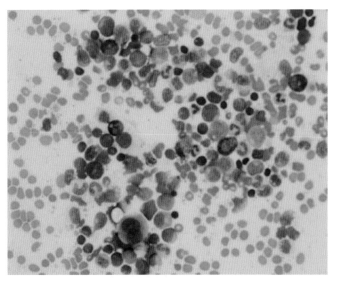

Figure 20.1. Bone marrow evaluation in DBA. This image from a bone marrow aspirate performed on a patient with Diamond Blackfan anemia reveals a paucity of later erythroid precursors. Image courtesy of Colin Sieff.

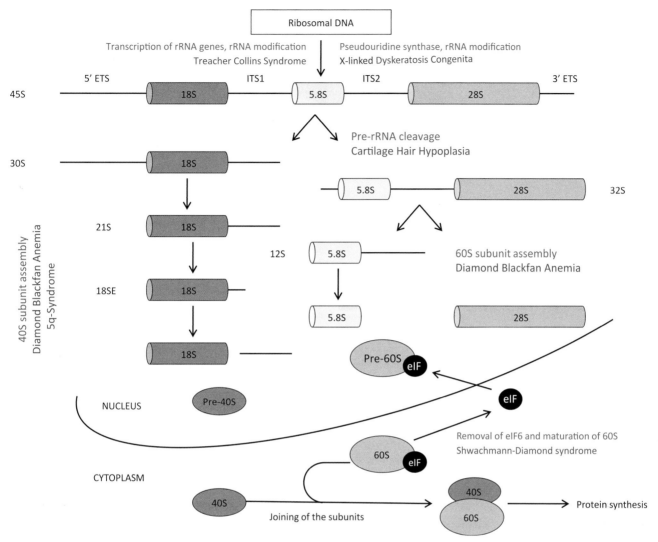

Figure 20.2. Overview of Ribosome Biogenesis. Simplified schematic of eukaryotic ribosome biogenesis. The step in ribosome biogenesis that is thought to be affected by each ribosomopathy is depicted in blue and purple, respectively. Adapted from Narla and Ebert.[3]

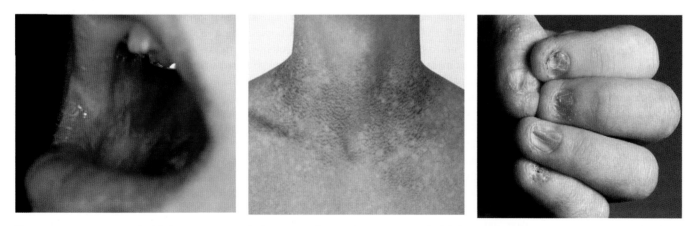

Figure 20.3. Diagnostic triad of dyskeratosis congenital. These panels illustrate the diagnostic triad of dyskeratosis congenita, including dystrophic fingernails, lacy/reticular pigmentation on neck and trunk, and oral leukoplakia (courtesy of Blanche Alter). Reprinted from *Hematology/Oncology Clinics of North America*, Volume 23/Edition 2, Savage SA and Alter BP, Dyskeratosis Congenita, Pages 215–231, Copyright 2009, with permission from Elsevier.[8]

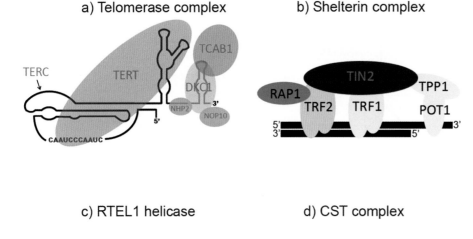

a) Telomerase complex

b) Shelterin complex

c) RTEL1 helicase

d) CST complex

Figure 20.4. Overview of the Telomere Disease States. Dyskeratosis congenita has been linked to germline mutations in nine genes that affect telomere homeostasis (each in red). These can be divided into four groups based on our current understanding: (a) telomerase components, (b) shelterin proteins, (c) the RTEL helicase and (d) the CST complex proteins. Figure courtesy of Steven Artandi. Reprinted from *Current Opinion in Genetics & Development*, Batista LF and Artandi SE, "Understanding telomere diseases through analysis of patient-derived iPS cells," 2013, 23:526–533. with permission from Elsevier.

variable age of onset. However, despite the wide spectrum of the disease ranging from classic DC to aplastic anemia, it is clear that the underlying pathology is due to defective telomere maintenance (the "telomeropathies"). In all characterized cases of DC, the causative mutations are in components of the telomerase complex (Figure 20.4). Mutations in seven telomerase-complex genes have been identified in DC: dyskerin (DKC1), TERT (telomerase), TERC (telomerase RNA component), TINF2 (Tin2, TRF1-interacting nuclear factor 2), WRAP53 (TCAB1), NOP10 (NOP10 ribonucleoprotein), and NHP2 (NHP2 ribonucleoprotein). Two additional candidate genes, also involved in telomere maintenance or elongation, have recently been identified by whole exome sequencing: CTC1 and RTEL1.[9] Therefore, functional assessment of telomere length, with the finding of telomere length to be less than the first percentile for age in leukocyte subsets, is highly sensitive and specific for the diagnosis.

Telomeres are specialized protein–RNA complexes, located at the ends of chromosomes, that help stabilize chromosome ends. This prevents premature shortening, end-to-end fusions, translocations, or breaks. Mutations in telomerase and shelterin components cause accelerated telomere loss. These mutations, in combination with environmental factors and possible second genetic hits, lead to premature cell death, stem cell depletion, and chromosome instability. Ultimately this cascade leads to the clinical phenotype of premature aging, bone marrow failure, nonhematologic abnormalities, and cancer.

The actuarial risk of cancer in patients with DC is 40% by age 50 years, with a particular risk for squamous cell carcinoma (head and neck, anogenital), MDS, and AML. Patients with DC are managed with supportive care and can respond to androgens and cytokines. The only long-term cure for the hematologic abnormalities is stem cell transplantation with a reduced intensity regimen. However, patients with DC have a much

higher incidence of transplant-related morbidity/mortality, primarily from pulmonary toxicity and veno-occlusive disease. In addition, the relatives of patients who have DC who are being considered as donors should themselves be evaluated carefully for DC.[10] The median overall survival of patients with DC is 43 years, although there is some correlation between genotype and both overall survival and age at cancer development.

Fanconi Anemia

Fanconi anemia (FA), the most common form of inherited bone marrow failure, was first described by Fanconi in 1927 in three brothers with pancytopenia and congenital abnormalities.[11] The disease typically progresses through several clinical stages, organized by age. In the first stage, in infancy and early childhood, congenital anomalies may be present, although they are not required for the diagnosis of FA and range from mild to severe. The most common malformations include short stature, hypopigmented or café au lait spots, thumb or radial ray abnormalities, micro- or hydrocephaly, structural renal anomalies, hypogonadism, and developmental delay. Within the first decade, patients may present with thrombocytopenia and macrocytosis before progressing to bone marrow failure when the diagnosis is often first made. During adolescence and adulthood, the risk of AML and MDS becomes very high. And in older adults, a range of solid tumors, particularly squamous cell carcinomas of the head/neck and GU tract, can be seen.[12] Throughout life, the hematopoietic phenotype can change because of genetic reversion or clonal evolution so a high index of suspicion and a careful history, including a family history of cancer predisposition, is essential.

The diagnosis of Fanconi anemia is based on the sensitivity of FA cells to DNA interstrand cross-links chemicals such as mitomycin C or diepoxybutane. In this assay, cells from

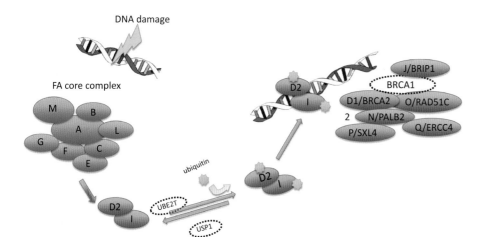

Figure 20.5. Overview of the FA/BRCA Damage Response Pathway. Following DNA damage, the proteins represented by A, B, C, E, F, G, L, and M form the core complex. This core complex is required for the ubiquitination of the I and D2 proteins, which are in turn required for the downstream complex to form foci for DNA repair (courtesy of Sharon Savage). Reprinted from *Seminars in Hematology*, Volume 50/Edition 4, Kincha PP and Savage SA, Genomic Characterization of the Inherited Bone Marrow Failure Syndromes, Pages 333–347, Copyright 2013, with permission from Elsevier.[28]

patients with FA develop characteristic chromosomal breaks that can be scored. Because of hematopoietic reversion, if the test is negative in lymphocytes but clinical suspicion is high, the test should be repeated on patient fibroblasts. Once the FA diagnosis is established, the *FANC* genes can be sequenced for mutations. Except for rare mutations in the *FANCB* gene, located on the X-chromosome, all other FA mutations are autosomal recessive. Mutations in 16 genes have been identified in FA, the most frequent of which are *FANCA, FANCC, FANCG*, and *FANCD2*.[13] Of note, FANCD1 is also known as BRCA2, conferring a powerful predisposition to breast and ovarian cancers.

The function of the Fanconi anemia proteins is to maintain genomic stability, mainly through repair of DNA interstrand crosslinks. Products of the FA genes function the FA/BRCA pathway, which is a DNA repair-signaling pathway (Figure 20.5). The encoded proteins can be subdivided into three groups: (1) proteins that make up the core complex, (2) proteins that compose the ID complex that is monoubiquitinated after DNA damage, and (3) downstream effector proteins that are thought to participate directly in DNA repair.[14] The FA gene products also participate in DNA damage response pathways involving other DNA repair proteins such as BRCA1, ATM and ATR.

The hypersensitivity of FA cells to DNA cross-linking agents, resulting in increased numbers of chromosomal abnormalities, has significant implications for the treatment of patients, whose median overall survival is only 33 years. Careful evaluation for congenital anomalies should be done, as well as routine monitoring for malignancy. Supportive care for marrow failure includes androgen therapy (oxymethalone), hematopoietic growth factors and transfusion support. HSCT is the only available curative treatment for the BMF of FA, and outcomes are better with matched sibs (who should be screened for FA), younger patients, and reduced intensity conditioning regimens. However, HSCT does not cure the nonhematopoietic manifestations of FA and may further increase the risk of solid tumors.[15] Gene therapy is being investigated for specific FA subtypes.

Schwachman-Diamond Syndrome

Schwachman-Diamond syndrome (SDS, also known as Schwachman-Diamond-Oski syndrome) was initially described in the early 1960s as a disorder of exocrine pancreatic dysfunction and bone marrow failure.[16] Patients generally present with steatorrhea, growth failure, and recurrent infections. The hematologic abnormalities are predominantly neutropenia, although anemia, thrombocytopenia, and pancytopenia can occur. Skeletal abnormalities (short stature, delayed appearance of normally shaped epiphyses, and progressive metaphyseal thickening/dysplasia) as well as poor growth are common in SDS patients. Patients without severe pancreatic disease may present later in childhood or as adults, and some patients may present with aplastic anemia or AML as the initial manifestation of the disease.[17]

The diagnosis of SDS relies on clinical findings. Exocrine pancreatic dysfunction, which can be subclinical, can be established by low serum trypsinogen in patients less than 3 years of age or low pancreatic isoamylase in patients greater than 3 years of age. In addition, patients may have low fecal elastase or a fatty pancreas that can be demonstrated by imaging. Genetic testing can be helpful to confirm the diagnosis (see what follows), but a negative test does not exclude the diagnosis.[17] It is essential to distinguish SDS from cystic fibrosis (the most common cause of exocrine pancreatic insufficiency in children), congenital neutropenia, and Pearson syndrome.

In 90% of affected patients, this autosomal recessive disorder is due to mutations in the Schwachman-Bodian-Diamond syndrome (SBDS) gene.[18] In the majority of cases, mutations are due to recombination of portions of an adjacent pseudogene with the SBDS gene. SBDS has been implicated in multiple biologic processes including ribosome biogenesis, stabilization of the mitotic spindle, and cell motility. Recent studies have confirmed that SDS is indeed a ribosomopathy caused by defective eIF6 recycling, with a subsequent decrease in levels of translationally active mature 80S ribosomes.[19] Developmental and tissue-specific gene expression or translational requirements may cause differential sensitivities to decreased expression of particular genes involved in ribosome function, but this remains to be elucidated.

Management of patients with SDS is directed at specific clinical manifestations. Clinically significant pancreatic dysfunction can be treated with oral enzyme replacement as well as supplemental ADEK vitamins. Pancreatic dysfunction improves with age in a subset of patients. Supportive care for the hematologic manifestations includes growth factors and transfusion support as well as aggressive management of infections in neutropenic patients.[17] Patients with SDS tend to do better than other IBMFs, and HSCT is generally reserved for severe persistent or symptomatic cytopenia(s) or development of MDS/AML.

Other Congenital Bone Marrow Failure Syndromes

Amegakaryocytic Thrombocytopenia

Congenital amegakaryocytic thrombocytopenia (CAMT) is a rare autosomal recessive disease characterized by an isolated, severe hypomegakaryocytic thrombocytopenia, which presents in infancy and progresses to pancytopenia and bone marrow failure in later childhood. Clinical manifestations can include petechiae at birth and intracranial hemorrhage, but unlike other IBMFs, congenital anomalies are rare.[20] CAMT is most commonly due to mutations in MPL, which encodes for the thrombopoietin (TPO) receptor.[21] In contrast to the activating *MPL* mutations seen in myeloproliferative neoplasms, CAMT mutations always lead to diminished or absent signaling of the TPO receptor. In general, loss-of-function mutations are associated with more severe thrombocytopenia and early onset pancytopenia (CAMT Type I). In cases with *MPL* gene missense mutations, patients have a transient increase in platelet counts in the first year of life (CAMT Type II).[22] The major treatment for bleeding is supportive care with platelet transfusions, and antifibrinolytic therapies for mucosal bleeding. Allogeneic HSCT is the only curative treatment option, but before this is considered, it is important to rule out Fanconi anemia and Dyskeratosis Congenita, both of which can initially present with isolated thrombocytopenia.[20] CAMT has been proposed to be an ideal target for gene therapy.

Pearson Syndrome

Pearson syndrome, also known as Pearson marrow-pancreas syndrome, is a multisystem disorder characterized by pancytopenia (anemia, neutropenia, and thrombocytopenia), ring sideroblasts in the marrow, and exocrine pancreatic insufficiency. Patients often present in infancy or early childhood with failure to thrive, although clinical variants and atypical presentations do occur.[23] The syndrome is caused by large deletions or rearrangements of mitochondrial DNA leading to the absence of many proteins normally encoded by the mitochondrial genome.[24] Heteroplasmy, the random distribution of mitochondrial DNA during cell division, is responsible for the high variability between patients and between different organs within the same patient.[25] The disease can be diagnosed by mitochondrial DNA sequencing, distinguishing Pearson syndrome from SDS, as does the presence of ringed sideroblasts and marrow cell vacuolization. About one half of patients die in infancy or early childhood due to severe lactic acidosis, sepsis, or liver failure. For patients who survive, the hematologic manifestations often resolve, while the neurological and myopathic issues appear or worsen.[23] Management is supportive and no specific therapy is currently available for individuals with Pearson syndrome or other mitochondriopathies.

Severe Congenital Neutropenia

Severe congenital neutropenia (SCN) is characterized by ANCs consistently less than $200/\mu L$ with recurrent severe infections, which often develop within the first few months of life. Evaluation of the bone marrow demonstrates a myeloid maturation arrest.[26] The disease can be autosomal recessive (Kostmann Syndrome), X-linked, or autosomal dominant. In Kostmann syndrome, mutations have been identified in the *HAX1*, *G6PC3*, and *GFI1* genes. In the X-linked disease, mutations have been found in the *WAS* gene. Finally, mutations in the *ELANE* gene are the most common cause of SCN and cause autosomal dominant disease. Mutations in *ELANE* are also found in cyclic neutropenia.[27]

Management of SCN includes aggressive treatment of infections and G-CSF to keep the ANC greater than 1,000. Consideration for HSCT is important, as patients with SCN are at an increased risk for MDS and AML. It remains to be resolved whether GCSF merely drives the clonal expansion of already damaged stem cells in SCN or whether it actively contributes to the leukemic process.

Thrombocytopenia Absent Radii Syndrome

Thrombocytopenia absent radius (TAR) syndrome is characterized by severe thrombocytopenia and bilateral absent radii. Other abnormalities of the upper limbs may occur, but the thumbs are always present. Patients may also have congenital heart disease, renal anomalies, and lower-limb defects. More than half of patients present within the first week of life, and morbidity and mortality are significant due to intracranial hemorrhage.[28] TAR is caused by dysmegakaryocytopoiesis with a differentiation blockage at an early precursor stage. Bone marrow evaluation shows normal erythroid and myeloid lineages but decreased or absent megakaryocytes. Genetically, TAR is associated with the compound inheritance of a low-frequency polymorphism and a rare null allele in RBM8A.[29] Management is supportive with platelet transfusion. Spontaneous resolution of the thrombocytopenia usually occurs after the first year of life, at which time orthopedic surgery can be performed without platelet coverage.

Conclusions

The inherited bone marrow failure syndromes (IBMFs) encompass a diverse collection of diseases. While they are rare causes of hematologic disorders, it is essential for the practicing hematologist to be aware of the IBMFs. These disorders have a wide phenotypic spectrum and may present cryptically in adult patients with cytopenias in one or more lineage. Furthermore, our evolving understanding of the pathophysiology of these disorders is critical to our general knowledge of the hematopoietic system.

References

1. Diamond LK, Blackfan KD. Hypoplastic anemia. *Am J Dis Child.* 1938; 15:307.

2. Lipton JM, Ellis SR. Diamond-Blackfan anemia: diagnosis, treatment, and molecular pathogenesis. *Hematol Oncol Clin North Am.* 2009; 23(2):261–282.

3. Narla A, Ebert BL. Ribosomopathies: human disorders of ribosome dysfunction. *Blood.* 2010; 115 (16):3196–205.

4. Sankaran V, Chazvinian R, Do R, et al. Exome sequencing identifies GATA1 mutations resulting in Diamond-Blackfan anemia. *J Clin Invest.* 2012; 122(7):2439–2443.

5. Fumagalli S, Thomas G. The role of p53 in ribosomopathies. *Semin Hematol.* 2011; 48(2):97–105.

6. Narla A, Vlachos A, Nathan DG. Diamond Blackfan anemia treatment: past, present, and future. *Semin Hematol.* 2011; 48(2):117–123.

7. Zinsser F. Atrophia cutis reticularis cum pigmentations, dystrophia unguium et leukoplakis oris (Poikioodermia atrophicans vascularis Jacobi). *Ikonogr. Dermatol.* 1910; 5:219–233.

8. Savage SA, Alter BP. Dyskeratosis congenita. *Hematol Oncol Clin North Am.* 2009; 23(2):215–231.

9. Ballew BJ, Savage SA. Updates on the biology and management of dyskeratosis congenital and related telomere biology disorders. *Expert Rev Hematol.* 2013; 6(3):327–337.

10. Alter B, Giri N, Savage S, et al. Malignancies and survival patters in the National Cancer Institute inherited bone marrow failure syndromes cohort study. *Br J Haematol.* 2010; 150(2):179–188.

11. Lobitz S, Velleuer E. Guido Fanconi: a jack of all trades. *Nat Rev Cancer.* 2006; 6(11):893–898.

12. Bagby GC, Alter BP. Fanconi anemia. *Semin Hematol.* 2006; 43(3):147–156.

13. Garaycoechea J, Patel KJ. Why does the bone marrow fail in Fanconi anemia. *Blood.* 2014; 123(1):26–34.

14. Kupfer GM. Fanconi anemia: a signal transduction and DNA repair pathway. *Yale J Biol Med.* 2013; 60(6):1291–1310.

15. Kee Y, D'Andrea D. Molecular pathogenesis and clinical management of Fanconi anemia. *J Clin Invest.* 2012; 122(11):3799–3806.

16. Schwachman H, Diamond LK, Oski FA, Khaw KT. The syndrome of pancreatic insufficiency and bone marrow dysfunction. *J Pediatr.* 1964; 65:645–663.

17. Myers KC, Davies SM, Shimamura A. Clinical and molecular pathophysiology of Schwachman-Diamond syndrome: an update. *Hematol Oncol Clin N Am.* 2013;(27):117–128.

18. Boocock GR, Morrioson JA, Popvic M, et al. Mutations in SBDS are associated with Schwachman-Diamond Syndrome. *Nat Genet.* 2003; 33(1):97–101.

19. Wong CC, Traynor D, Basse N, et al. Defective ribosome assembly in Shwachman-Diamond syndrome. *Blood.* 2011; 118(16):4305–4312.

20. Ballmaier M, Germeshausen M. Congenital amegakaryocytic thrombocytopenia: clinical presentation, diagnosis, and treatment. *Semin Thromb Hemost.* 2011; 37 (6):673–681.

21. Ballmaier M, Germeshausen M, Schulze H, et al. C-MPL mutations are the cause of congenital amegakaryocytic thrombocytopenia. *Blood.* 2001; 97:139–146.

22. Al-Qahtani. Congenital amegakaryocytic thrombocytopenia: a brief review of the literature. *Clin Med Insights Pathol.* 2010; 3:25–30.

23. DiMauro S, Hirano M. Mitochondrial DNA Deletion Syndromes. 2003 Dec 17 [Updated 2011 May 3]. In: Pagon RA, Adam MP, Bird TD, et al., editors. GeneReviews® [Internet]. Seattle, WA: University of Washington; 1993–2014. Available from: www.ncbi .nlm.nih.gov/books/ NBK1203/

24. Rotig A, Colonna M, Bonnefont JP, et al. A mitochondrial DNA deletion in Pearson's marrow pancreas syndrome. *Lancet.* 1989; 333:902–903.

25. Cherry AB, Gagne KE, McLoughlin EM, et al. Induced pluripotent stem cells with a mitochondrial DNA deletion. *Stem Cells.* 2013; 31(7):1287–1297.

26. Boxer LA. Severe congenital neutropenia: genetics and pathogenesis. *Trans Am Clin Climatol Assoc.* 2006; 117:13–32.

27. Horwitz MS, Corey SJ, Grimes HL, et al. ELANE mutations in cyclic and severe congenital neutropenia. *Hematol Oncol Clin N Am.* 2013; 27:19–41.

28. Khincha PP, Savage SA. Genomic characterization of the inherited bone marrow failure syndromes. *Semin Hematol.* 2013; 50(4):333–347.

29. Albers CA, Newbury-Ecob R, Ouwehand WH, et al. New insights into the genetic basis of TAR (thrombocytopenia-absent radii syndrome). *Curr Opin Genet Dev.* 2013; 23(3):316–323.

Anemia of Chronic Inflammation

21

Satish P. Shanbhag, MD, and Cindy N. Roy, PhD

Within any medical specialty, anemic patients are likely to be the most complex. Anemic patients are clearly vulnerable to untoward outcomes like increased morbidity, hospitalizations, and mortality. Current clinical and scientific evidence is not sufficient to demonstrate that anemia is the cause for such outcomes, but the presentation of anemia in a given patient should motivate the treating physician to be especially vigilant in assessing the course of the underlying disease, optimizing its treatment, and addressing the anemia. At minimum, the anemia can be viewed as a physiologic indicator of the severity of the initial stages of disease activity. In this chapter, we aim to provide the reader with the clinical context and physiologic causes of anemia in the setting of chronic inflammation (ACI). We will review current laboratory diagnostics that are useful in its evaluation and management during the patient's treatment course.

Etiology and Epidemiology

ACI is associated with various underlying disease states. Historically, this mild to moderate anemia has been associated with bacterial or fungal infections and poorly controlled autoimmune disorders.[1,2] In this chapter, we will focus on the anemia that develops in these contexts. Though the features of ACI are known to overlap with cancer-related anemia and the anemia associated with systemic diseases such as chronic kidney disease and chronic heart failure, those clinical contexts are addressed elsewhere.

It is important to note that while the World Health Organization (WHO) has loosely defined anemia as a hemoglobin concentration less than 13 g/dL for men and less than 12 g/dL for women,[3] much variability exists in the criteria used by investigators to document the prevalence of anemia in a given population. We have reported frequencies of ACI for specific populations as defined by the study authors (Table 21.1), even if they chose not to use WHO criteria.

ACI in the General Population

In the United States (US), the National Health and Nutrition Examination Surveys (NHANES) have provided data concerning the prevalence of ACI in a wide sampling of the general population.[4] Data from NHANES I indicated approximately 15% of anemic children less than 6 years of age have anemia associated with inflammation. In contrast, the same study concluded about one-third of anemia cases in women 18–44 years of age were associated with inflammation and nearly two-thirds of anemia cases were associated with inflammation for men and women 60–74 years of age. Thus, while iron deficiency is a more common cause of anemia in children and premenopausal women, inflammation is more common in the remainder of the adult population.

One limitation of these data is that ACI was defined as anemia with an elevated erythrocyte sedimentation rate. Adjudication of an underlying inflammatory disease was not feasible in this large study of more than 16,000 individuals. For NHANES III, ACI was defined with methods different than those used for the NHANES I study (low serum iron without absolute iron deficiency), but again without requiring diagnosis of a specific disease. The incidence of ACI in NHANES III was estimated to be 19.7% of all anemia in adults over 65 years of age, excluding those with renal insufficiency.[5]

Infections

With greater access to primary health care centers and the wide availability of antibiotics for treatment of infections in the US, there is less focus in current medical practice on anemia associated with infections that are expected to resolve rapidly. However, ACI has been demonstrated in pneumonia, cellulitis, osteomyelitis, chronic cholecystitis, bacterial endocarditis, genito-urinary infections. and other infections.[2]

Autoimmune Diseases

Rheumatoid arthritis (RA) is arguably the classic autoimmune condition associated with ACI. However, advances in the treatment of these patients with disease-modifying antirheumatic drugs has led to much better control of the disease, reducing the risk of anemia.[6] Like RA, other systemic autoimmune disorders such as SLE (systemic lupus erythematosus) and giant cell arteritis (GCA) cause a hypoproliferative anemia related to the inflammatory process. Among the autoimmune diseases, inflammatory bowel disease can present with a mixed picture including iron deficiency from gastrointestinal blood loss,[7] while SLE can be associated with autoimmune hemolysis (see Table 21.1). For these autoimmune diseases, anemia is more prevalent in patients hospitalized for their disease, a finding that is likely related to the increased severity of their autoimmune condition.[7]

Table 21.1. Incidence of anemia of chronic inflammation

| Population | Ages | ACI Incidence | | Anemia Definition | Complicating Features | References |
		% of Population	% of Anemic			
General Population						
NHANES I	<6 M/F	NM	~15	Defined by age, race, sex (see text and[25])	Iron deficiency	[4]
	18–44 F		~35			
	60–74 F		~60			
	60–74 M		~65			
Older Adults						
Community (NHANES III)	65 and over	2.1	19.7	M: Hgb <13 g/dL F: Hgb <12 g/dL	Unexplained anemia, gastrointestinal blood loss	[5]
Outpatient hematology (Stanford/VA)		ND	6			[26]
Anemia referral (Chicago)		ND	9.8			[27]
Autoimmune						
Rheumatoid arthritis	Adult	17–59	N/A	Variable		[6]
Inflammatory bowel disease	Pediatric to adult	8.8–73.7			Folate deficiency, gastrointestinal blood loss	[7]
Systemic lupus erythematosus		38.3	37.1	M: Hgb <13.5 g/dL F: Hgb <12 g/dL	Iron deficiency, autoimmune hemolytic anemia	[28]
Giant cell arteritis	Older adult	18–21	N/A	Hgb <12 g/dL		[29]
Acute Care						
Inpatient (County Hospital)	19–91	54.5	ND	M: Hct <40% F: Hct <37%	Acute blood loss, renal failure	[21]
Critically ill (Western European ICU)	NM	63		Hgb < 12 g/dL		[30]

NM, not mentioned; ND, not determined; N/A, not applicable

Critically Ill

While patients in the acute care, critical care, or intensive care settings may have rapid, traumatic blood loss that contributes to their anemia at admission, these patients often experience declining hemoglobin during their hospital stay, despite transfusions. Additionally, many patients discharged from these critical care settings remain anemic 6 months after their discharge.[8] These findings would suggest that the same mechanisms that drive anemia in chronic inflammatory states without blood loss could contribute to persistent anemia in critical care patients.[9,10]

Pathophysiology

The pathophysiology of ACI is multifactorial (Figure 21.1) and varies according to the underlying disease. We will delineate each of the primary pathways that have been implicated here, but only selected pathways may contribute to the presentation of ACI in an individual patient, depending upon the specific disease pathology.

Inflammatory Cytokines and Hypoproliferative Effects

The common feature of all cases of ACI is an inflammatory process, whether it is derived from the innate immune response to a pathogen or the adaptive response involved in autoimmune disease. At the molecular level, these disease processes result in the elaboration of inflammatory cytokines of various kinds, which have pleiotropic effects on the development of erythroid progenitors.

Committed erythroid progenitors require signaling through the erythropoietin receptor (EpoR) for survival and growth, but in the context of ACI, inflammatory cytokines can impair production of EPO.[11] In addition to an effect on EPO production, inflammation can impair erythroid progenitor

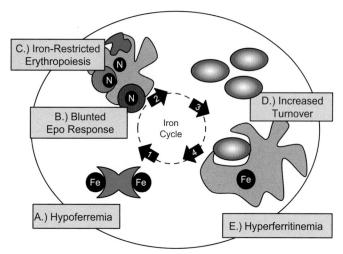

Figure 21.1 Pathophysiology of anemia of chronic inflammation (ACI). Transferrin-bound iron[1] is the primary iron source for developing erythrocytes, which produce hemoglobin.[2] The iron from heme in hemoglobin of senescent red blood cells[3] must be recovered by macrophages after erythrocytosis.[4] The recycled iron is released to transferrin, completing the iron cycle (represented by the dashed, inner circle). In addition to hypoferremia (A), the blunted Epo response (B) impairs survival of erythroid progenitors. Furthermore, iron-restricted erythropoiesis (C) may result in reduced erythrocyte mean cell volume if the severity or timing of iron sequestration exceeds the extent of the suppression of erythropoiesis. Poorly formed erythrocytes with increased reactive oxygen species are removed from the circulation more rapidly (D). Increased erythrocyte turnover and hepcidin-mediated iron restriction result in the accumulation of iron in macrophages and hyperferritinemia (E).

responsiveness to available EPO. A number of inflammatory cytokines [interferon γ, interleukin (IL)-1β, IL-6, tumor necrosis factor α] have been shown to directly impair formation of erythroid colony forming units or blast forming units under culture conditions,[12] but thorough clinical data supporting these in vitro observations are currently lacking. Similar effects of cytokines are likely to be active in anemia related to cancer and chronic kidney disease and may contribute to the persistence of anemia in these patients despite treatment with erythroid stimulating agents.

Iron-restricted Erythropoiesis

Hemoglobin production occurs at the erythroblast stage, largely independent of Epo.[13] Here, transferrin receptors expressed on the erythroblast cell surface acquire iron from serum transferrin. Serum iron concentration and transferrin saturation is often low in the context of ACI. This hypoferremia is thought to be a key feature of ACI that prevents the proliferation of iron-requiring pathogens.[1] In light of the suppression of erythropoiesis reviewed earlier, it might also be an adaptive response to prevent the saturation of serum transferrin in the face of declining erythropoietic output. Hypoferremia withholds iron from erythroid precursors and limits hemoglobin production, thereby contributing to ACI. However, ACI differs from iron deficiency anemia. Cartwright emphasized that ACI is only rarely microcytic and hypochromic.[2,14]

Hepcidin antimicrobial peptide is a peptide hormone, produced in the liver, that regulates serum iron levels. Hepcidin is induced in response to inflammation and binds its receptor, ferroportin, the only transporter known to facilitate cellular iron egress. With induction of hepcidin, ferroportin on the surface of macrophages and enterocytes is internalized and degraded.[15–17] This leads to decreased serum iron, accumulation of iron in macrophages, and increased serum ferritin. Ferroportin degradation also results in impaired iron absorption from duodenal enterocytes. Hepcidin is such a potent regulator of iron availability that molecules that target hepcidin are being vigorously pursued for their potential therapeutic value for ACI in multiple disease settings including chronic kidney disease and cancer.[18,19]

Turnover

In addition to impaired erythroid production, erythrocyte turnover may be increased in ACI. Poorly vascularized solid tumors and hemodialysis can physically harm erythrocytes and contribute to anemia in patients with cancer or kidney disease. Furthermore, ACI erythrocytes may have cell-intrinsic deficiencies that reduce their survival in circulation, such as increased reactive oxygen species or poorly formed membrane or cytoskeleton. Macrophages of the spleen, which survey circulating erythrocytes for aged or damaged cells, may also be overly active in response to inflammatory cytokines or infection.

While macrophages may be responsible for increased erythrocyte turnover, they also contribute to the hyperferritinemia observed in ACI. Macrophages secrete ferritin as part of the acute phase response.[20] This may be the direct result of inflammation-mediated transcriptional control or related to hepcidin-mediated iron accumulation.

Clinical Presentation

For epidemiologic studies, ACI has often been broadly defined as anemia in the setting of inflammation. In clinical practice, however, it is most often diagnosed in the context of a defined disease process. The anemia is usually hypoproliferative (evidenced by low reticulocytes); normocytic and normochromic; accompanied by low serum iron despite normal iron stores; with normal to elevated serum ferritin.[1] ACI is most likely to be detected in the most severely affected patients at the initial disease presentation. It usually resolves with effective treatment of the underlying disease but may reappear with relapse.

An important 1989 study by Cash and Sears in hospitalized patients illustrates some common uncertainty in regard to the presentation and diagnosis of ACI. Beyond the 90 patients in their study admitted to the hospital with defined ACI, an additional 48 patients in their study had anemia and infections, inflammatory disease, malignancies, or renal insufficiency but lacked laboratory values consistent with their definition of ACI. Twenty-seven patients had laboratory values inconsistent with ACI, iron deficiency anemia, renal insufficiency, or malignancy but had nonclassical underlying inflammatory conditions, such as congestive heart failure. While these patients were not followed to determine whether the anemia improved after resolution of the underlying inflammatory insult, it suggests some canonical features of ACI, such as hypoferremia or hyperferritinemia, may be transient over the disease course or limited to a subset of underlying diseases.[21]

Diagnostic Evaluation and Lab Findings

A complete blood count with red blood cell indices is instrumental for the assessment of ACI. Hemoglobin should be evaluated in light of the patient's age, sex, and race. ACI is most often normocytic and normochromic. In the absence of very long-standing disease, hypochromia and microcytosis suggest iron deficiency or ACI mixed with iron deficiency. Reticulocyte hemoglobin content and soluble transferrin receptor can also be useful when evaluating overlap with iron deficiency.[22] Soluble transferrin receptor is produced when erythroid progenitors have completed hemoglobin production and shed transferrin receptor from their cell surface. It is increased in response to iron deficiency and in cases of expanded erythropoiesis related to hemolysis or the use of erythroid stimulating agents.[23] Serum ferritin will be normal to elevated in ACI.[1] The ratio of soluble transferrin receptor to the log of ferritin is useful to discriminate between anemia related to iron deficiency and anemia related to chronic inflammation, because iron deficiency will result in increased soluble transferrin receptor and decreased ferritin, while ACI will result in increased soluble transferrin receptor and increased ferritin. We have included several common clinical diagnostics and their utility in Table 21.2.

Treatment and Prognosis

Treatment of the underlying inflammatory disease should be the first step in the management of ACI. However, for patients with multiple chronic disorders, very severe or refractory disease, this can be a difficult task. Neither oral nor parenteral iron has proven to be of much benefit in ACI unless there is significant overlap of absolute or functional iron deficiency. Modulation of iron availability through the use of hepcidin antagonists awaits adequate clinical trial data in relevant populations. Such treatments may put subjects at increased risk for infections. A critical evaluation of infection rates with the use of these treatments will be highly important.

Several small studies have assessed the utility of erythroid stimulating agents (ESAs) to improve hemoglobin during ACI. A Cochrane review of ESA use for anemic RA patients found no significant improvement in hemoglobin concentration or quality of life.[24] Similarly, the data for transfusion or ESA treatment of critically ill patients has not provided convincing evidence that these treatments improve survival or functional outcomes.[10]

Table 21.2. Clinical diagnostics

Diagnostic	Findings for ACI [1,22]	Overlaps with
Hemoglobin (g/dL)	Mild to moderately reduced	Any anemia
Red cell count (M/mcL)	Low	Hypoproliferative anemias (e.g., aplastic anemia, myelodysplastic syndrome)
Mean cell volume (fL)	Normocytic to mildly microcytic	Iron deficiency anemia
Reticulocytes (%)	Inappropriately low on correction	All hypoproliferative anemias
Reticulocyte hemoglobin content (pg)	Early indicator of iron-restricted erythropoiesis (<28)	Iron deficiency anemia
Transferrin saturation (%)	Hypoferremia (<16)	Iron deficiency anemia
Serum ferritin (ng/ml)	Normal (>30) to high	Thalassemia
Soluble transferrin receptor/log serum ferritin	Low, reflects reduced erythroid response (<0.8–1)	Hypoproliferative anemias

Case Study

A 79-year-old African American female is referred to a hematology clinic for evaluation of progressive anemia over several years. She has multiple medical comorbidities including hypertension, diabetes managed with oral medications, chronic obstructive pulmonary disease, and mild congestive heart failure with preserved ejection fraction requiring intermittent diuretics.

A review of her labs shows a normal baseline hemoglobin of 13 g/dL about 6 years ago, but it dropped to around 10–11 g/dL 3 years prior to presentation and now runs in the 8.5–9.5 g/dl range. Her Hemoglobin A1C was 7.5% at last check, indicating poor blood sugar control. Additional laboratory workup demonstrates normal serum vitamin B12 and folate levels, liver, kidney, and thyroid function. The total white cell count, differential, and platelet counts are within normal limits. The MCV has been running in the low 80 fL range more recently, a significant reduction from a baseline in the low 90 fL when her hemoglobin was normal. Recent iron studies have revealed low serum iron of 36 mcg/dL, while serum transferrin saturation has also been low at just 8% despite more than a year of daily oral iron prescribed by her internist. The ferritin was 128 ng/ml (normal 30–150); therefore not indicative of depleted total body marrow iron stores.

(a)　　　　　　　　　　　　　　　　　　　　(b)

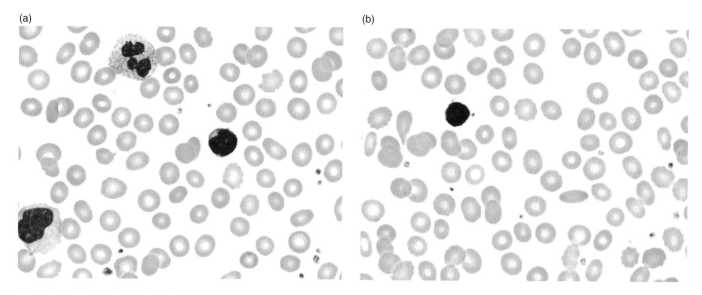

Figure 21.2 Case study: Peripheral blood smear. Two separate fields (a) and (b), in the blood smear show reticulocytopenia, anisopoikilocytosis with few echinocytes. The red cells are a mixture of mildly microcytic to normocytic forms (compare with size of a normal lymphocyte), while the white cell and platelet populations are unremarkable.

(cont.)

On exam, the patient exhibits mild conjunctival pallor, and no source of bleeding has been found on prior upper and lower gastrointestinal endoscopies. Her hematologist conducts additional lab testing to elucidate the etiology of the anemia and finds a hypoproliferative process, with reticulocytes comprising just 1% (uncorrected) of her red cell population and an inappropriately low absolute reticulocyte count of just 40k/cu mm. A gammopathy evaluation proves unremarkable.

The blood smear (Figure 21.2) shows reticulocytopenia and mild anisopoikilocytosis (red cell distribution width 15%). The red cells are a mixture of mildly microcytic to normocytic forms, while the white cell and platelet populations are unremarkable.

Acknowledgments

We regret that, due to space limitations, we were unable to cite the majority of the primary literature that has contributed to the advancements in our understanding of the pathogenesis, diagnosis, and treatment of ACI. We encourage the reader to seek additional information in the references of the many reviews cited here.

References

1. Weiss G, Goodnough LT. Anemia of chronic disease. *N Engl J Med.* 2005; 352 (10):1011–1023.

2. Cartwright GE, Lauritsen MA, Jones PJ, Merrill IM, Wintrobe MM. The anemia of infection. I. Hypoferremia, hypercupremia, and alterations in porphyrin metabolism in patients. *J Clin Invest.* 1946; 25(1):65–80.

3. Blanc B, et al. Nutritional anaemias. Report of a WHO scientific group. *World Health Organization Technical Report Series.* 1968; 405:5–37.

4. Yip R, Dallman PR. The roles of inflammation and iron deficiency as causes of anemia. *Am J Clin Nutr.* 1988; 48(5):1295–1300. Epub 1988/11/01.

5. Guralnik JM, Eisenstaedt RS, Ferrucci L, Klein HG, and Woodman RC. Prevalence of anemia in persons 65 years and older in the United States: evidence for a high rate of unexplained anemia. *Blood.* 2004; 104(8):2263–2268.

6. Masson C. Rheumatoid anemia. *Joint Bone Spine.* 2011; 78(2):131–137. Epub 2010/09/21.

7. Wilson A, Reyes E, Ofman J. Prevalence and outcomes of anemia in inflammatory bowel disease: a systematic review of the literature. *Am J Med.* 2004; 116 Suppl 7A:44S–49S.

8. Piagnerelli M, Vincent JL. The use of erythropoiesis-stimulating agents in the intensive care unit. *Crit Care Clin.* 2012; 28(3):345–362, v. Epub 2012/06/21.

9. van Iperen CE, van de Wiel A, Marx JJ. Acute event-related anaemia. *Br J Haematol.* 2001; 115(4):739–743. Epub 2002/02/15.

10. Sihler KC, Napolitano LM. Anemia of inflammation in critically ill patients. *J Intensive Care Med.* 2008; 23(5): 295–302. Epub 2008/08/15.

11. Baer AN, Dessypris EN, Goldwasser E, Krantz SB. Blunted erythropoietin response to anaemia in rheumatoid arthritis. *Br J Haematol.* 1987; 66(4): 559–564.

12. Means RT, Jr., Krantz SB. Progress in understanding the pathogenesis of the anemia of chronic disease. *Blood.* 1992; 80(7):1639–1647.

13. Koury MJ, Ponka P. New insights into erythropoiesis: the roles of folate, vitamin B12, and iron. *Annu Rev Nutr.* 2004; 24:105–131.

14. Cartwright GE, Lee GR. The anaemia of chronic disorders. *Br J Haematol.*

1971; 21(2):147–152. Epub 1971/08/01.

15. Nemeth E, et al. Hepcidin regulates cellular iron efflux by binding to ferroportin and inducing its internalization. *Science*. 2004; 306(5704): 2090–2093.

16. Qiao B, et al. Hepcidin-induced endocytosis of ferroportin is dependent on ferroportin ubiquitination. *Cell Metab*. 2012; 15(6):918–924. Epub 2012/06/12.

17. Ross SL, et al. Molecular mechanism of hepcidin-mediated ferroportin internalization requires ferroportin lysines, not tyrosines or JAK-STAT. *Cell Metab*. 2012; 15(6):905–917. Epub 2012/06/12.

18. Ganz T, Nemeth E. The hepcidin-ferroportin system as a therapeutic target in anemias and iron overload disorders. *Hematol Am Soc Hematol Educ Program*. 2011; 2011:538–542. Epub 2011/12/14.

19. Schwoebel F, et al. The effects of the anti-hepcidin Spiegelmer NOX H94 on inflammation-induced anemia in cynomolgus monkeys. *Blood*. 2013; 121(12):2311–2315. Epub 2013/01/26.

20. Wang W, Knovich MA, Coffman LG, Torti FM, Torti SV. Serum ferritin: past, present and future. *Biochim Biophys Acta*. 2010; 1800(8):760–769. Epub 2010/03/23.

21. Cash JM, Sears DA. The anemia of chronic disease: spectrum of associated diseases in a series of unselected hospitalized patients. *Am J Med*. 1989; 87(6):638–644.

22. Roy CN. Anemia of inflammation. *Hematology Am Soc Hematol Educ Program*. 2010; 30:276–280.

23. Skikne BS. Serum transferrin receptor. *Am J Hematol*. 2008; 83(11):872–85.

24. Marti-Carvajal AJ, Agreda-Perez LH, Sola I, Simancas-Racines D. Erythropoiesis-stimulating agents for anemia in rheumatoid arthritis. *Cochrane Database Syst Rev*. 2013; 2: CD000332. Epub 2013/03/02.

25. Dallman PR, Yip R, Johnson C. Prevalence and causes of anemia in the United States, 1976 to 1980. *Am J Clin Nutr*. 1984; 39(3):437–445. Epub 1984/03/01.

26. Price EA, Mehra R, Holmes TH, Schrier SL. Anemia in older persons: etiology and evaluation. *Blood Cells Mol Dis*. 2011; 46(2):159–165. Epub 2011/01/07.

27. Artz AS, Thirman MJ. Unexplained anemia predominates despite an intensive evaluation in a racially diverse cohort of older adults from a referral anemia clinic. *J Gerontol A Biol Sci Med Sci*. 2011; 66(8):925–932. Epub 2011 Jun 9.

28. Voulgarelis M, Kokori SI, Ioannidis JP, Tzioufas AG, Kyriaki D, Moutsopoulos HM. Anaemia in systemic lupus erythematosus: aetiological profile and the role of erythropoietin. *Ann Rheum Dis*. 2000; 59(3):217–222.

29. Martinez-Lado L, et al. Relapses and recurrences in giant cell arteritis: a population-based study of patients with biopsy-proven disease from northwestern Spain. *Medicine (Baltimore)*. 2011; 90(3):186–193. Epub 2011/04/23.

30. Vincent JL, et al. Anemia and blood transfusion in critically ill patients. *J Am Med Assoc*. 2002; 288 (12):1499–1507. Epub 2002/09/24.

Chapter

22

Myelodysplasia

Ida Wong-Sefidan, MD, and Rafael Bejar, MD, PhD

Case: *Mr. Jones is a 67-year-old man experiencing fatigue and dyspnea on exertion. He is found to have a macrocytic anemia, leukopenia, and thrombocytopenia. His primary care physician is concerned this might be due to a myelodysplastic syndrome.*

Introduction

Myelodysplastic syndromes (**MDS**) are a diverse group of clonal hematologic disorders characterized by ineffective production of blood cells in the bone marrow, cytopenias of the peripheral blood, and increased risk of progression to acute myeloid leukemia (AML). MDS patients often suffer from anemia but can have neutropenia and/or thrombocytopenia. Diagnosing MDS can be challenging because dysplasia of the marrow can be observed in a variety of benign conditions as well as in other bone marrow failure syndromes (Figure 22.1).

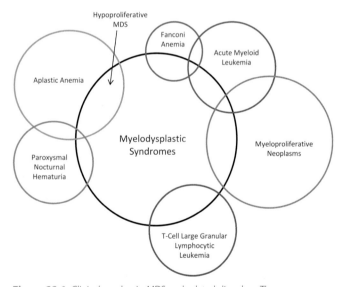

Figure 22.1 Clinical overlap in MDS and related disorders. The myelodysplastic syndromes (MDS) are a diverse collection of disorders that can clinically overlap with other clonal diseases, bone marrow failure syndromes, and immune-mediated cytopenias.

Epidemiology

MDS are largely diseases of older individuals. Approximately 86% of cases are diagnosed in patients over 60 years of age, with a median age of 72 years.[1] Men are more frequently affected than women (1.7:1 ratio).[2] There are an estimated 45,000 new cases of MDS diagnosed per year, making it the most common myeloid disorder in the elderly.[3] This incidence appears to be growing as our population ages.[2]

The etiology of *de novo*, or primary, MDS is not well understood. Environmental risk factors for MDS include smoking and exposure to solvents and agricultural chemicals. Prior exposures to ionizing radiation or chemotherapy are well-established risk factors for the development of therapy-related, or secondary MDS (t-MDS). Therapy-related MDS can occur at a much younger age and carries a worse prognosis compared with primary disease. Median time to onset varies upon the type and dose of exposure but typically occurs 1 to 7 years after treatment.[4]

MDS are uncommon in children and adolescents and may represent a different etiology in this population. Pediatric MDS account for less than 10% of childhood hematological malignancies and are frequently heritable or associated with other disorders (Table 22.1). Variable risks of myelodysplasia are seen in congenital syndromes such as Fanconi anemia, dyskeratosis congenita, and MonoMAC syndrome.[5–7] Therefore, obtaining a detailed family history, performing a careful physical exam, and testing for inherited bone marrow failure syndromes is mandatory in younger MDS patients (age <40) prior to treatment with chemotherapy or stem cell transplantation.

Pathophysiology

MDS are clonal disorders of genetically abnormal hematopoietic stem cells. Genetic abnormalities are acquired and promote the clonal expansion of disease stem cells. Somatic mutations drive clonal dominance and result in impaired differentiation, while secondary immune, cytokine, and stromal responses can alter the bone marrow microenvironment and suppress the function of normal hematopoietic stem cells and their differentiating progeny.[8] Subsequent evolution of disease subclones with additional mutations can lead to progression or transformation into acute leukemia.[9]

Table 22.1. Risk factors for the development of MDS

Environmental
　Increasing age
　DNA alkylating agents
　Topoisomerase II inhibitors
　Ionizing radiation
　Occupational exposures (benzene, hydrocarbons)
　Agricultural chemicals (pesticides)
　Smoking

Antecedent Hematologic Disorders
　Aplastic anemia
　Paroxysmal nocturnal hemoglobinuria

Congenital Bone Marrow Failure and Myeloid Malignancy Predisposition Syndromes
　Dyskeratosis congenita (*DKC1, TERC, TERT, TINF2* mutations)
　Shwachman-Diamond syndrome (*SBDS* mutations)
　Severe congenital neutropenia (*ELANE, HAX1, GFI1, G6PC3, WAS* mutations)
　MonoMAC syndrome (*GATA2* mutations)
　Fanconi anemia (*FANC* gene family mutations)
　Familial platelet disorders (*RUNX1, ANKRD26* mutations)
　Late-onset familial MDS/AML (*DDX41* mutations)
　Telomere deficiency–associated familial MDS (*TERC, TERT* mutations)
　Li-Fraumeni syndrome (*TP53* abnormalities)
　Bloom syndrome (*BLM* mutations)
　Ataxia-telangiectasia (*ATM* mutations)

Table 22.2. Common genetic abnormalities in MDS

Chromosomal Abnormalities	Freq. (%)	Prognostic Association
Normal	49	Favorable
Isolated del(5q)	6	Favorable
+8	5	Intermediate
−7/del(7q)	4	Poor
del(20q)	2	Favorable
-Y	2	Favorable
Others (2 chromosomal abnormalities)	11	Intermediate
Complex (≥3 chromosomal abnormalities, no chromosome 5 and/or 7 abnormalities)	4	Poor
Complex (≥3 chromosomal abnormalities, chromosome 5 and/or 7 abnormalities)	15	Very poor

Gene mutations	Freq. (%)	Prognostic Association
TET2	25	Neutral
SF3B1	25	Favorable
ASXL1	15	Poor
SRSF2	14	Poor
U2AF1	12	Poor
RUNX1	9	Poor
TP53	8	Very poor
EZH2	6	Very poor
NRAS	4	Poor
JAK2	3	Neutral
ETV6	3	Poor
CBL	2	Neutral

Acquired chromosomal abnormalities can be identified in 50% of *de novo* MDS and 80% of those with therapy-related disease.[10] Recurrent chromosomal abnormalities are most often deletions of chromosomes or chromosome segments, suggesting that loss of genes located at these sites contributes to abnormal differentiation and clonal dominance. Many karyotype abnormalities have prognostic and predictive value. For example, loss of the long arm of chromosome 5 (del[5q]) is associated with a more favorable prognosis and predicts response to the oral immunomodulatory agent lenalidomide.[11] (Table 22.2).

The large number of potential chromosomal abnormalities and the number of patients with normal karyotypes indicate that there is no single molecular mechanism that leads to MDS. More sensitive techniques can identify additional abnormalities not detectable with a standard karyotype. Microdeletions and point mutations of single genes are common in MDS, with more than 90% of patients carrying a mutation in one or more of the most frequently mutated genes.[12–14]

Recurrently mutated genes have implicated several molecular mechanisms in the development of MDS. These include changes in epigenetic regulating enzymes and alterations to mRNA splicing factors. Each of these pathways is mutated in more than 50% of patients (Table 22.2).[15,16] The *TP53* gene is mutated or deleted in 10–15% of cases, particularly those with prior exposure to alkylating agents or radiation. *TP53* abnormalities are strongly associated with the presence of multiple cytogenetic abnormalities and may drive the negative prognosis associated with these highly abnormal karyotypes.[17] While not yet standard of care, testing for somatic mutations in MDS genes is increasingly available to clinicians and can be used to aid in the diagnosis, prediction of prognosis, and classification of MDS.

Clinical Presentation

Presenting symptoms for MDS patients, like those experienced by Mr. Jones in our example, are often nonspecific and depend upon the type and severity of their cytopenias. Anemia is the most common cytopenia. Anemic patients may complain of fatigue, exercise intolerance, and lightheadedness. Neutropenic patients may have recurrent or unusually severe infections. Thrombocytopenic patients may complain of easy bruising or, in rare cases, spontaneous bleeding. However, many patients do not have severe symptoms and are identified by routine blood counts.[6]

Diagnostic Evaluation

The goal of the initial evaluation is to identify elements of the diagnosis as well as to exclude alternative, and often reversible, causes of cytopenias. A comprehensive history of medications, toxin exposures, alcohol use, radiation, and prior chemotherapy should be obtained. A physical exam is necessary but generally nonrevealing. Hepatomegaly and splenomegaly are uncommon in MDS compared with myeloproliferative neoplasms.[6]

Initial laboratory findings can be variable, as MDS encompass a heterogeneous group of diseases. Abnormalities can range from a slowly progressing anemia over years to multiple cytopenias developing after only a few months (Table 22.3).[6] While specific cutpoints for cytopenias are useful for predicting prognosis, any blood count that is below the lower limit of normal is sufficient to meet the cytopenia criteria for an initial diagnosis of MDS. (18) When anemia is present, the reticulocyte count is inappropriately low, indicating ineffective RBC production. Anemias of inadequate production, such as iron deficiency, B12 or folate deficiency, and erythropoietin deficiency from chronic renal disease ,must be excluded.[6]

Case: *Repeat blood tests one week later confirm that Mr. Jones has a low hemoglobin (9.8 g/dL), low white blood cell count (3.1 × 10⁹/L, 47% neutrophils), and a low platelet count (77 × 10⁹/L).*

Table 22.3. Minimal diagnostic criteria for MDS

Minimal Diagnostic Criteria for MDS

Prerequisite criteria[a]	Constant cytopenia (value below the lower limit of normal) in one or more cell lineages
	Exclusion of all other hematopoietic or nonhematopoietic disorders as primary reason for cytopenia/dysplasia
MDS-related (decisive) criteria	Dysplasia in at least 10% of erythroid, neutrophilic, or megakaryocytic cells in the bone marrow aspirate, or
	>15% ring sideroblasts (iron stain), or
	5–14% ring sideroblasts and a typical *SF3B1* mutation, or
	5–19% blast cells in bone marrow smears, or
	Typical chromosomal abnormality (by karyotyping or FISH)

[a] Both prerequisite criteria and at least one decisive criterion are required

Case: *His reticulocyte count is low, and tests for common causes of anemia are unremarkable. He is not taking any suspect medications and denies alcohol use. Dysplastic cells similar to those shown in Figure 22.2 are noted on his blood smear.*

A peripheral blood smear may sometimes demonstrate dysplasia. The most common red blood cell findings are anisocytosis, poikilocytosis, and oval macrocytes. Occasionally, microcytic red blood cells or a dimorphic population of macrocytic and microcytic cells can be seen. Hypogranular neutrophils can be present, as can dysplastic, hypolobated neutrophils, such as pseudo-Pelger-Huet cells. An increased%age of eosinophils or basophils is not uncommon. Platelets can demonstrate hypogranulation (Figure 22.2).[19]

After excluding reversible causes of cytopenias, patients are typically referred to a hematologist for further evaluation and to obtain bone marrow biopsy and aspiration, if indicated. The biopsy and aspirate are required to make the diagnosis of MDS and can identify other causes of cytopenias such as aplastic anemia and myelofibrosis, which may present clinically like MDS.[19]

Case: *Mr. Jones's bone marrow biopsy is 80% cellular. The aspirate shows dysplasia in myeloid, erythroid, and megakaryocyte lineages similar to that shown in Figure 22.3. Bone marrow blasts are elevated at 8% of cells and demonstrate abnormal antigen expression by flow cytometry. Trisomy 8 is noted in 12 out of 20 metaphases.*

The bone marrow is typically hypercellular for age, although it can be normocellular or even hypocellular in 20% of patients. Dysplasia involving >10% of cells in a myeloid lineage in the bone marrow aspirate is the decisive criterion for MDS (Table 22.3, Figure 22.3).[6,20] An increase in the proportion of myeloblasts can be observed in the aspirate and is important for both the classification and risk assessment of MDS. A myeloblast % age of ≥20% is diagnostic of AML and is not considered MDS even if dysplasia is present.

The aspirate is used to determine the karyotype of diseased cells. Acquired chromosomal abnormalities indicate the presence of clonal hematopoiesis and can support the diagnosis, although more than 50% of patients with MDS have a normal disease karyotype.

Several cytogenetic changes, including del(5q), −7, del(7q), and idic(X)(q13), are considered presumptive evidence of MDS, while others, such as del(20q) and +8, are also found in related disorders and not considered diagnostic of MDS by themselves.[20]

Gene mutations are frequent and important to the progression and outcomes of MDS. Germline predisposition mutations are not infrequent and should be considered in those with a family history, young at age of diagnosis, or associated syndromic features. However, most mutations are acquired. By

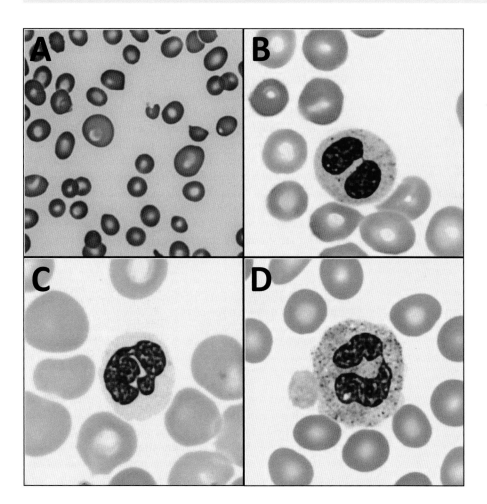

Figure 22.2 Peripheral blood dysplasia.
(A) Dimorphic red cell populations with marked poikilocytosis and anisocytosis. (B) Neutrophil with hypolobated nuclei, resulting in the pseudo-Pelger-Huet anomaly. (C) Hypogranular neutrophil. (D) Hypogranular platelet (next to a normally granulated neutrophil).

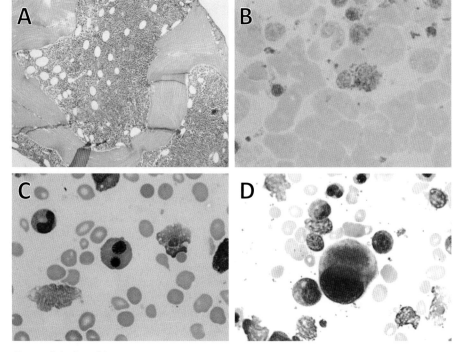

Figure 22.3 Bone marrow dysplasia.
(A) Hypercellular bone marrow biopsy. (B) Ringed sideroblasts visible on iron stain. (C) Bone marrow aspirate with erythroid multinucleation. (D) Micromegakaryocyte with an eccentric, hypolobulated nucleus.

Hypercellular Bone Marrow
Ring Sideroblasts
Erythroid Dysplasia
Megakaryocyte Dysplasia

Table 22.4. World Health Organization (WHO) classification for MDS and MDS/MPN

Myelodysplastic Syndromes (MDS)

MDS with single-lineage dysplasia (MDS-SLD)

MDS with ring sideroblasts (MDS-RS):
 MDS-RS and single-lineage dysplasia (MDS-RS-SLD)
 MDS-RS and multilineage dysplasia (MDS-RS-MLD)

MDS with multilineage dysplasia (MDS-MLD)

MDS with excess blasts:
 MDS with excess blasts-1 (MDS-EB-1)
 MDS with excess blasts-2 (MDS-EB-2)

MDS with isolated del(5q)

MDS, unclassifiable (MDS-U)

Provisional entity: Refractory cytopenia of childhood

Myeloid neoplasms with germline predisposition

Myelodysplastic/Myeloproliferative Neoplasms (MDS/MPN)

Chronic myelomonocytic leukemia (CMML)

Atypical chronic myeloid leukemia, *BCR-ABL1*–negative (aCML)

Juvenile myelomonocytic leukemia (JMML)

MDS/MPN with ringed sideroblasts and thrombocytosis (MDS/MPN-RS-T)

MDS/MPN, unclassifiable

current criteria, somatic mutations are not considered diagnostic of MDS, with the sole exception of mutations in the splicing factor *SF3B1*. Typical mutations of *SF3B1* in cytopenic patients with at least 5% ring sideroblasts are considered diagnostic of MDS.[20,21]

Additional tests on the aspirate that may be useful in certain clinical settings include flow cytometry to assess for paroxysmal nocturnal hemoglobinuria and large granular lymphocytic disease. *JAK2* mutation testing in patients with thrombocytosis and genetic testing for younger patients with a history of familial cytopenias may also be appropriate.[22]

The diagnosis of MDS occasionally can be problematic due to the subjective nature of the morphologic diagnostic criteria. Nearly 40% of patients with unexplained cytopenias who do not meet morphologic criteria for MDS will have somatic mutations common in MDS and can be described as having clonal cytopenias of undetermined significance (CCUS). These patients may be at high risk of progressing to MDS or AML. Detection of CCUS merits careful observation and may allow for future intervention to prevent progression.[23,24]

Classification and Prognosis

The overall survival of MDS patients is poor, with an estimated 3-year survival rate of 35%. Those who are diagnosed at a later age have an appreciably inferior survival. However, survival rates vary widely by clinical subtype and risk features.

MDS subtypes are defined by the 2016 revision to the World Health Organization (WHO) classification of myeloid neoplasms and acute leukemia. The WHO classification is largely based on the type of morphologic dysplasia present, the number of lines affected, and the proportion of blasts in the aspirate. It classifies patients into MDS subtypes that may share molecular and clinically important features such as prognosis and risk of transformation to AML. Patients with both dysplastic and proliferative features, like those seen in chronic myelomonocytic leukemia (CMML), are considered to have MDS/MPN overlap syndromes that should be distinguished from those with MDS (Table 22.4).[20]

> **Case:** *Based on his bone marrow findings, Mr. Jones is diagnosed with the MDS-EB-I subtype of MDS. His clinical and cytogenetic features place him in the Intermediate-2 risk group of the original International Prognostic Scoring System (IPSS) and in the high-risk group of the revised IPSS (IPSS-R).*

Treatments for MDS are tailored to the predicted prognosis of each patient, making accurate risk stratification a critical component of care. The criteria considered by the WHO classification for MDS are prognostic risk factors.[20] However, the WHO classification does not include all of the potentially prognostic information available to clinicians. Therefore, separate risk-assessment tools for MDS have been developed.

The International Prognostic Scoring System (IPSS) was developed in 1997 and has been the standard for MDS risk assessment. It was used to define patient populations in clinical trials and is the basis for risk-adapted therapy in consensus practice guidelines. The IPSS considers three risk factors: bone marrow blast proportion, cytogenetic abnormalities, and the number of peripheral cytopenias present. Based on these features, patients are assigned to one of four risk groups (Table 22.5).[25] Despite its utility, the IPSS has several recognized limitations, including the potential to underestimate disease risk in many IPSS "lower-"risk patients.[26,27]

A revision to the IPSS (IPSS-R) that addresses some of these limitations was released in 2012. The IPSS-R considers the same features as the IPSS, but in greater detail. Many more chromosomal abnormalities are explicitly included and are more finely stratified according to their associated risk. Blast proportions were revised to exclude patients with $\geq 20\%$ blasts (redefined as AML by WHO criteria). Cytopenias are considered individually, with additional weight given for increased severity. Finally, patients are assigned to one of five risk groups with cutoffs adjusted for patient age (Table 22.6).[28] It is important to note that both the IPSS and IPSS-R were created by examining cohorts of patients that never

Table 22.5. International Prognostic Scoring System (IPSS)(25)

Prognostic Variable	Point Values				
	0	0.5	1	1.5	2.0
Bone marrow blasts (%)	<5	5–10		11–20	21–30
Karyotype *	Good	Intermediate	Poor		
Cytopenias **	0–1	2–3			

* Karyotype definitions:
   Good: Normal; -Y; del(5q); del(20q)
   Poor: Complex (≥3 abnormalities); abnormal chromosome 7
   Intermediate: All others
** Cytopenia definitions:
   Hemoglobin <10 g/dL (100 g/L)
   Absolute neutrophil count <1.8×10^9/L
   Platelet count <100×10^9/L

Risk Categories	Total Points	Median Survival (Years)	Time Until 25% Develop Leukemia (Years)
Low	0	5.7	9.4
Intermediate-1	0.5–1	3.5	3.1
Intermediate-2	1.5–2	1.2	1.1
High	≥2.5	0.4	0.2

Table 22.6. Revised International Prognostic Scoring System (IPSS-R)(28)

Prognostic Variable	Point Values						
	0	0.5	1.0	1.5	2.0	3.0	4.0
Cytogenetics *	Very good		Good		Intermediate	Poor	Very poor
Bone marrow blast (%)	≤2		>2 to <5		5 to 10	>10	
Hemoglobin (g/dL)	≥10		8 to <10	<8			
Platelets (×10^9/L)	≥100	50 to 100	<50				
Absolute neutrophil count (×10^9/L)	≥0.8	<0.8					

* Cytogenetic definitions:
   Very good: -Y, del(11q)
   Good: Normal, del(5q), del(12p), del(20q), double including del(5q)
   Intermediate: del(7q), +8, +19, i(17q), any other single or double independent clones
   Poor: -7, inv[3]/t(3q)/del(3q), double including -7/del(7q), complex: 3 abnormalities
   Very poor: Complex: >3 abnormalities

Risk Categories	Total Points	Median Survival (years)	Time Until 25% Develop Leukemia (Years)
Very low	≤1.5	8.8	>14.5
Low	>1.5 to 3.0	5.3	10.8
Intermediate	>3.0 to 4.5	3.0	3.2
High	>4.5 to 6	1.6	1.4
Very high	>6	0.8	0.7

received disease-modifying agents such as immunomodulatory drugs, hypomethylating agents, chemotherapy, or stem cell transplantation. Therefore the estimates of overall survival are useful to understand the risks of not treating patients with these agents but may not be accurate estimates of outcomes for patients who are treated.

Somatic mutations can have independent prognostic implications that refine how patients are risk stratified. Mutations in several genes, like *TP53*, are consistently adverse, while *SF3B1* mutations indicate more favorable risk. Mutations may be prognostically additive to clinically based risk assessment tools like the IPSS and IPSS-R and will be included in clinical guidelines in the future.[21,29]

Treatment

Subtype classification and determination of a patient's risk category form the basis for selecting a treatment plan. Other factors such as age, performance status, and co-morbidities must also be taken into consideration, as these factors may limit certain treatments. In addition to a higher risk of developing AML, patients with MDS have a greater prevalence of diabetes, cardiac events, and infections when age-adjusted and compared to the general population.[3]

All patients should receive appropriate supportive care tailored to their needs (Figure 22.4). This includes packed red blood cell (pRBC) and platelet transfusions for symptomatic anemia and bleeding prophylaxis, respectively. Leukocyte-reduced blood products are recommended for MDS patients, and those who are potentially transplant candidates should receive leukocyte-reduced, irradiated products.[22] Prophylactic antibiotics are not routinely used for neutropenic patients, although they may be appropriate in cases of recurrent infections and during treatment with hypomethylating agents or high-dose intensive therapy.

Lower-Risk Patients (IPSS Low and Intermediate-1)

Many patients with lower-risk disease are asymptomatic and do not need treatment. A "watch-and-wait" strategy of monitoring blood counts at regular intervals or when symptoms arise would be most appropriate for these patients. Treatment of lower-risk MDS should be considered when there are clinically significant cytopenias requiring frequent transfusions, or neutropenia or thrombocytopenia resulting in complications such as recurrent infections or bleeding, respectively. The main goal in lower-risk patients is to improve quality of life by minimizing symptoms caused by cytopenias and the interventions required to address them.

Lenalidomide is an oral immunomodulatory derivative of thalidomide that is highly active in MDS patients that carry a del(5q) abnormality. More than 70% of del(5q) patients will respond to lenalidomide, with many demonstrating a major cytogenetic marrow response and normalization of their peripheral blood counts. The median duration of transfusion independence in responding patients is 2 years, and side effects are typically transient (neutropenia, thrombocytopenia) or manageable (gastrointestinal, rash, fatigue). As a single agent, lenalidomide is less effective in del(5q) patients with multiple additional cytogenetic abnormalities or higher-risk disease and in patients without del(5q).[11]

For lower-risk patients without del(5q), the first line of treatment often involves an erythropoiesis-stimulating agent

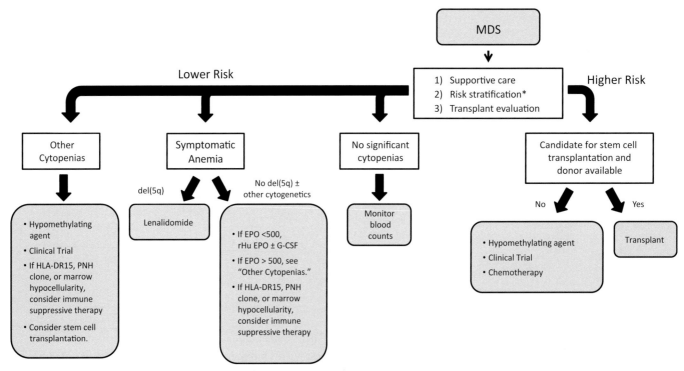

Figure 22.4 Risk-adjusted schema for management of MDS.
* Risk stratification can be based on IPSS or IPSS-R: Lower Risk = Low or Intermediate-1 by IPSS or Very Low, Low, or Intermediate by the IPSS-R.

(ESA). These synthetic erythropoietins (EPOs) are effective in nearly 75% of patients requiring <2 units of pRBCs per month and with endogenous EPO levels <500 U/L. Therefore, it is valuable to check EPO levels in patients before they are first transfused. More heavily transfused patients with EPO levels >500 U/L have less than a 10% likelihood of response.[30] Adequate iron stores are required for a response to ESAs and should be checked before these drugs are first administered. A significant fraction of patients who fail to respond or lose their response to ESAs can achieve a response with the addition of a granulocyte colony–stimulating factor (G-CSF).[31] G-CSF is not routinely used to treat neutropenia but may be used in patients with fungal or recurrent bacterial infections.

The next treatment to consider in lower-risk MDS is immune suppressive therapy (IST) with anti-thymocyte globulin (ATG) and cyclosporine.[32] Some patients with MDS will have disease features suggestive of autoimmune disruption of hematopoiesis like that seen in aplastic anemia. These features include a hypocellular bone marrow and the presence of a paroxysmal nocturnal hemoglobinuria (PNH) clone. Other factors that may predict a favorable response to IST include having the HLA-DR15 haplotype, younger age, and recent onset of transfusion dependence. ATG is given with glucocorticoids in the inpatient setting, followed by daily cyclosporine dosed to appropriate blood levels. Meaningful responses may take several months to manifest and can be expected in about 30% of cases.

Thrombopoietin (TPO)-receptor agonists such as romipolostim and eltrombopag are FDA-approved stimulators of platelet production currently being studied in lower-risk MDS patients but are not yet part of the standard of care.

Lower-risk patients with longer life expectancy and transfusion dependence are at risk of developing iron overload. Iron overload can impair hepatic, cardiac, and endocrine function and is a risk factor for shorter overall survival and adverse outcomes after HSCT. If iron overload is not just a marker of more advanced disease but contributes directly to the risk of death from MDS, chelation may be able to improve outcomes for patients with elevated iron levels. Recent studies have suggested both a survival advantage and hematologic benefit in some patients after several months of chelation therapy.[33] Deferoxamine (intramuscular or subcutaneous injections), deferasirox (oral), and deferiprone (oral) are iron chelators approved for use in MDS. Barriers to their use include bothersome side effects, cost, and the potential for various organ toxicities. Which patients to treat and when to start are not well defined. National Comprehensive Cancer Network (NCCN) guidelines recommend that iron chelation be considered for low- or intermediate-risk patients who have or will likely be receiving >20 units of packed red blood cells or have a ferritin >2,500. The goal is to bring the ferritin down to <1,000.[22]

Higher-Risk Patients (IPSS Intermediate-2 and High Risk)

Given the poor prognosis and higher risk of AML transformation, the treatment goal for higher-risk patients is to increase overall survival. Treatment options for higher-risk patients include HSCT, high-dose cytotoxic agents, hypomethylating agents, and clinical trials. Studies examining the optimal timing for HSCT predict a net benefit for immediate transplantation in selected higher-risk patients but not in lower-risk patients.[34,35] Clinical features that influence eligibility for transplantation include age, performance status, comorbidities, psychosocial status, donor availability, social support, and patient preference. Advances in supportive care and the increased use of reduced-intensity conditioning allow for patients in their early 70s to be considered for HSCT.

Case: *Mr. Jones is evaluated for hematopoietic stem cell transplantation with reduced-intensity conditioning. While a donor is sought, he begins treatment with IV azacitidine. For the first two cycles, his blood counts fall further, and he requires two pRBC transfusions. By the beginning of cycle 4, he is no longer transfusion dependent, his platelet count rises to over 100×10^9/L, and his WBC normalizes.*

If HSCT is not an option or will be delayed, treatment with a hypomethylating agent, like azacitidine or decitabine, should be considered. Both agents are associated with similar overall response rates of nearly 50%, but only azacitidine has demonstrated a prolongation of survival in a randomized clinical trial.[36] Hypomethylating agents may take 12–16 weeks to generate a response and can worsen cytopenias before a response is seen. Observed survival in patients who do not respond or stop responding to hypomethylating agents is dismal at around 6 months.[37] High-intensity chemotherapy can be effective in certain populations; however, response and survival rates are still low. Clinical trials often represent the best option for patients with higher-risk disease.

Conclusion

MDS is a complex and heterogeneous disease with a rising incidence among our aging population. Complications from cytopenias are the most significant contributors to morbidity and mortality in MDS patients along with progression to AML for some. Risk stratification is the basis for selecting among various treatment options. Newer treatments and advances in transplantation have increased the therapeutic options for MDS patients. However, most therapies are palliative and offer only temporary responses at best. Recent discoveries about the genetic basis of MDS have improved our understanding of the pathogenesis of these disorders and can help inform clinical care decisions. These findings will help better classify and risk stratify MDS patients while building the foundation for more targeted treatments.

References

1. Sekeres MA, Schoonen WM, Kantarjian H, List A, Fryzek J, Paquette R, et al. Characteristics of US patients with myelodysplastic syndromes: results of six cross-sectional physician surveys. *Journal of the National Cancer Institute.* 2008; 100(21):1542–1551.

2. Rollison DE, Howlader N, Smith MT, Strom SS, Merritt WD, Ries LA, et al. Epidemiology of myelodysplastic syndromes and chronic myeloproliferative disorders in the United States, 2001–2004, using data from the NAACCR and SEER programs. *Blood.* 2008; 112(1):45–52.

3. Goldberg SL, Chen E, Corral M, Guo A, Mody-Patel N, Pecora AL, et al. Incidence and clinical complications of myelodysplastic syndromes among United States Medicare beneficiaries. *Journal of Clinical Oncology: Official Journal of the American Society of Clinical Oncology.* 2010; 28(17): 2847–2852.

4. Pedersen-Bjergaard J, Daugaard G, Hansen SW, Philip P, Larsen SO, Rorth M. Increased risk of myelodysplasia and leukaemia after etoposide, cisplatin, and bleomycin for germ-cell tumours. *Lancet.* 1991; 338(8763):359–363.

5. Liew E, Owen C. Familial myelodysplastic syndromes: a review of the literature. *Haematologica.* 2011; 96(10):1536–1542.

6. Hoffman R. *Hematology: Basic Principles and Practice.* 5th ed. Philadelphia, PA: Churchill Livingstone/Elsevier; 2009:xxvii, 2523.

7. Hsu AP, Sampaio EP, Khan J, Calvo KR, Lemieux JE, Patel SY, et al. Mutations in GATA2 are associated with the autosomal dominant and sporadic monocytopenia and mycobacterial infection (MonoMAC) syndrome. *Blood.* 2011; 118(10): 2653–2655.

8. Bejar R, Levine R, Ebert BL. Unraveling the molecular pathophysiology of myelodysplastic syndromes. *Journal of Clinical Oncology: Official Journal of the American Society of Clinical Oncology.* 2011; 29(5):504–515.

9. Walter MJ, Shen D, Ding L, Shao J, Koboldt DC, Chen K, et al. Clonal architecture of secondary acute myeloid leukemia. *The New England Journal of Medicine.* 2012; 366(12): 1090–1098.

10. Haase D, Germing U, Schanz J, Pfeilstocker M, Nosslinger T, Hildebrandt B, et al. New insights into the prognostic impact of the karyotype in MDS and correlation with subtypes: evidence from a core dataset of 2124 patients. *Blood.* 2007; 110(13): 4385–4395.

11. List A, Dewald G, Bennett J, Giagounidis A, Raza A, Feldman E, et al. Lenalidomide in the myelodysplastic syndrome with chromosome 5q deletion. *The New England Journal of Medicine.* 2006; 355(14):1456–1465.

12. Bejar R, Stevenson KE, Caughey BA, Abdel-Wahab O, Steensma DP, Galili N, et al. Validation of a prognostic model and the impact of mutations in patients with lower-risk myelodysplastic syndromes. *Journal of Clinical Oncology: Official Journal of the American Society of Clinical Oncology.* 2012; 30(27):3376–3382.

13. Papaemmanuil E, Gerstung M, Malcovati L, Tauro S, Gundem G, Van Loo P, et al. Clinical and biological implications of driver mutations in myelodysplastic syndromes. *Blood.* 2013; 122(22):3616–3627; quiz 99.

14. Haferlach T, Nagata Y, Grossmann V, Okuno Y, Bacher U, Nagae G, et al. Landscape of genetic lesions in 944 patients with myelodysplastic syndromes. *Leukemia.* 2014; 28(2): 241–247.

15. Bejar R, Stevenson K, Abdel-Wahab O, Galili N, Nilsson B, Garcia-Manero G, et al. Clinical effect of point mutations in myelodysplastic syndromes. *The New England Journal of Medicine.* 2011; 364 (26):2496–2506.

16. Yoshida K, Sanada M, Shiraishi Y, Nowak D, Nagata Y, Yamamoto R, et al. Frequent pathway mutations of splicing machinery in myelodysplasia. *Nature.* 2011; 478(7367):64–69.

17. Christiansen DH, Andersen MK, Pedersen-Bjergaard J. Mutations with loss of heterozygosity of p53 are common in therapy-related myelodysplasia and acute myeloid leukemia after exposure to alkylating agents and significantly associated with deletion or loss of 5q, a complex karyotype, and a poor prognosis. *Journal of Clinical Oncology: Official Journal of the American Society of Clinical Oncology.* 2001; 19(5): 1405–1413.

18. Greenberg PL, Tuechler H, Schanz J, Sanz G, Garcia-Manero G, Sole F, et al. Cytopenia levels for aiding establishment of the diagnosis of myelodysplastic syndromes. *Blood.* 2016; 128(16):2096–2067.

19. Valent P. Low blood counts: immune mediated, idiopathic, or myelodysplasia. *Hematology/the Education Program of the American Society of Hematology American Society of Hematology Education Program.* 2012; 2012:485–491.

20. Arber DA, Orazi A, Hasserjian R, Thiele J, Borowitz MJ, Le Beau MM, et al. The 2016 revision to the World Health Organization classification of myeloid neoplasms and acute leukemia. *Blood.* 2016; 127(20):2391–2405.

21. Bejar R, Greenberg PL. The impact of somatic and germline mutations in myelodysplastic syndromes and related disorders. *Journal of the National Comprehensive Cancer Network.* 2017; 15(1):131–135.

22. Network NCC. National Comprehensive Cancer Network Guidelines: Myelodysplatic Syndromes Version 2.2014 275 Commerce Drive, Suite 300, Fort Washington, PA 190342013 Version 2.2014: Available from: www.nccn.org.

23. Cargo CA, Rowbotham N, Evans PA, Barrans SL, Bowen DT, Crouch S, et al. Targeted sequencing identifies patients with preclinical MDS at high risk of disease progression. *Blood.* 2015; 126(21):2362–2365.

24. Kwok B, Hall JM, Witte JS, Xu Y, Reddy P, Lin K, et al. MDS-associated somatic mutations and clonal hematopoiesis are common in idiopathic cytopenias of undetermined significance. *Blood.* 2015; 126(21):2355–2361.

25. Greenberg P, Cox C, LeBeau MM, Fenaux P, Morel P, Sanz G, et al. International scoring system for evaluating prognosis in myelodysplastic syndromes. *Blood.* 1997; 89(6): 2079–2088.

26. Garcia-Manero G, Shan J, Faderl S, Cortes J, Ravandi F, Borthakur G, et al. A prognostic score for patients with lower risk myelodysplastic syndrome. *Leukemia: Official Journal of the Leukemia Society of America, Leukemia Research Fund, UK.* 2008; 22(3):538–543.

27. Bejar R, Stevenson KE, Caughey BA, Abdel-Wahab O, Steensma DP, Galili N,

et al. Validation of a prognostic model and the impact of mutations in patients with lower-risk myelodysplastic syndromes. *Journal of Clinical Oncology.* 2012; 30(27):3376–3382.

28. Greenberg PL, Tuechler H, Schanz J, Sanz G, Garcia-Manero G, Sole F, et al. Revised international prognostic scoring system for myelodysplastic syndromes. *Blood.* 2012; 120(12): 2454–2465.

29. Greenberg PL, Stone RM, Al-Kali A, Barta SK, Bejar R, Bennett JM, et al. Myelodysplastic Syndromes, Version 2.2017, NCCN Clinical Practice Guidelines in Oncology. *Journal of the National Comprehensive Cancer Network.* 2017; 15(1):60–87.

30. Hellstrom-Lindberg E, Gulbrandsen N, Lindberg G, Ahlgren T, Dahl IM, Dybedal I, et al. A validated decision model for treating the anaemia of myelodysplastic syndromes with erythropoietin + granulocyte colony-stimulating factor: significant effects on quality of life. *British Journal of Haematology.* 2003; 120(6): 1037–1046.

31. Greenberg PL, Sun Z, Miller KB, Bennett JM, Tallman MS, Dewald G, et al. Treatment of myelodysplastic syndrome patients with erythropoietin with or without granulocyte colony-stimulating factor: results of a prospective randomized phase 3 trial by the Eastern Cooperative Oncology Group (E1996). *Blood.* 2009; 114(12): 2393–2400.

32. Passweg JR, Giagounidis AA, Simcock M, Aul C, Dobbelstein C, Stadler M, et al. Immunosuppressive therapy for patients with myelodysplastic syndrome: a prospective randomized multicenter phase III trial comparing antithymocyte globulin plus cyclosporine with best supportive care–SAKK 33/99. *Journal of Clinical Oncology: Official Journal of the American Society of Clinical Oncology.* 2011; 29(3):303–309.

33. Malcovati L, Porta MG, Pascutto C, Invernizzi R, Boni M, Travaglino E, et al. Prognostic factors and life expectancy in myelodysplastic syndromes classified according to WHO criteria: a basis for clinical decision making. *Journal of Clinical Oncology: Official Journal of the American Society of Clinical Oncology.* 2005; 23(30): 7594–7603.

34. Cutler CS, Lee SJ, Greenberg P, Deeg HJ, Perez WS, Anasetti C, et al. A decision analysis of allogeneic bone marrow transplantation for the myelodysplastic syndromes: delayed transplantation for low-risk myelodysplasia is associated with improved outcome. *Blood.* 2004; 104(2):579–585.

35. Koreth J, Pidala J, Perez WS, Deeg HJ, Garcia-Manero G, Malcovati L, et al. Role of reduced-intensity conditioning allogeneic hematopoietic stem-cell transplantation in older patients with de novo myelodysplastic syndromes: an international collaborative decision analysis. *Journal of Clinical Oncology: Official Journal of the American Society of Clinical Oncology.* 2013; 31(21): 2662–2670.

36. Silverman LR, Demakos EP, Peterson BL, Kornblith AB, Holland JC, Odchimar-Reissig R, et al. Randomized controlled trial of azacitidine in patients with the myelodysplastic syndrome: a study of the cancer and leukemia group B. *Journal of Clinical Oncology: Official Journal of the American Society of Clinical Oncology.* 2002; 20(10): 2429–2440.

37. Kadia TM, Jabbour E, Kantarjian H. Failure of hypomethylating agent-based therapy in myelodysplastic syndromes. *Seminars in Oncology.* 2011; 38(5): 682–692.

HIV and Anemia

23

Owen Seddon, MB BCh, Andrew Freedman, MD, and David T. Scadden, MD

Etiology and Epidemiology

Anemia is the most common cytopenia associated with HIV infection. Its incidence increases with disease progression, with one review demonstrating a yearly incidence of 3% in asymptomatic HIV infection, 12% in patients with CD4 counts less than 200 who were otherwise asymptomatic, and 37% in patients with AIDS-related illnesses.[1] Large population studies have also shown the risk of death in patients with anemia to increase independently of the baseline CD4 count, age, or clinical stage of HIV.[1,2]

As it may be encountered as the initial presentation of an otherwise asymptomatic patient, physicians should be alert to the possibility of HIV in the investigation of any cytopenia.

The prevalence of severe anemia in the HIV population has decreased in the era of combined antiretroviral therapy (cART) but mild to moderate anemia continues to be common, and even after 6 months of treatment, estimates place the prevalence at around 50%.[2]

As with anemia in the general population, HIV-related anemia has a female preponderance, with a 71% greater prevalence, reflecting the impact of menstrual blood loss, pregnancy, and delivery on hemoglobin levels in women.[3]

There are numerous mechanisms by which an HIV-infected individual may develop anemia, and it is likely that in most cases the cause is multifactorial, reflecting the cumulative effects of malnutrition, medication, malignancy, autoimmune processes, and infection (both by HIV itself and with associated opportunistic infections). The pathophysiology of these will be discussed in turn.

Pathophysiology

Nutritional Deficiencies

Nutritional deficiencies are common in HIV patients. Anorexia can result from factors including HIV infection itself and the gastrointestinal disturbances of antiretroviral medication. Secondary infection may also be significant, particularly oral and esophageal complications such as candidiasis and aphthous ulcers, which may reduce voluntary food intake and result in hematinic deficiencies. Folate deficiency may result from both decreased dietary intake and poor absorption.[4] Vitamin B12 deficiency has an estimated prevalence of 10% in this population, reflecting malabsorption in the distal ileum, achlorhydria, and resultant decreased intrinsic factor production, and an alteration in the functioning of cobalamin transport proteins.[5,6] Iron deficiency will less commonly be attributable to reduced intake and more frequently reflect gastrointestinal blood loss from intestinal ulceration, infection, or malignancy.

Hypogonadism

Hypogonadism occurs frequently in advanced HIV infection, and decreased testosterone has been observed in cross-sectional studies of HIV-related anemia. Additionally, the use of androgen medications is inversely correlated with the presence of anemia in studies.[7] Testosterone deficiency is therefore likely to be a clinically relevant contributor to anemia in HIV through decreased production of hematopoietic growth factors and possible effects on iron bioavailability.

Marrow Suppression

As well as gastrointestinal disturbance, HIV medication may induce anemia through marrow-suppressive effects. Zidovudine (AZT) is a nucleoside analogue reverse transcriptase inhibitor and was the first antiretroviral medication available. Its marrow-suppressive side effects have been well documented, and cytopenia is the most common side effect of treatment. Trials have shown that 25% of patients treated with higher doses of AZT develop anemia, sufficient to require transfusion in 21%.[8] This effect can be ameliorated by dose modification, but most patients will still develop a macrocytosis secondary to inhibition of nucleic acid synthesis, although this may not develop into anemia.

Other current antiretroviral therapies are more rarely associated with bone marrow suppression sufficient to cause anemia. However, several other drugs used to treat HIV-related opportunistic infections may suppress red cell production. These include the antiviral agents ganciclovir, foscarnet, and cidofovir, the antifungal agents flucytosine and amphotericin, anti-*Pneumocystis jiroveci* agents TMP-SMX, pentamidine and pyrimethamine, and antineoplastic agents of multiple classes used in HIV-related malignancies.

Table 23.1 Medications that may cause marrow suppression

Antifungals	Antivirals	Anti-PCP/Opportunistic infection	Antiretrovirals	Cytotoxics
Amphotericin	Ganciclovir	Co-trimoxazole (Trimethoprim/Sulfamethoxazole)	Zidovudine	Of multiple classes
Flucytosine	Foscarnet	Pyrimethamine		
	Cidofovir	Pentamidine		
	Ribavirin	Dapsone		
	Interferon			

Hemolysis

HIV medications may also induce anemia through hemolysis. Dapsone and primaquine therapy may cause severe, life-threatening hemolysis in the presence of G6PD deficiency, which should be excluded prior to treatment initiation. In patients with normal G6PD levels, mild reductions in hemoglobin values may still be expected. In the treatment of coinfected individuals with hepatitis C, ribavirin therapy is commonly associated with the development of a hemolytic anemia. One study found concomitant therapy with zidovudine to be a significant predicator of severe hematological toxicity in patients receiving treatment for hepatitis C with interferon- and ribavirin-based regimens,[9] and zidovudine should be excluded from the antiretroviral therapy regimens of these patients.

Infiltration

In advanced HIV, malignancy and lymphoproliferative disorders may cause anemia through direct infiltration of the bone marrow. This is most commonly associated with Burkitt-like non-Hodgkin's lymphoma, but other lymphomas have been recorded, and rarely, the effect has been seen in Kaposi's sarcoma. It should be noted that Kaposi's sarcoma may also cause anemia via other mechanisms, including bleeding, depending on the anatomic site of the lesion.

A dysregulated autoimmune response, with a generalized hypergammaglobulinemia, is a hallmark of HIV infection and may produce antibodies to red cell antigens. The most common antibodies detected are directed against U and I red cell antigens, and most studies estimate the prevalence of this laboratory finding at around 20%.[10] Their presence is more common as an incidental finding, however, than in the setting of hemolysis.[11] In the rare cases in which hemolysis is seen, it occurs as a typical warm autoimmune hemolytic anemia. One caveat to this is that it is possible that mild hemolysis is underdiagnosed due to the relative reticulocytopenia frequently seen in HIV.

Opportunistic Infections

Opportunistic infections are capable of causing anemia through marrow suppression, direct marrow invasion, and blood loss.

Marrow suppression may be associated with acute viral infections including CMV and EBV, which cause a mild to moderate anemia in acute infection. Parvovirus B19 infects and lyses early erythroid precursors and in immunodeficient patients can cause a life-threatening anemia. Persistent viremia with parvovirus appears to be rare, although in the investigation of HIV-infected individuals with a severe unexplained anemia it may be present in as many as 50%.[12]

Direct marrow invasion by mycobacteria and fungi can lead to loss of the normal marrow architecture and inhibit the maturation of progenitor cells necessary for erythropoiesis. *Mycobacterium avium* complex is diagnosed in up to 18% of subjects with advanced HIV and usually involves the bone marrow, causing an anemia out of proportion to other cytopenias.[13] Marrow function may not improve even with appropriate treatment. *Mycobacterium tuberculosis* and *Histoplasma capsulatum* are other common infectious causes of marrow infiltration, whilst rarer causes include *Pneumocystis jiroveci, Cryptococcus neoformans,* and *Penicillium marneffei.*[14]

Infectious causes of gastrointestinal blood loss include CMV-induced colitis, *Campylobacter, Entamoeba histolytica,* and *Shigella.* Candidal infections can cause a severe, erosive esophagitis, and rarely histoplasmosis can lead to colonic ulcerations that bleed.

Direct Effects of HIV

Last, HIV itself appears to be a major contributor to abnormal hematopoiesis. The mechanisms by which this occurs are the subject of ongoing research. While HIV infection can be demonstrated in a variety of differentiated cell types,[15] the most primitive types of bone marrow progenitor cells, stem cells, appear highly resistant to infection despite expressing HIV receptor proteins.[16] That does not appear to be the case for lineage-committed progenitor cells. *In vitro*, CD34+ cells (which include progenitor as well as stem cells) show evidence of HIV infection in the form of viral inclusions on microscopy and through nucleic acid amplification,[17,18] but amplifying HIV-derived DNA from these cells has proved more difficult.[19] *In vivo*, CD34+ cells have been found to be HIV+ in infected individuals,[20] and lineage-committed progenitor cells have been shown to survive and harbor proviral DNA in a xenotransplant model.[21] However, it does not appear that this population of cells represents a reservoir of persistent virus, as analysis of a limited cohort of patients after effective anti-HIV therapy did not detect any residual virus in CD34+ cells[22]

The consequences of progenitor infection in vivo are unclear, but HIV-1 subtype C is more commonly found in Southern Africa, appears to have increased tropism for progenitor cells, and is associated with higher levels of anemia in these populations.[23]

Whether the effects of HIV infection are direct may remain controversial, but the presence of disordered hematopoiesis in HIV infection in HIV disease is not. Morphologic abnormalities are often seen in multiple lineages that resemble myelodysplasia and include megaloblastic changes and marrow hypercellularity.[24] There are often abnormalities in megakaryocyte morphology, but the micromegakaryocytes that characterize the myelodysplastic syndrome (MDS) are generally not present.[25] Functional assays have revealed high levels of the most primitive erythroid precursor – the erythroid burst-forming unit (BFU-E), in the bone marrow of HIV infected-individuals, and the subsequent normalization of the BFU-E levels in HIV patients who have been treated with cART.[26]

HIV and Anemia of Inflammation

A minority of patients remain anemic despite initiation of cART with effective virologic suppression. In addition to effects on hematopoiesis, some evidence suggests the existence of a proinflammatory state in chronic HIV may contribute toward anemia in a manner similar to the pathophysiology of chronic anemia in other inflammatory conditions (formerly described as anemia of chronic disease, now "anemia of inflammation"). There is evidence that a proinflammatory state may persist after initiation of cART.

Two examples are that HIV has been shown to be associated with dysregulation of hepcidin, an acute-phase reactant that is a critical regulator of iron stores and iron-limited erythropoiesis. Dysregulation of hepcidin is thought to be a key driver of anemia in chronic inflammation associated with increased levels of IL-6.[27] Second, leptin, a protein studied principally for its association with body mass, is known to induce hepcidin, and decreased levels of leptin also correlate with a blunted response to erythropoietin in the elderly. Polymorphisms in the leptin gene promoter have been shown to correlate with the development of anemia in an HIV-positive population.[28]

Research is ongoing as to whether polymorphisms in other key mediators of inflammatory pathways may play a role in contributing to anemia in patients with HIV, and the clinical impact remains unclear.[29]

Clinical Presentation

As with anemia in any other setting, patients may be symptomatic or asymptomatic. Asymptomatic patients may find their anemia come to light as part of routine testing for known HIV patients, the investigation of an unrelated disorder, or in the investigation of symptoms of other cytopenias.

In the symptomatic patient, the typical symptoms of fatigue, dyspnea, reduced exercise tolerance, and diminished functional capacity are commonly reported. Fatigue is a common symptom in HIV and is associated with impaired physical function, psychological distress, and poor quality of life. Studies have shown a positive correlation between the presence of a decreased hemoglobin level and self-reporting of fatigue in HIV-positive individuals.[30] There is an independent relationship between overall quality of life and decreased baseline hemoglobin, and correction of anemia has been shown to lead to statistically significant improvements in measures of quality of life and physical function.[31]

Diagnostic Evaluation

Due to the multifactorial nature of anemia in HIV, a careful assessment is necessary to elucidate underlying causes. The initial evaluation should attempt to identify treatable deficiencies as an underlying cause, including hematinics and hypogonadism as discussed earlier. However, routine hematological investigations for anemia may be misleading, for example the falsely low reticulocyte count associated with HIV infection and macrocytosis associated with zidovudine therapy already mentioned.

The stage of progression of immunodeficiency due to HIV is an important issue and can be assessed from history, CD4 count, and the presence or absence of HIV complications. The medication list should be carefully considered for potentially suppressive agents.

The presence of malignancy or coinfection with opportunistic organisms should be investigated by way of culture, serology, and relevant imaging and guided by an experienced HIV physician according to the relevant symptoms and signs of the patient.

Bone marrow aspiration and trephine biopsy may reveal the etiology of the anemia by demonstrating infiltration with malignancy or disseminated infection. It may also demonstrate characteristic giant pronormoblasts seen in parvovirus B19 infection. Other diagnostic findings may include the megaloblastic changes associated with AZT or B12 and folate deficiencies.[32]

However, the evidence does not currently support the routine use of bone marrow sampling in the diagnosis of HIV-related anemia. Studies have shown that the most frequent finding is a normocellular marrow (up to 70%),[33] and bone marrow culture performs no better than peripheral blood culture in time to diagnosis of mycobacterial infections.[34] The use of bone marrow aspirate and biopsy should be withheld except in cases of a rapidly changing clinical picture, when atypical cells are seen on peripheral blood smear, when there is a strong suspicion of underlying hematological malignancy (for example, with the presence of unexplained constitutional or "B" symptoms), or for staging as appropriate in a diagnosed malignancy. Most HIV physicians would continue to recommend bone marrow culture routinely in the investigation of a fever of unknown origin in an HIV patient.

Treatment and Prognosis

Correction of reversible causes is the initial step in the management of HIV-related anemia. Infectious etiologies should be treated appropriately and aggressively, deficiencies in testosterone, B12, folate, or iron should be corrected, and attempts should be made to dose-reduce or discontinue contributory medications.

Hemolysis appears to respond to steroid therapy, and intravenous immunoglobulin remains the therapy of choice for parvovirus B19-associated pure red cell aplasia.

Once these have been excluded, the introduction of cART has been shown to reduce both the incidence and the degree of anemia in all groups of HIV-infected patients. The women's interagency HIV study (WIHS) showed that cART was associated with a statistically significant improvement in hemoglobin levels after 6 months of treatment and that levels continued to improve with longer periods of therapy. Resolution of anemia is statistically less likely in patients with an MCV less than 80, a CD4+ lymphocyte count less than 200 cells/μl, a viral load above 50,000 copies/ml or zidovudine therapy in the preceding 6 months.[35] Recent studies in patients initiating cART indicate a correlation both between short-term mortality and anemia at baseline and between longer-term mortality and persistent anemia.[36]

Multiple studies have shown recombinant erythropoietin to be safe and effective in the treatment of HIV-associated anemia. In patients with reduced serum levels of erythropoietin (<500 IU/l), it has been shown to reduce transfusion requirements and increase hematocrit.[37] No effect has been demonstrated on mortality. The two dosing regimens most commonly used are 40,000 units once weekly, or 100 to 300 units per kilogram thrice weekly, and no significant difference has been demonstrated in tolerability, hemoglobin responses, or quality-of-life measures.[38] For obvious reasons, the once weekly dosing regime performs better on patient estimations of impact on quality of life, and it is a useful alternative to transfusion in patients meeting criteria.

When transfusion is required, the consensus opinion is that CMV-negative blood should be given to CMV-seronegative HIV patients, although this is rarely necessary due to high numbers of HIV patients displaying evidence of past infection. Some studies have suggested that transfusion with blood or blood products may "activate" HIV replication and result in a fall in CD4 count and decreased survival[39]. This is controversial, and insufficient data exist at present to make recommendations. Leukocyte-depleted blood transfusion appears to have no benefit or impact on HIV progression, the development of opportunistic infections, or death and does not appear to be necessary.

Conclusion

Anemia continues to have a significant impact on the health and healthcare of the HIV population. Treatment strategies should focus on identifying reversible causes and, once excluded, on appropriate initiation of cART, supportive transfusion if necessary, and consideration of erythropoietin therapy for suitable patients. In addition, HIV should be considered in the differential diagnosis of any patient presenting with an unexplained cytopenia.

References

1. Sullivan PS, Hanson DL, Chu SY, et al. *Epidemiology of anemia in human immunodeficiency virus (HIV)-infected persons: results from the multistate adult and adolescent spectrum of HIV disease surveillance project. Blood.* 1998; 91:301.

2. Mocroft A, Kirk O, Barton SE, et al. *Anaemia is an independent predictive marker for clinical prognosis in HIV-infected patients from across Europe. EuroSIDA Study Group. AIDS.* 1999; 13:943.

3. Creagh T, Mildvan D. Greater prevalence of anemia in women and African Americans with HIV/AIDS in the CART era: a study of 10,000 patients. The Anemia Prevalence Study Group, In: *Program and Abstracts of the 40th Annual Meeting of the Infectious Diseases Society of America (Chicago).* Alexandria, VA: Infectious Diseases Society of America; 2002:127.

4. Revell P, O'Doherty MJ, Tang A, Savidge GF. *Folic acid absorption in patients infected with the human immunodeficiency virus. J Intern Med.* 1991; 230:227.

5. Burkes RL, Cohen H, Krailo M, et al. *Low serum cobalamin levels occur frequently in the acquired immune deficiency syndrome and related disorders. Eur J Haematol.* 1987; 38:141.

6. Harriman GR, Smith PD, Horne MK, et al. *Vitamin B12 malabsorption in patients with acquired immunodeficiency syndrome. Arch Intern Med.* 1989; 149:2039.

7. Behler C, Shade S, Gregory K, et al. *Anemia and HIV in the antiretroviral era: potential significance of testosterone. AIDS Res Hum Retroviruses.* 2005; 21:200.

8. Richman DD, Fischl MA, Grieco MH, et al. *The toxicity of azidothymidine (AZT) in the treatment of patients with AIDS and AIDS-related complex. A double-blind, placebo-controlled trial. N Engl J Med.* 1987; 317:192.

9. Mira JA, López-Cortés LF, Merino D, et al. *Predictors of severe haematological toxicity secondary to pegylated interferon plus ribavirin treatment in HIV-HCV-coinfected patients. Antivir Ther.* 2007; 12:1225.

10. McGinniss MH, Macher AM, Rook AH, Alter HJ. *Red cell autoantibodies in patients with acquired immune deficiency syndrome. Transfusion.* 1986; 26:405.

11. Lai M, Visconti E, D'Onofrio G, et al. *Lower hemoglobin levels in human immunodeficiency virus-infected patients with a positive direct antiglobulin test (DAT): relationship*

with DAT strength and clinical stages. *Transfusion*. 2006; 46:1237.

12. Abkowitz JL, Brown KE, Wood RW, et al. *Clinical relevance of parvovirus B19 as a cause of anemia in patients with human immunodeficiency virus infection. J Infect Dis*. 1997; 176:269.

13. Hawkins CC, Gold JW, Whimbey E, Kiehn TE, Brannon P, Cammarata R, Brown AE, Armstrong D. *Mycobacterium avium complex infections in patients with the acquired immunodeficiency syndrome. Ann Intern Med*. 1986 Aug;105(2):184–188.

14. Mootsikapun P, Srikulbutr S. *Histoplasmosis and penicilliosis: comparison of clinical features, laboratory findings and outcome. Int J Infect Dis*. 2006; 10:66.

15. Scadden DT, Zon LI, Groopman JE. *Pathophysiology and management of HIV-associated hematologic disorders. Blood*. 1989; 74:1455.

16. Shen H, et al. Intrinsic human immunodeficiency virus type 1 resistance of hematopoietic stem cells despite coreceptor expression. *J Virol*. 1999; 73:728.

17. Folks TM, Kessler SW, Orenstein JM, et al. *Infection and replication of HIV-1 in purified progenitor cells of normal human bone marrow. Science*. 1988; 242:919.

18. Chelucci C, Hassan HJ, Locardi C, et al. *In vitro human immunodeficiency virus-1 infection of purified hematopoietic progenitors in single-cell culture. Blood*. 1995; 85:1181.

19. Molina JM, Scadden DT, Sakaguchi M, et al. *Lack of evidence for infection of or effect on growth of hematopoietic progenitor cells after in vivo or in vitro exposure to human immunodeficiency virus. Blood*. 1990; 76:2476.

20. Carter CC, et al. *HIV-1 infects multipotent progenitor cells causing cell death and establishing latent cellular reservoirs. Nat Med*. 2010; 16:446.

21. Nixon CC, Vatakis DN, et al. *HIV-1 infection of hematopoietic progenitor cells in vivo in humanized mice. Blood*. 2013; 122:2195.

22. Josefsson L, et al. *Hematopoietic precursor cells isolated from patients on long-term suppressive HIV therapy did not contain HIV-1 DNA. JID*. 2012; 206:28.

23. Redd AD, Avalos A, Essex M. *Infection of hematopoietic progenitor cells by HIV-1 subtype C, and its association with anemia in southern Africa. Blood*. 2007; 110:3143.

24. Karcher DS, Frost AR. *The bone marrow in human immunodeficiency virus (HIV)-related disease. Morphology and clinical correlation. Am J Clin Path*. 1991; 95:63.

25. Thiele J, et al. *Megakaryocytopoiesis in bone marrow biopsies of patients with acquired immunodeficiency syndrome (AIDS). An immunohistochemical and morphometric evaluation with special emphasis on myelodysplastic features and precursor cells. Pathol Res Pract*. 1992; 188:722.

26. Costantini A, Giuliodoro S, Butini L, et al. *Abnormalities of erythropoiesis during HIV-1 disease: a longitudinal analysis. J Acquir Immune Defic Syndr*. 2009; 52:70.

27. Vanasse GJ. Berliner N. *Anemia in elderly patients: an emerging problem for the 21st century. Hematology Am Soc Hematol Educ Program*. 2010: 271–275.

28. Vanasse GJ. Jeong JY. Tate J. *A polymorphism in the leptin gene promoter is associated with anemia in patients with HIV disease. Blood*. 2011;118(20):5401–5408.

29. Redig A. Berliner N. *Pathogenesis and clinical implications of HIV-related anemia in 2013. Hematology*. 2013; 1 377–381.

30. Darko DF. McCutchan JA. Kripke DF. Gillin JC. Golshan S. *Fatigue, sleep disturbance, disability, and indices of progression of HIV infections. Am J Psychiatry*. 1992; 149:514–520.

31. Abrams DL. Steinhart C. Frascino R. *Epoetin alfa therapy for anaemia in HIV-infected patients: impact on quality of life. Int J STD AIDS*. 2000; 11:659–665.

32. Spivak JL, Bender BS, Quinn TC. *Hematologic abnormalities in the acquired immune deficiency syndrome. Am J Med*. 1984; 77:224.

33. Castella A, Croxson TS, Mildvan D, et al. *The bone marrow in AIDS. A histologic, hematologic, and microbiologic study. Am J Clin Pathol*. 1985; 84:425.

34. Kilby JM, Marques MB, Jaye DL, et al. *The yield of bone marrow biopsy and culture compared with blood culture in the evaluation of HIV-infected patients for mycobacterial and fungal infections. Am J Med*. 1998; 104:123.

35. Berhane K, Karim R, Cohen MH, et al. *Impact of highly active antiretroviral therapy on anemia and relationship between anemia and survival in a large cohort of HIV-infected women: Women's Interagency HIV Study. J Acquir Immune Defic Syndr*. 2004; 37:1245.

36. Fregonese F, Collins IJ, Jourdain G, et al. Predictors of 5-year mortality in HIV-infected adults starting highly actrive antiretroviral therapy in Thailand. *J Acquir Immune Defic Syndr*. 2012; May 1; 60 91–98.

37. Phair JP, Abels RI, McNeill MV, Sullivan DJ. *Recombinant human erythropoietin treatment: investigational new drug protocol for the anemia of the acquired immunodeficiency* syndrome. *Overall Results. Arch Intern Med*. 1993; 153:2669.

38. Grossman HA, Goon B, Bowers P, et al. *Once-weekly epoetin alfa dosing is as effective as three times-weekly dosing in increasing hemoglobin levels and is associated with improved quality of life in anemic HIV-infected patients. J Acquir Immune Defic Syndr*. 2003; 34:368.

39. Mudido PM, Georges D, Dorazio D, et al. *Human immunodeficiency virus type 1 activation after blood transfusion. Transfusion*. 1996; 36:860.

Anemia in the Patient with Cancer

Murat O. Arcasoy, MD, FACP

Definition and Epidemiology

Anemia is the most frequently encountered hematologic abnormality in patients with cancer, diagnosed either at presentation of the malignancy or during the trajectory of the illness. Anemia in the cancer patient is often multifactorial and secondary, occurring as a result of the combined effect on the host of the underlying malignancy, comorbid conditions, and antineoplastic treatments such as myelosuppressive chemotherapy. Cancer is among the most common causes of secondary anemia due to the condition known as "anemia of chronic inflammation," also encountered in patients with infectious or autoimmune disorders. Anemia of chronic inflammation in the cancer patient (or cancer-related anemia) denotes an underlying immune-mediated mechanism leading to cytokine-induced perturbation of iron metabolism and erythropoiesis. Regardless of its etiology and pathogenesis, anemia frequently potentiates cancer-related fatigue, dyspnea on exertion, and decline in quality of life, the amelioration of which may require red blood cell transfusions. Furthermore, anemia has been implicated in impaired tumor response to radiotherapy and constitutes an adverse survival factor independent of tumor type.[1]

Estimates of anemia prevalence and incidence in cancer patients vary depending on the threshold hemoglobin for anemia definition, tumor type, cancer stage, patient age, and type and intensity of cancer treatment. Anemia is encountered often in newly diagnosed patients with hematologic malignancies such as multiple myeloma and leukemia. Among patients with nonhematologic malignancies, a high incidence is reported in lung, gynecologic, breast, and gastrointestinal cancer. The European Cancer Anemia Survey reported anemia prevalence of 31.7% (defined as hemoglobin <12 g/dL) among patients not receiving cancer treatment at survey enrollment (10% had hemoglobin <10 g/dL). Anemia prevalence increased to 67% during the 6-month survey (39% had hemoglobin <10 g/dL). The incidence of anemia during follow-up among patients who were not anemic at enrollment was 53.7% (hemoglobin <10 g/dL in 15.2%). The highest incidence (62.7%) was in patients receiving chemotherapy.[2] In a large cohort of cancer patients not receiving recombinant human erythropoietin (rhEPO), 39% of patients required transfusions.[3] The incidence and severity of chemotherapy-related anemia depends on the specific tumor type and stage as well as the type, schedule, and intensity of myelosuppressive therapy.[4] A grading system is commonly used (Table 24.1) to assess severity of therapy-related anemia.[5]

Etiology and Pathogenesis

The major pathophysiologic mechanisms that affect erythropoiesis regulation and cause anemia in cancer patients are listed in Table 24.2. Factors related to the patient's comorbidities, the cancer itself, or its treatment are involved. Bleeding may occur as a complication of malignancy or during surgical procedures to stage or treat cancer. Red cell survival may be shortened due to hemolytic anemia associated with malignancy or antineoplastic drugs. Cancer-related anemia may also contribute to decreased red cell survival. Impaired red cell production in bone marrow is typically multifactorial, associated with direct cytokine-mediated suppression of erythropoiesis as a result of immune system activation, reduced renal EPO production in response to anemia, blunted EPO responsiveness of bone marrow erythroid precursors, and iron-restricted erythropoiesis due to iron sequestration.[6] Figure 24.1 illustrates the multifactorial etiology and pathogenesis of anemia in the cancer patient and effects of inflammatory stress. The role of cytokines and the acute-phase peptide hepcidin in cancer-related anemia was investigated in several studies. For instance, in patients with anemia associated with advanced ovarian cancer, hemoglobin levels

Table 24.1. Therapy-related toxicity grading for anemia

Severity*	Hemoglobin (g/dL)
Grade 0 (normal)	>12 in women and >14 in men
Grade 1 (mild)	10–LLN
Grade 2 (moderate)	8–9.9
Grade 3 (serious/severe)	6.5–7.9
Grade 4 (life-threatening)	<6.5
Grade 5	Death

* National Cancer Institute Common Terminology for Adverse Events version 4.03 June 14, 2010, NCI publication No 09-5410. LLN: lower limit of normal.

correlated negatively with serum levels of IL-1, IL-6, and TNF-α.[7] In patients with Hodgkin's lymphoma, plasma hepcidin was elevated compared to healthy controls, strongly correlated with IL-6 and ferritin levels, and inversely correlated with hemoglobin in anemic patients.[8] In patients with diffuse large B-cell lymphoma, plasma hepcidin levels were significantly higher than in healthy controls, correlated with ferritin and IL-6 levels but not with hemoglobin.[9] In patients

with multiple myeloma, urinary hepcidin levels were higher than in normal controls, correlated with serum ferritin, and exhibited significant inverse correlation with hemoglobin levels.[10]

Evaluation and Diagnosis

Anemia evaluation in the cancer patient requires careful review of medical, surgical, and oncologic history, with attention to the type (hematologic malignancy or solid tumor), stage, and treatment modality of cancer. The baseline hemoglobin level preceding cancer diagnosis, if available, may indicate a preexisting hematologic disorder associated with anemia. Family history may provide clues to an inherited anemia. Surgical procedures for tumor resection or cancer staging cause blood loss anemia. Chronic gastrointestinal or genitourinary hemorrhage caused by primary or metastatic lesions contributes to absolute iron deficiency. Review of the type and intensity of antineoplastic treatment is indicated to establish a temporal relationship to the development and progression of anemia. Chemotherapy-related anemia occurs

Table 24.2. Major pathophysiologic mechanisms of anemia in cancer patients

Blood loss

Shortened red cell survival

Decreased red cell production
   Direct suppression of erythropoiesis
   Iron-restricted erythropoiesis
   EPO deficiency

Blunted EPO responsiveness

Poor nutritional status

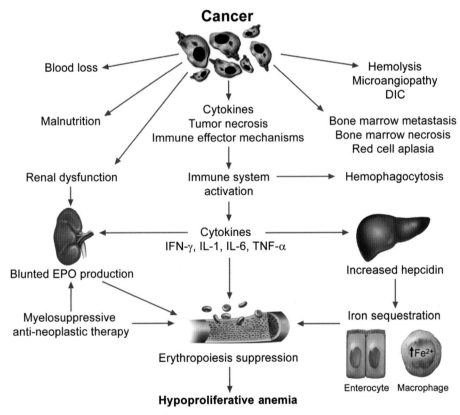

Figure 24.1 Pathophysiology of anemia in the cancer patient. Multiple factors contribute to the development of anemia. Cancer-related anemia, a form of anemia of chronic inflammation, plays a significant role in most cancer patients, particularly in those with advanced disease, due to a distinct pathophysiology involving deranged iron homeostasis as a result of immune system activation and inflammatory cytokines (interferon-γ, interleukin-1, interleukin-6, tumor necrosis factor-α). Interactions between cancer cells and immune effector cells, tumor necrosis, or aberrant gene expression in cancer cells trigger cytokine production and an inflammatory response, leading to increased production of hepcidin in the liver. Hepcidin binds to the cell membrane iron transport protein ferroportin in tissue macrophages (bone marrow, liver, spleen) and in enterocytes, thereby blocking the egress of iron from macrophages and intestinal iron absorption, respectively. Limitation of storage or dietary iron availability gives rise to iron-restricted erythropoiesis and contributes to anemia. Inflammatory cytokines also lead to impaired EPO production in the kidney and direct suppression of erythropoiesis to potentiate cancer-related anemia. DIC: disseminated intravascular coagulation.

due to myelosuppression, particularly with platinum-containing regimens. External beam radiation therapy involving the pelvis or spine, especially in combination with chemotherapy, may cause myelosuppression and anemia. Androgen deprivation therapy in patients with prostate cancer may be associated with mild to moderate anemia. The tyrosine kinase inhibitor imatinib that targets BCR-ABL1 and c-KIT was associated with any-grade anemia in the majority of patients with chronic myeloid leukemia (83%) and gastrointestinal stromal tumors (94%), with grade 3/4 anemia incidence of 10% and 13%, respectively.[11,12] Sunitinib, the antivascular endothelial growth factor receptor agent that also inhibits FLT-3 and c-KIT, was associated with any-grade anemia in 44% and grade 3/4 anemia in 10% of patients with renal cell cancer.[13]

The differential diagnostic considerations during anemia evaluation in the cancer patient are outlined in Table 24.3. Multiple factors often contribute in the same patient. Laboratory evaluation begins with measurement of reticulocyte count, review of red cell indices including mean corpuscular volume (MCV), and examination of the peripheral blood smear. Inappropriately low reticulocyte response is typical in cancer-related anemia, accompanied by normochromic, normocytic (MCV 80–100 fL), or sometimes microcytic indices (MCV <80 fL) and normal red cell morphology. Significant hypochromic and microcytic anemia mimicking iron deficiency anemia may be encountered in some patients presenting with Hodgkin's or non-Hodgkin's lymphoma and renal cell carcinoma. Elevated reticulocytes and polychromasia on smear suggest bleeding or hemolysis. Schistocytes in peripheral blood and associated thrombocytopenia indicate possibility of DIC or microangiopathy due to cancer or chemotherapeutic drugs. Peripheral blood leukoerythroblastosis, especially when associated with elevated serum lactate dehydrogenase, may indicate myelophthisis and trigger consideration of a bone marrow biopsy.

Assessment of iron parameters is indicated when evaluating suspected iron deficiency as well as cancer-related anemia, conditions that often occur concurrently. Absolute iron deficiency is readily diagnosed when transferrin saturation is <15% and serum ferritin is <30 ng/ml. Cancer-related anemia is usually mild to moderate (hemoglobin 9–11 g/dL) and characterized by low serum iron, reduced transferrin saturation, and normal or elevated ferritin level, no longer a reliable indicator of storage iron in the presence of inflammation. In contrast to isolated iron deficiency, transferrin level and total iron-binding capacity are normal or decreased in cancer-related anemia. Soluble transferrin receptors released by erythroid precursors are typically increased in isolated iron deficiency anemia. However, cancer patients with concomitant iron deficiency and cancer-related anemia often have normal soluble transferrin receptor levels due to erythropoiesis suppression.

Functional iron deficiency is a form of iron-restricted erythropoiesis in iron-replete individuals, typically associated with rhEPO administration in patients with inflammation. The release of storage iron from macrophages is inadequate to support the demands of erythropoiesis. These patients

Table 24.3. Differential diagnosis of anemia in cancer patients

Mechanism and Etiology	Clinical Scenario/Diagnosis
Blood loss, acute or chronic	
Surgery	Resection and staging of cancer
Hemorrhage	Gastrointestinal or genitourinary tract tumors
Iatrogenic	Phlebotomy for tests; vascular catheter flushes
Bone marrow suppression/ impaired erythropoiesis	
Marrow involvement with metastatic tumor	Breast, prostate, small-cell cancer; lymphoma
Bone marrow necrosis	Hematologic malignancies
Cytokine-mediated	Cancer-related anemia
Red cell aplasia	Thymoma
Therapy-related	Chemotherapy; radiation therapy; androgen deprivation; tyrosine kinase inhibitors
Shortened red cell survival	
Hemolytic anemia	Autoimmune in lymphoma; drug-induced (e.g., fludarabine)
Hypersplenism	Massive splenomegaly in hematologic malignancy
Microangiopathy	DIC; drug-induced (e.g., mitomycin C, gemcitabine)
Hemophagocytosis	Hematologic malignancies
Iron-restricted erythropoiesis	
Absolute iron deficiency	Chronic blood loss; malabsorption; poor nutrition
Functional iron deficiency	Associated with rhEPO
Iron-sequestration anemia	Cancer-related anemia
EPO deficiency	
Renal dysfunction	Obstructive uropathy; chemotherapy-induced (cisplatin)
Blunted EPO production	Cancer-related anemia; chemotherapy
Nutritional deficiency (poor intake or malabsorption)	Folate, cobalamin, iron deficiency; protein-calorie malnutrition

typically have normal or elevated serum ferritin and transferrin saturation <20%. Other laboratory markers have been investigated to improve diagnosis of functional iron deficiency. Detection of newly formed iron-deficient red cells that reflect early changes of iron-restricted erythropoiesis is feasible using flow cytometry. Reticulocyte hemoglobin content <28 pg or proportion of hypochromic red cells >10% are consistent with functional iron deficiency, although these tests are not routinely used in the clinic.[14]

Plasma EPO level measurement may be considered in selected cases if hemoglobin is <10 g/dL and renal function is normal. Patients with cancer-related anemia or those receiving chemotherapy typically exhibit impaired EPO production for the degree of anemia.[6] However, plasma EPO levels in patients with nonmyeloid malignancies have not been shown to predict rhEPO treatment response. Direct antiglobulin test is indicated when autoimmune hemolytic anemia is suspected. In patients with macrocytic anemia, poor nutritional status, or malabsorption due to gastrointestinal surgery, measurement of serum B12 and folate levels is indicated.

Management

General Considerations

Choice of anemia treatment options in the cancer patient involves consideration of the type of malignancy, comorbid conditions, the cause, severity, and symptoms of anemia, and goals of antineoplastic and supportive therapies, as well as patient and physician preferences. Identification of correctable anemia causes such as B12, folate, or absolute iron deficiency, is an indication for replenishment as appropriate. In patients with hematologic malignancies such as multiple myeloma, leukemia, or lymphoma with bone marrow involvement, antineoplastic treatment frequently leads to amelioration of anemia as remission is achieved, although many patients require supportive transfusions during treatment course. Asymptomatic patients with solid tumors and stable, mild-moderate cancer-related anemia (hemoglobin >8 g/dL) often do not require transfusions. In patients with cancer therapy–related symptomatic anemia, treatment options for consideration include red cell transfusions, and specifically in patients receiving chemotherapy, rhEPO with or without intravenous iron supplementation. In patients with cancer-related anemia who are not receiving concomitant myelosuppressive chemotherapy, rhEPO use is contraindicated. In this clinical setting, randomized, placebo-controlled trials reported worse survival associated with rhEPO use targeting near-normal hemoglobin levels.[15,16]

The decision to transfuse red cells depends on specific clinical circumstances for each cancer patient rather than a threshold hemoglobin level. The main benefit of transfusion therapy is rapid hemoglobin rise and improved oxygen-carrying capacity, particularly in patients with severe or symptomatic anemia and in those with limited cardiopulmonary reserve who require immediate correction of anemia. The risks of transfusion therapy include transfusion-related acute reactions, volume overload, infectious agent transmission, alloimmunization, and iron overload. In a retrospective study, red cell transfusions were associated with increased thrombotic events and in-hospital mortality in cancer patients, although this association has not been shown to be causal. It is possible that transfusion need is a marker of relatively severe anemia due to more advanced cancer or higher intensity antineoplastic therapy.[17]

Cancer Therapy–Related Anemia

Management options for patients with symptomatic chemotherapy-related anemia include transfusions and rhEPO, given with or without iron supplementation for suspected functional iron deficiency. Table 24.4 summarizes the

Table 24.4. Summary of clinical practice guidelines for rhEPO use in cancer patients

American Society of Hematology/American Society of Clinical Oncology (ASH/ASCO) – 2010[27]

Evaluate for correctable causes of anemia before initiating therapy

Consider in patients receiving chemotherapy and hemoglobin <10 g/dL

Avoid use in cancer patients not receiving concurrent chemotherapy

Discuss potential harms and benefits of rhEPO and red cell transfusions

Administer lowest dose possible to avoid transfusions

Follow FDA-approved labeling for starting doses and dose modifications

In nonresponders, discontinue after 6–8 weeks

Iron supplementation is not routinely recommended

National Comprehensive Cancer Network (NCCN) – 2016[28]

Evaluate anemia (hemoglobin <11 g/dL or ≥2 g/dL below baseline) to delineate the origin

rhEPO should not be used when the anticipated outcome is cure

Use lowest dose necessary to avoid transfusion

Iron studies should be monitored to detect functional iron deficiency during rhEPO use

European Society for Medical Oncology (ESMO) – 2010[31]

All causes of anemia should be taken into account and, if possible, corrected before use

Consider for treatment of patients with symptomatic chemotherapy-related anemia

Use according to European Medicines Agency (EMEA) label

In patients with hemoglobin ≤10 g/dL, to increase hemoglobin or prevent further decline

There is no indication in patients not treated with chemotherapy

In patients treated with curative intent, caution is advised

In absence of response, continuation beyond 6–8 weeks is not beneficial*

Patients with solid tumors on platinum-based chemotherapy seem to benefit more than others

National Institute for Health and Clinical Excellence (NICE) – 2014[32]

Epoetins are recommended, within their marketing authorizations, as options for treating anemia in people with cancer who are having chemotherapy, when hemoglobin concentrations are 10 g/dL or lower, and target values up to 12 g/dL.

* Absence of response defined as hemoglobin rise <1–2 g/dL or no diminution in transfusion requirement.

spectrum of clinical practice guidelines for rhEPO use. The decision to embark should be individualized following a risk–benefit discussion and informed consent. In 2011, the United States Food and Drug Administration (US FDA) had required implementation of a Risk Evaluation and Mitigation Strategy to prescribe rhEPO products, a requirement that was discontinued in 2017.

The efficacy of rhEPO preparations (epoetin-alfa, epoetin-beta, and darbepoetin-alfa) to significantly reduce transfusion risk by 30–40% in cancer patients has been documented in clinical trials. In a systematic review, 25 of 100 persons receiving epoetin or darbepoetin underwent transfusions, compared to 39 of 100 persons not receiving rhEPO (risk ratio 0.65; 95% confidence interval [CI] 0.62–0.68, 70 trials, $N = 16,093$ patients). On average, patients in rhEPO cohort received one red cell unit less than the control group, who received a mean of 3.65 units.[3]

Improvement in health-related quality of life and cancer-related fatigue after rhEPO use was reported in several single-arm and randomized clinical trials using various instruments of Functional Assessment of Cancer Therapy. A comparative effectiveness review concluded that treating to high hemoglobin targets (>12/dL) was accompanied by improved quality-of-life scores but that the magnitude of any beneficial effect and its clinical significance are likely to be small.[18] The impact on quality of life when rhEPO is used at doses just sufficient to avoid transfusions according to revised clinical practice guidelines remains less certain.

The major risks associated with rhEPO use in cancer patients, particularly when targeting high hemoglobin levels, include increased mortality, tumor progression, and thromboembolism reported in a series of randomized, controlled trials involving patients with diverse tumor types (head-neck, breast, non–small cell lung, uterine cervix, lymphoproliferative and mixed nonmyeloid malignancies) and meta-analyses prompting warnings and use restrictions by the US FDA.[19] A systematic review and a comparative effectiveness update reported increased mortality associated with rhEPO use in cancer patients during active study period.[3,18] A large individual-patient-data meta-analysis reported mortality increase (hazard ratio [HR] 1.17, 95% CI 1.06–1.30, $p = 0.003$) and worsened overall survival (HR = 1.06, 1.00–1.12, $p = 0.046$, $N = 13,933$) during and shortly following rhEPO use (active study period).[20] In the subgroup of patients on chemotherapy, the effect on mortality increase and survival was not statistically significant, with hazard ratio for mortality 1.10 (0.98–1.24, $p = 0.12$) and for overall survival 1.04 (0.97–1.11, $p = 0.263$, $N = 10,441$). In patients with chronic kidney disease and cancer, rhEPO administration to target hemoglobin 13 g/dL was associated with higher cancer-related mortality compared to placebo.[21]

The overall effect of rhEPO on tumor control and progression is uncertain across clinical trials and in a systematic review.[3] Several studies involving patients with head-neck cancer (treated by primary radiotherapy) and breast cancer

(palliative or neoadjuvant chemotherapy) targeting high hemoglobin levels raised concern for increased tumor progression and relapse in cancer patients with significant tumor burden at time of rhEPO exposure.[22–24] A recent study has concluded that rhEPO use should be avoided in patients with metastatic breast cancer receiving standard chemotherapy.[25] The potential mechanisms for increased mortality and tumor progression associated with rhEPO reported in some studies have been investigated and debated in the literature. A complex interplay of direct EPO effects on cancer cells and the tumor microenvironment as well as indirect systemic effects are likely involved.[26,27]

Thromboembolic complication risk in cancer patients is consistently increased during rhEPO use compared to controls across several clinical trials and meta-analyses. In a systematic review involving 15,498 patients, 7 of 100 patients receiving rhEPO developed thromboembolic complications compared to five of 100 patients (HR 1.52, 95% CI 1.34–1.74, 57 trials) not receiving these agents.[3] In cancer patients at high risk for thromboembolic complications, thromboprophylaxis is considered when embarking on a course of rhEPO during chemotherapy.

rhEPO use may be considered if anemia (hemoglobin <10 g/dL) is due to concomitant myelosuppressive chemotherapy, and upon initiation, there is a minimum of 2 additional months of planned chemotherapy (Table 24.4). Epoetin-alfa, epoetin-beta, and darbepoetin-alfa are the available EPO analogues with similar efficacy and adverse effect profile. Darbepoetin-alfa is a hyperglycosylated form with a longer *in vivo* half-life, allowing less frequent administration. Typical dosing regimens for epoetins are 150 units/kg subcutaneously three times a week or 40,000 units/week until completion of chemotherapy course. Darbepoetin-alfa regimens are 2.25 µg/kg/week, 200 µg every 2 weeks, or 500 µg every 3 weeks. The US FDA-approved label recommends using the lowest rhEPO dose needed to avoid transfusions. Discontinuation is recommended if there is no hemoglobin response, if transfusions are still required after 8 weeks, and when chemotherapy is completed. Dose reduction by 25% is recommended if hemoglobin increases by >1 g/dL in any 2-week period or if hemoglobin reaches a level at which transfusion is not required.

In cancer patients receiving curative chemotherapy, rhEPO use is not recommended according to most recent National Comprehensive Cancer Network Clinical Practice guidelines[28] and US FDA-approved medication label. The effect of rhEPO has been investigated in randomized controlled clinical trials in the curative chemotherapy setting for specific types of malignancy. For instance, in a cohort of Hodgkin's lymphoma patients receiving intensive curative chemotherapy, epoetin use did not affect treatment failure or survival compared to placebo.[29] In a randomized trial involving high-risk breast cancer patients receiving adjuvant dose-dense chemotherapy, rhEPO was not associated with an adverse effect on relapse-free and overall survival.[30] In cancer patients undergoing radiotherapy alone, rhEPO use is not indicated for treatment or prevention of anemia. The role of rhEPO in treatment of anemia associated with tyrosine kinase inhibitors has not been investigated in prospective studies. In anemic patients with chronic myeloid leukemia treated with imatinib, a retrospective review reported that rhEPO use led to hemoglobin increase >2 g/dL in 80% of patients without adverse effect on survival but increased incidence of thromboembolic events.[11]

Iron Supplementation in rhEPO-Treated Patients

A significant hemoglobin response to rhEPO administration is not achieved in approximately 30–50% of cancer patients. Baseline assessment of iron parameters and correction of absolute iron deficiency are indicated. In some cases, iron-restricted erythropoiesis due to inflammation may limit storage iron availability to meet erythropoietic demand. In dialysis patients, intravenous iron supplementation has been reported to improve hemoglobin response and reduce rhEPO dose requirement, even in some patients with normal or elevated ferritin level. In patients with nonmyeloid malignancies receiving chemotherapy, a series of randomized clinical trials investigated the role and route of iron supplementation during rhEPO administration. In patients with absolute or functional iron deficiency, improved hemoglobin response was reported in intravenous iron-treated patients compared to oral iron or no iron.[28] It remains uncertain whether intravenous iron supplementation may allow rhEPO dose reduction in cancer patients undergoing chemotherapy. In the absence of absolute iron deficiency, the pretreatment iron parameters that reliably identify patients most likely to respond to intravenous iron supplementation and the optimal dose of intravenous iron have not been identified.[27] The long-term safety of intravenous iron in cancer patients has not been studied. Potential safety issues with intravenous iron include susceptibility to infections, increased oxidative stress, iron overload (a "safe" upper level of ferritin has not been determined), and modulation of tumor biology.

Currently, the National Comprehensive Cancer Network recommends consideration of intravenous iron supplementation (e.g., low-molecular-weight iron dextran, ferric gluconate, or iron sucrose) in the presence of functional iron deficiency suggested by serum ferritin 30–500 ng/ml and transferrin saturation <50%.[28]

Summary

Anemia occurs frequently in cancer patients due to multifactorial etiology, including blood loss, poor nutritional status, blunted EPO production and response, myelosuppressive therapy, and cancer-related anemia due to cytokine release, increased hepcidin, and defective iron metabolism. Anemia potentiates cancer-related fatigue and it is associated with inferior survival. A systematic clinical and laboratory evaluation is indicated to identify treatable anemia causes and to assess the contribution of cancer-related anemia. In addition to identifying and treating reversible anemia causes, effective treatment of the underlying malignancy is the mainstay of anemia management. Supportive interventions to improve anemia during cancer treatment are generally reserved for symptomatic patients and those at risk for transfusions during myelosuppressive chemotherapy. Treatment of anemia using EPO analogues focusing on hemoglobin level improvement is associated with deleterious effects when targeting high hemoglobin levels. In anemic patients receiving palliative chemotherapy, concurrent rhEPO use reduces transfusion risk in some patients and appears not to be associated with increase in mortality when used within drug label recommendations. The quality-of-life benefits of rhEPO are less certain, especially when dosing is restricted according to revised guidelines to avoid transfusions. Concomitant intravenous iron supplementation may augment hemoglobin response in some patients, although further study is required to identify the patient subpopulation that benefits most, to determine the effect on rhEPO dose reduction, the optimal iron dose, and long-term safety. Rigorous clinical trials will be required to investigate newer erythropoiesis-stimulating agents with novel mechanisms of action – such as upregulation of endogenous EPO production – to ensure efficacy and safety in the supportive treatment of anemia in cancer patients.

References

1. Caro JJ, Salas M, Ward A, Goss G. Anemia as an independent prognostic factor for survival in patients with cancer: a systemic, quantitative review. *Cancer*. 2001; **91**: 2214–2221.

2. Ludwig H, Van Belle S, Barrett-Lee P, et al. The European Cancer Anaemia Survey (ECAS): a large, multinational, prospective survey defining the prevalence, incidence, and treatment of anaemia in cancer patients. *European Journal of Cancer*. 2004; **40**:2293–2306.

3. Tonia T, Mettler A, Robert N, et al. Erythropoietin or darbepoetin for patients with cancer. *Cochrane Database of Systematic Reviews*. 2012; **12**:CD003407.

4. Knight K, Wade S, Balducci L. Prevalence and outcomes of anemia in cancer: a systematic review of the literature. *The American Journal of Medicine*. 2004; **116** Suppl 7A: 11S–26S.

5. Groopman JE, Itri LM. Chemotherapy-induced anemia in adults: incidence and treatment. *Journal of the National Cancer Institute*. 1999; **91**:1616–1634.

6. Spivak JL. The anaemia of cancer: death by a thousand cuts. *Nature Reviews Cancer*. 2005; **5**:543–555.

7. Maccio A, Madeddu C, Massa D, et al. Hemoglobin levels correlate with interleukin-6 levels in patients with advanced untreated epithelial ovarian cancer: role of inflammation in cancer-related anemia. *Blood*. 2005; **106**:362–367.

8. Hohaus S, Massini G, Giachelia M, et al. Anemia in Hodgkin's lymphoma: the role of interleukin-6 and hepcidin. *Journal of Clinical Oncology: Official Journal of the American Society of*

Clinical Oncology. 2010; **28**: 2538–2543.

9. Tisi MC, Bozzoli V, Giachelia M, et al. Anemia in diffuse large B cell non-Hodgkin Lymphoma: the role of IL-6, hepcidin and erythropoietin. *Leukemia & Lymphoma.* 2013.

10. Sharma S, Nemeth E, Chen YH, et al. Involvement of hepcidin in the anemia of multiple myeloma. *Clinical Cancer Research: An Official Journal of the American Association for Cancer Research.* 2008; **14**:3262–3267.

11. Santos FP, Alvarado Y, Kantarjian H, et al. Long-term prognostic impact of the use of erythropoietic-stimulating agents in patients with chronic myeloid leukemia in chronic phase treated with imatinib. *Cancer.* 2011; **117**:982–991.

12. Van Glabbeke M, Verweij J, Casali PG, et al. Predicting toxicities for patients with advanced gastrointestinal stromal tumours treated with imatinib: a study of the European Organisation for Research and Treatment of Cancer, the Italian Sarcoma Group, and the Australasian Gastro-Intestinal Trials Group (EORTC-ISG-AGITG). *European Journal of Cancer.* 2006; **42**:2277–2285.

13. Funakoshi T, Latif A, Galsky MD. Risk of hematologic toxicities in cancer patients treated with sunitinib: A systematic review and meta-analysis. *Cancer Treatment Reviews.* 2013; **39**:818–830.

14. Goodnough LT, Nemeth E, Ganz T. Detection, evaluation, and management of iron-restricted erythropoiesis. *Blood.* 2010; **116**:4754–4761.

15. Wright JR, Ung YC, Julian JA, et al. Randomized, double-blind, placebo-controlled trial of erythropoietin in non-small-cell lung cancer with disease-related anemia. *Journal of Clinical Oncology: Official Journal of the American Society of Clinical Oncology.* 2007; **25**:1027–1032.

16. Smith RE, Jr., Aapro MS, Ludwig H, et al. Darbepoetin alpha for the treatment of anemia in patients with active cancer not receiving chemotherapy or radiotherapy: results of a phase III, multicenter, randomized, double-blind, placebo-controlled study. *Journal of Clinical Oncology: Official Journal of the American Society of Clinical Oncology.* 2008; **26**:1040–1050.

17. Khorana AA, Francis CW, Blumberg N, et al. Blood transfusions, thrombosis, and mortality in hospitalized patients with cancer. *Archives of Internal Medicine.* 2008; **168**:2377–2381.

18. Grant MD, Piper M, Bohlius J, et al. *Epoetin and Darbepoetin for Managing Anemia in Patients Undergoing Cancer Treatment: Comparative Effectiveness Update.* AHRQ Comparative Effectiveness Reviews. Rockville (MD); 2013.

19. FDA Briefing Document Oncologic Drugs Advisory Committee. 2008 [accessed May 26, 2017]. Available from: www.fda.gov/ohrms/dockets/ac/08/briefing/2008-4345b2-01-FDA.pdf.

20. Bohlius J, Schmidlin K, Brillant C, et al. Recombinant human erythropoiesis-stimulating agents and mortality in patients with cancer: a meta-analysis of randomised trials. *Lancet.* 2009; **373**:1532–1542.

21. Pfeffer MA, Burdmann EA, Chen CY, et al. A trial of darbepoetin alfa in type 2 diabetes and chronic kidney disease. *The New England Journal of Medicine.* 2009; **361**:2019–2032.

22. Henke M, Laszig R, Rube C, et al. Erythropoietin to treat head and neck cancer patients with anaemia undergoing radiotherapy: randomised, double-blind, placebo-controlled trial. *Lancet.* 2003; **362**:1255–1260.

23. Leyland-Jones B, Semiglazov V, Pawlicki M, et al. Maintaining normal hemoglobin levels with epoetin alfa in mainly nonanemic patients with metastatic breast cancer receiving first-line chemotherapy: a survival study. *Journal of clinical oncology: official journal of the American Society of Clinical Oncology.* 2005; **23**:5960–5972.

24. Untch M, von Minckwitz G, Konecny GE, et al. PREPARE trial: a randomized phase III trial comparing preoperative, dose-dense, dose-intensified chemotherapy with epirubicin, paclitaxel, and CMF versus a standard-dosed epirubicin-cyclophosphamide followed by paclitaxel with or without darbepoetin alfa in primary breast cancer–outcome on prognosis. *Annals of Oncology: Official Journal of the European Society for Medical Oncology/ESMO.* 2011; **22**:1999–2006.

25. Leyland-Jones B, Bondarenko I, Nemsadze G, et al. A Randomized, Open-Label, Multicenter, Phase III Study of Epoetin Alfa Versus Best Standard of Care in Anemic Patients With Metastatic Breast Cancer Receiving Standard Chemotherapy. *Journal of Clinical Oncology: Official Journal of the American Society of Clinical Oncology.* 2016; **34**:1197–1207.

26. McKinney M, Arcasoy MO. Erythropoietin for oncology supportive care. *Experimental Cell Research.* 2011; **317**:1246–1254.

27. Rizzo JD, Brouwers M, Hurley P, et al. American Society of Hematology/American Society of Clinical Oncology clinical practice guideline update on the use of epoetin and darbepoetin in adult patients with cancer. *Blood.* 2010; **116**:4045–4059.

28. National Comprehensive Cancer Network Clinical Practice Guidelines in Oncology: Cancer- and Chemotherapy-Induced Anemia, updated November 16, 2016 [accessed May 26, 2017]. Version 2.2017. Available from: www.nccn.org/professionals/physician_gls/pdf/anemia.pdf.

29. Engert A, Josting A, Haverkamp H, et al. Epoetin alfa in patients with advanced-stage Hodgkin's lymphoma: results of the randomized placebo-controlled GHSG HD15EPO trial. *Journal of Clinical Oncology: Official Journal of the American Society of Clinical Oncology.* 2010; **28**:2239–2245.

30. Moebus V, Jackisch C, Schneeweiss A, et al. Adding epoetin alfa to intense dose-dense adjuvant chemotherapy for breast cancer: randomized clinical trial. *Journal of the National Cancer Institute.* 2013; **105**:1018–1026.

31. Schrijvers D, De Samblanx H, Roila F, E.G.W. Group. Erythropoiesis-stimulating agents in the treatment of anaemia in cancer patients: ESMO Clinical Practice Guidelines for use. *Annals of Oncology: Official Journal of the European Society for Medical Oncology/ESMO.* 2010; **21**(Suppl)5: v244–v247.

32. Erythropoiesis-stimulating agents (epoetin and darbepoetin) for treating anaemia in people with cancer having chemotherapy: National Institute for Health and Clinical Excellence technology appraisal guidance TA323; 2014 [accessed May 26, 2017]. Available from: www.nice.org.uk/guidance/ta323.

Secondary Anemias Associated with Hematopoietic Stem Cell Transplantation

Joseph H. Antin, MD

Ironically, while hematopoietic stem cell transplantation (HSCT) is typically undertaken for diseases that are associated with anemia, persistent anemia can be one of the most vexing problems of otherwise successful transplantation. Conventional approaches to the evaluation and management of anemia are often quite successful after HSCT, but there are some unique, transplant-related issues that require special attention. Moreover, the diagnostic criteria applied to anemic patients who were not transplanted may not apply after HSCT, and the approach to management of anemia is often quite different.

What Defines Anemia after HSCT?

It is reasonable to expect that many people will have some degree of anemia after HSCT, since the transplantation involves the transfer of a very small population of stem cells to the donor. In conventional marrow transplantation, it is estimated that the donor provides about 5% of his stem cell pool. In umbilical cord blood transplantation, the number of stem cells is even smaller. While erythropoiesis may be completely restored after a successful transplantation, many patients remain mildly or moderately anemic by standard criteria. This may be more problematic if the donor is older and there is a smaller pool of stem cells, perhaps with shorter telomeres, that are expected to reconstitute hematopoiesis permanently in a large young adult. One should distinguish anemia from limiting stem cell numbers from other causes of anemia that may be more amenable to correction. Thus, even with excellent restoration of the stem cell pool, some patients may continue to be anemic related to bleeding, shortened RBC survival, nutritional deficiencies, relapse, infection, or failure of erythropoietin production. The value of RBC parameters such as MCV, MCHC, and RDW may be diminished by limiting stem cell numbers. One must also consider intrinsic features of donor erythropoiesis, for instance, using a donor with β-thalassemia minor. Thus, more so than in nontransplant hematology, the determination of the cause of the anemia and its clinical importance must be considered in the context of the transplant.

Pathophysiology of Anemia after Transplantation

The pathophysiologic classification of anemia after transplantation is similar to that of nontransplanted patients. The major categories of decreased production, increased destruction, maturation defects, and bleeding apply, although the universe of differential diagnoses is much smaller, since most of the congenital and acquired hematopoietic defects that might be present in the donor will have been avoided. The RBC indices can be helpful, although a mild to moderate macrocytosis is common for months or years after transplantation and is not necessarily indicative of nutritional deficiency, abnormal DNA synthesis, or reticulocytosis. The reticulocyte count is a very good friend in evaluating anemias, and this applies in transplantation as well. An approach to anemia in patients after allogeneic transplantation based on reticulocytosis is shown in Figure 25.1.

Graft Failure

One of the principle causes of erythropoietic insufficiency after HSCT is failure of the graft. Graft failure can reflect several underlying causes: graft rejection, insufficient stem cells, or damaged stem cells. It may also occur early, at the time of anticipated engraftment, or later after a graft appeared to be stable.

Normally primary graft failure is defined by global failure of hematopoiesis by day 28–40 depending on the stem cell source. Cord blood transplants have notoriously late engraftment thought to be related to the limiting numbers of infused stem cells. Typically, the absolute neutrophil count (ANC) is used as the primary measure of engraftment; however, if reticulocytes are monitored as well as ANC, there will be a failure of reticulocytosis. A hemoglobin level of ≥ 8 g/dL without transfusion support is an accepted threshold for red cell engraftment. If the criteria for engraftment have been met and there is late decline in blood counts (normally at least 2 lines) the patient is thought to have late graft failure.

Possible causes of graft failure are varied. Graft rejection can be mediated by residual host T cells or NK cells or by preexistent anti-HLA antibodies in patients with mismatched transplants. There may be underlying microenvironment defects that fail to support normal hematopoiesis (e.g., myelofibrosis), low stem cell dose, drug toxicity (e.g., trimethoprim-sulfamethoxazole, valganciclovir, linezolid), infection (e.g., HHV-6, cytomegalovirus, parvovirus), cryopreservation problems resulting in damaged stem cells, and, rarely, donor hematopoietic problems that were unrecognized prior to

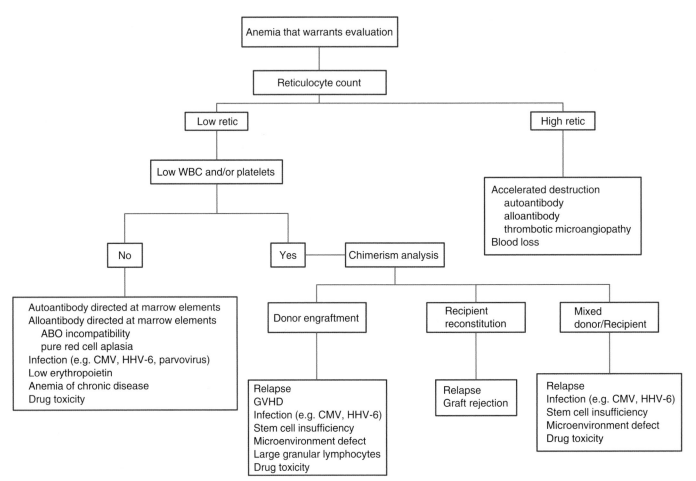

Figure 25.1 Approach to anemia after transplantation.

transplantation. We have observed graft failure using donors with undiagnosed short telomere syndromes. In autologous transplantation, very heavily treated patients may have chemotherapy-induced stem cell damage that results in poor engraftment and increases the risk of the late development of myelodysplasia. Older donors may have clonal hematopoiesis of indeterminate potential (CHIP), which can result in poor graft function and secondary myelodysplasia.[1,2] There appear to be patients with insufficient stem cell numbers resulting in poor graft function, termed stem cell exhaustion, and it often can be rectified with an infusion of CD34-selected stem and progenitor cells.[3] In aplastic anemia, graft failure is more common. The intensity of the conditioning regimen is less, and, importantly, graft failure can be mediated by *both* allogeneic T cell recognition of minor histocompatibility antigen as well as residual, conditioning-resistant T cells that recognize autologous stem cell antigens that were responsible for the aplastic anemia in the first place.

There may be a relative decrease in erythropoietin production after conditioning that may reflect injury to the renal epithelium. Moreover, nephrotoxic drugs given either before the transplantation (e.g., cisplatin) or after transplantation (e.g., cyclosporine) may reduce the responsiveness of the kidney to anemia and result in relative insufficiency of red cell numbers compared with neutrophils and platelets.[4,5]

In order to distinguish graft rejection from other causes, of stem cell failure measurements of blood chimerism are helpful. Several approaches to measurement of chimerism are in wide use, but most commonly we obtain DNA from the patient and donor and evaluate the short tandem repeat (STR) genomic polymorphisms. The proportion of recipient and donor cells can be quantified either in unfractionated blood or in specifically isolated leukocyte populations. If donor STRs are identified, then a graft is present. If there is complete lympho-hematopoietic chimerism, it is difficult to invoke rejection, while if donor cells are not identified, graft rejection is likely. In some instances, for instance reduced-intensity transplantation for sickle cell disease, there may be stable mixed chimerism in the erythroid compartment in which the donor erythron predominates.[6,7] Thus, complete chimerism is not necessary for functional recovery of erythropoiesis.

Graft-versus-Host Disease (GVHD)

Anemia may be a prominent feature in patients with active acute or chronic GVHD, but in this context, it typically does not reflect failure of erythropoiesis or accelerated red cell destruction. GVHD is a systemic inflammatory syndrome, typically associated with high levels of inflammatory cytokines. Hepcidin levels have not been reported in GVHD, but it is likely that anemia in the setting of GVHD will have a similar pathophysiology to the anemia of chronic inflammation. Gastrointestinal blood loss is common with gut GVHD. As discussed elsewhere, drugs used to treat GVHD may be associated with renal insufficiency, thrombotic microangiopathy, or direct myelosuppression. Treatment of chronic GVHD with extracorporeal photopheresis may result in enough blood loss to cause an iron deficiency. Finally, nutritional deficiencies may result from poor oral intake or from poor vitamin B12 absorption due to involvement of the terminal ileum. Thus anemia may be polyfactorial.

ABO Incompatibility

Donor selection is based on MHC compatibility, and ABO matching is a separate issue. While efforts are made to minimize the complications associated with ABO mismatching, exigencies of donor selection result in mismatching in 30–40% of allogeneic transplants. The number may be even higher with umbilical cord procedures. ABO mismatch is divided into three categories – major, minor, and major-minor – as described in Table 25.1.

In a major mismatch, the stem cell products must be red cell depleted to avoid immediate antibody-mediated hemolysis. Once hematopoiesis is restored, reticulocytes or late red cell precursors expressing the disparate antigen may hemolyze in the marrow, resulting in failure of mature red cells to leave the marrow, or they may hemolyze shortly after release into the circulation. Especially after reduced-intensity conditioning, there may be a prolonged transfusion requirement until antibody titers diminish. This reflects the lower degree of conditioning-related depletion of endogenous antibody-producing B cells. The failure of erythropoiesis may persist until offending B cells are eliminated and until the antibody is either completely adsorbed and reduced in titer or until it is removed by strategies such as plasmapheresis, rituximab, or possibly daratumomab therapy. This manifests as a form of pure red cell aplasia, since neutrophils and platelets may recover normally.

In minor mismatched transplantation, the infusion of the product is safe. However, the plasma accompanying the stem cells contains preformed antibody. If the antibody titers in the donor are high, immediate hemolysis may result. Even if the titers are not particularly elevated, antibody-antigen complexes may form that are initially clinically benign but can result in tissue damage that increases the risk of transplant-related toxicity such as veno-occlusive disease of the liver.[8,9] In addition, there may be plasma cells or isohemagglutinin-producing B lymphoblasts that can be stimulated by exposure to host A or B substance. This "passenger lymphocyte syndrome" can result in a delayed acute hemolytic reaction that

Table 25.1 ABO incompatibility in transplantation

Donor	Recipient	Antibodies	Type of Mismatch
A, B, AB	O	Preformed recipient anti-A and/or anti-B	Major
AB	A or B	Preformed recipient anti-A or anti-B	Major
A	B	Bidirectional antibodies	Major-minor
B	A	Bidirectional antibodies	Major-minor
O	A, B or AB	Preformed donor anti-A and anti-B	Minor
A or B	AB	Preformed donor anti-A or anti-B	Minor

can at times be severe.[10] This can be avoided by transfusing the patient with type O or donor type–specific blood. A similar passenger lymphocyte syndrome can be seen in organ transplantation where the isohemagglutinin producing cells are passively transferred with the transplanted organ.[11]

In major-minor mismatches, both scenarios may occur. ABO antigens are the most common targets, but hemolysis has also been reported against Rh, Jk(a), Kidd, and Lewis blood group antigens.[12] Disparities for these minor antigens may be more apparent in cord blood transplantation or when the donor and recipient are different ethnicities. Stem cell products are not typically typed for minor RBC antigens.

Thrombotic Microangiopathic Hemolytic Anemia

Coombs negative red cell fragmentation after HSCT was previously called hemolytic uremic syndrome (HUS) or thrombotic thrombocytopenic purpura (TTP) or a combination called TTP/HUS. However, the hallmarks of those illnesses – Shiga toxin–induced endothelial damage (e.g., from *E. coli* O:157 or O:104 serotypes) or loss of ADAMTS-13 is rarely encountered after HSCT. Some patients do have genetic susceptibility to TMA based on mutations in complement control proteins.[13] Renal and neurologic toxicity is common after HSCT and does not define the syndrome as TTP. It is important to recognize that the same end result may derive from several different causes in transplantation, which may remain obscure. Therefore, the syndrome of endothelial injury with associated hemolytic anemia after transplantation is called thrombotic microangiopathic hemolytic anemia (TMA).

All of these entities share the characteristics of microvascular obstruction and red cell fragmentation, although the stimulus triggering the injury differs. Calcineurin inhibitors (CNI) may trigger TMA by two mechanisms. First, there may be direct endothelial toxicity with associated production of fibrin stranding and thrombosis in the microvasculature. Such injury can also be caused by the mTOR inhibitor sirolimus,

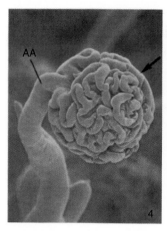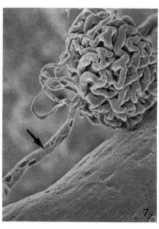

Figure 25.2 On the left is a scanning EM of a normal rat glomerulus. On the right, after 14 days of cyclosporine, there is arteriolar narrowing that may contribute to red cell fragmentation. English J, Evan A, Houghton DC, Bennett WM. Cyclosporine-induced acute renal dysfunction in the rat. Evidence of arteriolar vasoconstriction with preservation of tubular function. *Transplantation.* 1987; 44(1):135–141.

Table 25.2 Criteria for the diagnosis of TMA

BMT-CTN Toxicity Committee	EBMT International Working Group
RBC fragmentation and ≥ 2 schistocytes per high-power field on peripheral smear	>4% schistocytes
–	De novo, prolonged, or progressive thrombocytopenia ($<50 \times 10^3$, or 50% decline)
Concurrent increased serum LDH above institutional baseline	Sudden and persistent increase in LDH
Concurrent renal* and/or neurologic dysfunction without other explanations	–
–	Decrease in Hb or increase transfusion requirement
–	Decreased haptoglobin
Negative direct and indirect Coombs test results	–

*Doubling of serum creatinine from baseline (baseline = creatinine before hydration and conditioning) or 50% decrease in creatinine clearance from baseline

and indeed the endothelial toxicity of sirolimus may be additive or synergistic with CNI. CNI can also cause spasm of the afferent arteriole of the kidney, resulting in azotemia, hypertension, and hemolysis as a nonthrombotic complication (Figure 25.2).[14]

Total body irradiation may cause radiation nephritis. This is characterized by azotemia, hypertension, and TMA. [15] Kidney biopsy shows loss of glomeruli. Although total body irradiation is rarely used in autologous HSCT any more, the observation of this syndrome in autologous HSCT where calcineurin and mTOR inhibitors are not used allowed the distinction to be made from CNI-induced injury. In allogeneic transplantation, TBI may similarly cause kidney injury, but in this instance the concomitant use of tacrolimus, cyclosporine, or sirolimus may cause additive injury.

Finally, graft-v-host disease (GVHD) has a vasculopathic component that interacts with the mechanisms described already, increasing the risk of TMA. Moreover, there is some evidence that complement dysregulation may be involved, much along the lines of what can be observed in atypical HUS.[16]

The Bone Marrow Transplant Clinical Trials Network (BMT-CTN)[17] and the European Group for Blood and Marrow Transplantation International Working Group[18] have established useful criteria for diagnosing TMA. The BMT-CTN criteria focus more on organ dysfunction and do not include thrombocytopenia, reflecting the observation that there are varied causes for low platelets after HSCT. Although plasma exchange has been used in the management of TMA, no convincing studies have demonstrated that it is more effective than blood pressure control and reduction of offending agents.

Autoimmune Hemolytic Anemia

There is a tendency for some patients with chronic GVHD to develop autoantibodies. Often there is no particular pathology

associated with autoantibody production, but sometimes they are clinically significant.[19,20] Warm autoimmune hemolytic anemia is a rarely reported complication that presumably reflects dysfunctional immune regulation, since it occurs without known autoantibody production in the donor. It may occur concomitantly with autoimmune thrombocytopenia. Risk factors are difficult to enumerate accurately, but there is a sense that GVHD is associated with the development of these antibodies and that they may be triggered by an infection. Normally it is seen within 6 months of transplantation, and it can result in serious hemolytic anemia that at times is life threatening. The standard therapy is prednisone, but it tends to be resistant to treatment. Rituximab, cyclophosphamide, high-dose IgG, alemtuzumab, mycophenolate, bortezomib, calcineurin inhibition, plasmapheresis, and splenectomy have all been used with variable outcomes.

Other Causes

Perhaps the most frequent cause of failure of erythropoiesis after transplantation is relapse of the underlying disease. The frequency of relapse is highly dependent on the disease, stage at transplantation, the intensity of conditioning, the GVHD prophylactic regimen utilized, and stem cell source. In general, the use of unrelated donors and the development of chronic GVHD are associated with fewer relapses. In autologous transplantation, relapse is a common cause of count depression, but one must also consider the risk of secondary myelodysplastic syndrome (MDS). The risk of secondary MDS is dependent on several factors.[21] Prior chemotherapy or radiotherapy will often induce stem cell injury that may be unrecognized at the time of stem cell collection for transplantation, as can the chemotherapy used for stem cell mobilization. The use of total body irradiation as part of the conditioning regimen is also strongly implicated in the late development of MDS.[22] There is often an increase in MCV and RDW that presages the development of more significant marrow dysfunction. Thus, the late development of anemia after otherwise successful autologous marrow transplantation should prompt a marrow evaluation with cytogenetics. A devastating complication of HSCT is the development of leukemia in the transplanted marrow. This does not reflect relapse since the cells are of donor origin.[23] The diagnosis is generally made when chimerism analysis of leukemic blasts demonstrates residual host elements.

Rarely, hemophagocytic lymphohistiocytosis (HLH) can complicate marrow transplantation.[24] It is usually associated with viral infection, such as EBV, CMV, or adenovirus.

However, there are some cases in which the underlying trigger cannot be identified. Most commonly, this syndrome occurs less than 30 days after transplantation, and it is associated with fever, hemophagocytosis, and elevation of serum ferritin and serum soluble IL-2 receptor, much like HLH that occurs in the absence of HSCT. Epstein-Barr virus infection can be associated with HLH, or it can initiate a post-transplant lymphoproliferative disorder (EBV-PTLD) that can result in anemia as well.[25]

Conclusion

Anemia after stem cell transplantation is common. It may be inconsequential or indicative of severe problems with hematopoiesis. It may or may not be correctable. In general, a logical approach to diagnosis of anemia will result in a reasonable idea of the underlying cause; however, often the etiology of the anemia can only be inferred.

References

1. Gibson CJ, Kennedy JA, Nikiforow S, Kuo FC, Alyea EP, Ho V, Ritz J, Soiffer R, Antin JH, Lindsley RC. Donor-engrafted CHIP is common among stem cell transplant recipients with unexplained cytopenias. *Blood.* 2017;130:91–94.

2. Gibson CJ, Lindsley RC, Tchekmedyian V, Mar BG, Shi J, et al. Clonal hematopoiesis associated with adverse outcomes after autologous stem-cell transplantation for lymphoma. *Journal of Clinical Oncology.* 2017;35:1598–1605.

3. Larocca A, Piaggio G, Podesta M, et al. Boost of CD34+-selected peripheral blood cells without further conditioning in patients with poor graft function following allogeneic stem cell transplantation. *Haematologica.* 2006; 91:935–940.

4. Schapira L, Antin JH, Ransil BJ, et al. Serum erythropoietin levels in patients receiving intensive chemotherapy and radiotherapy. *Blood.* 1990; 76:2354–2359.

5. Miller CB, Lazarus HM. Erythropoietin in stem cell transplantation. *Bone Marrow Transplantation.* 2001; 27:1011–1016.

6. Wu CJ, Gladwin M, Tisdale J, et al. Mixed haematopoietic chimerism for sickle cell disease prevents intravascular haemolysis. *British Journal of Haematology.* 2007; 139:504–507.

7. Wu CJ, Krishnamurti L, Kutok JL, et al. Evidence for ineffective erythropoiesis

in severe sickle cell disease. *Blood.* 2005; 106:3639–3645.

8. Benjamin RJ, Antin JH. ABO-incompatible bone marrow transplantation: the transfusion of incompatible plasma may exacerbate regimen-related toxicity. *Transfusion.* 1999; 39:1273–1274.

9. Benjamin RJ, McGurk S, Ralston MS, Churchill WH, Antin JH. ABO incompatibility as an adverse risk factor for survival after allogeneic bone marrow transplantation. *Transfusion.* 1999; 39:179–187.

10. Bolan CD, Childs RW, Procter JL, Barrett AJ, Leitman SF. Massive immune haemolysis after allogeneic peripheral blood stem cell transplantation with minor ABO incompatibility. *British Journal of Haematology.* 2001; 112: 787–795.

11. Nadarajah L, Ashman N, Thuraisingham R, Barber C, Allard S, Green L. Literature review of passenger lymphocyte syndrome following renal transplantation and two case reports. *American Journal of Transplantation: Official Journal of the American Society of Transplantation and the American Society of Transplant Surgeons.* 2013; 13:1594–1600.

12. Young PP, Goodnough LT, Westervelt P, Diersio JF. Immune hemolysis involving non-ABO/RhD alloantibodies following hematopoietic stem cell transplantation. *Bone Marrow Transplantation.* 2001; 27:1305–1310.

13. Jodele S, Zhang K, Zou F, Laskin B, Dandoy CE, Myers KC, Lane A, Meller J, Medvedovic M, Chen J, Davies SM. The genetic fingerprint of susceptibility for transplant-associated thrombotic microangiopathy. *Blood.* 2016;127:989–996.

14. English J, Evan A, Houghton DC, Bennett WM. Cyclosporine-induced acute renal dysfunction in the rat. Evidence of arteriolar vasoconstriction with preservation of tubular function. *Transplantation.* 1987; 44:135–141.

15. Guinan EC, Tarbell NJ, Niemeyer CM, Sallan SE, Weinstein HJ. Intravascular hemolysis and renal insufficiency after bone marrow transplantation. *Blood.* 1988; 72:451–455.

16. Mii A, Shimizu A, Kaneko T, et al. Renal thrombotic microangiopathy associated with chronic graft-versus-host disease after allogeneic hematopoietic stem cell transplantation. *Pathology International.* 2011; 61:518–527.

17. Ho VT, Cutler C, Carter S, et al. Blood and marrow transplant clinical trials network toxicity committee consensus summary: thrombotic microangiopathy after hematopoietic stem cell transplantation. *Biology of Blood and Marrow Transplantation: Journal of the American Society for Blood and Marrow Transplantation.* 2005; 11:571–575.

18. Ruutu T, Barosi G, Benjamin RJ, et al. Diagnostic criteria for hematopoietic stem cell transplant-associated

microangiopathy: results of a consensus process by an International Working Group. *Haematologica.* 2007; 92:95–100.

19. Daikeler T, Labopin M, Ruggeri A, et al. New autoimmune diseases after cord blood transplantation: a retrospective study of EUROCORD and the Autoimmune Disease Working Party of the European Group for Blood and Marrow Transplantation. *Blood.* 2013; 121:1059–1064.

20. Rovira J, Cid J, Gutierrez-Garcia G, et al. Fatal Immune Hemolytic Anemia Following Allogeneic Stem Cell Transplantation: report of 2 Cases and Review of Literature. *Transfusion Medicine Reviews* 2013; 27:166–170.

21. Krishnan A, Bhatia S, Slovak ML, et al. Predictors of therapy-related leukemia and myelodysplasia following autologous transplantation for lymphoma: an assessment of risk factors. *Blood.* 2000; 95:1588–1593.

22. Friedberg JW, Neuberg D, Stone RM, et al. Outcome in patients with myelodysplastic syndrome after autologous bone marrow transplantation for non-Hodgkin's lymphoma. *Journal of Clinical Oncology: Official Journal of the American Society of Clinical Oncology.* 1999; 17:3128–3135.

23. Hertenstein B, Hambach L, Bacigalupo A, et al. Development of leukemia in donor cells after allogeneic stem cell transplantation – a survey of the European Group for Blood and Marrow Transplantation (EBMT). *Haematologica.* 2005; 90:969–975.

24. Asano T, Kogawa K, Morimoto A, et al. Hemophagocytic lymphohistiocytosis after hematopoietic stem cell transplantation in children: a nationwide survey in Japan. *Pediatric Blood & Cancer.* 2012; 59:110–114.

25. van Esser JW, van der Holt B, Meijer E, et al. Epstein-Barr virus (EBV) reactivation is a frequent event after allogeneic stem cell transplantation (SCT) and quantitatively predicts EBV-lymphoproliferative disease following T-cell–depleted SCT. *Blood.* 2001; 98:972–978.

The Anemia of Aging

Amanda J. Redig, MD, PhD and Nancy Berliner, MD

Anemia is among the most common hematologic abnormalities seen in elderly patients. There are many factors that likely play a role in this disorder, including dietary deficiencies, the accumulation of physical comorbidities, and an age-related decline in the regulation of normal hematopoietic parameters. However, although anemia is widely recognized as a condition associated with aging, the mechanisms by which advancing age contributes to a decline in erythrocyte production remain unclear. Anemia has been clearly established as a contributing factor to frailty, morbidity, and mortality in the aging population;[1] thus a greater understanding of the unique features of anemia in the elderly is likely to have significant public health benefits. As more and more individuals worldwide live into old age, the anemia of aging will continue to remain an area of active clinical and research interest.

Epidemiology

The most widely used definition of anemia is that established by the World Health Organization, notably a hemoglobin concentration of <13 g/dL for men and <12 g/dL for non-pregnant women.[2] The Third National Health and Nutritional Examination Survey (NHANES) assesses health and nutritional status of sequential cohorts of United States citizens, combining interviews, physical examinations, and comprehensive laboratory evaluation. Guralnik et al. documented that the overall incidence of anemia in NHANES III was 10% in women and 11% in men.[3] From census data from 2010, this translates to just over three million anemic, elderly individuals in the United States alone.[4] Several interesting trends emerge upon closer evaluation of the epidemiologic data. First, the increased frequency of anemia seen in younger women compared to younger men disappears in the aging population, likely a reflection of menopause. Older men and older women both develop anemia in association with advancing age,[5] but the age-associated prevalence increases more rapidly in older men than in older women.[6] In older men, there is some suggestion that decreasing levels of testosterone are associated with anemia, while increasing levels of estradiol are associated with a higher hematocrit.[7]

There is also a significant ethnic disparity in the prevalence of anemia in the aging population, as multiple studies have demonstrated that older non-Hispanic black individuals are up to three times as likely as non-Hispanic whites to develop anemia.[8] This difference persists despite correcting for the frequency of thalassemia, iron deficiency, and socioeconomic factors. In addition, such ethnic differences in hemoglobin levels are also seen in nonelderly populations.[6] There is some suggestion that non-Hispanic whites may be less likely to suffer from nutritional deficiencies associated with anemia,[9] but this alone is unlikely to account for the full extent of the clinical differences noted across ethnicities. Although there are fewer data evaluating anemia in aging patients of Hispanic ethnicity, it appears that the distribution of hemoglobin in this population parallels that seen in a white population even though socioeconomic factors may be more similar to a those of black population.[6] Interestingly, when mortality and anemia are evaluated in these patient cohorts, an increase in mortality in non-Hispanic black patients was seen with a drop in Hgb of 0.7 g/dL below WHO-defined anemia, while an increase in mortality was seen in non-Hispanic white patients with a drop in Hgb of only 0.2 g/dL below WHO-defined anemia.[10] Overall, it is clear that differences in ethnicity may influence the biology and clinical outcomes of the anemia of aging. Further evaluation of the mechanisms responsible for such differences may provide important clues about the genetic regulation of erythropoiesis.

Large-scale epidemiologic studies have also demonstrated intriguing insights into the multifactorial mechanisms of anemia in the aging population. The NHANES III study as well as the Women's Health and Aging Study I both evaluated the etiology of the anemia noted in study participants and found strikingly concordant results. In NHANES III, approximately one-third of patients had nutritional deficiencies linked to anemia (iron, B12, folate); one-third of patients were determined to have anemia of inflammation based on iron studies not consistent with iron deficiency; and one-third of patients had anemia of unexplained etiology.[3,11] In the Women's Health and Aging Study, an estimated third of study participants also had unexplained anemia.[11] Overall, most large studies in elderly patients find that an estimated 30% of those with anemia do not have a readily identifiable cause. Understanding the mechanisms behind this so-called "unexplained anemia" remains an important research question. While most studies find that anemia of any type in patients over age 65 predisposes to increased morbidity and mortality,[12–14] it is interesting that in a study from the Netherlands of adults age 85 or older, increased mortality was seen only in the population with explained anemia;[15] as the incidence of anemia exceeds 40% in patients over the age of 80,[16] it is possible that pathways leading to anemia in the extreme elderly are more complex and less morbid.

Inflammation, Aging, and Anemia

The aging process has been linked to increased expression of multiple markers of inflammation, including the cytokines IL-1, IL-6, tumor necrosis factor alpha (TNF-α), and macrophage migratory inhibitory factor (MIF).[1] The large InCHIANTI study evaluating the aging process in 1,300 individuals in the Chianti region of Italy demonstrated that all study participants over age 65 had detectable elevations in IL-1 receptor antagonist, IL-6, IL-18, CRP, and fibrinogen.[17] The development of a proinflammatory state in older patients may reflect a physiologic trend inherent to the aging process or may be associated with comorbidities seen in older populations such as diabetes, heart disease, or autoimmune disorders. The clinical development of "frailty," a syndrome described in elderly patients characterized by weight loss, weakness, and impaired balance, is strongly linked to both a proinflammatory state and anemia.[1] What is less certain is the precise causal relationship between inflammation, aging, and anemia. However, many proinflammatory mediators have specific effects upon the hematopoietic system, which may help o explain the pathogenesis of the anemia of aging and may contribute to the development of clinical frailty with its associated increase in morbidity and mortality.

Both MIF and TNF-α are associated with impaired erythroid colony formation in the laboratory setting, and multiple studies have identified MIF and TNF genetic polymorphisms that play a critical role in the severity of anemia associated with malarial infection (1). TNF-α upregulation has also been suggested to contribute to bone marrow failure seen in anemia syndromes such as Fanconi anemia, while patients with autoimmune disorders treated with anti-TNF-α antibodies demonstrate a statistically significant increase in hemoglobin.[18] IL-6 may play a particularly significant role in potentiating anemia through its role in regulating hepcidin, an acute-phase reactant that is now known to be a critical regulator of iron stores and iron-limited erythropoiesis.[1]

Leptin, a protein associated with body mass and energy metabolism, has also been shown to induce hepcidin, providing a further link between the regulation of iron metabolism and inflammation. There has also been speculation that the proinflammatory state found in both elderly patients and the HIV+ population may lead to a similar etiology for the anemia seen in both groups. A recent study analyzing a cohort of more than 2,000 HIV+ patients with matched controls revealed that a functional high-expressing polymorphism in the leptin gene promoter is associated with the development of anemia in HIV + but not HIV− individuals.[19] Overall, the shift towards a proinflammatory milieu that occurs with age is likely to contribute to the concurrent development of anemia noted in elderly patients. Complementary studies have suggested leptin can play a role in the decreased responsiveness to EPO in elderly patients[20] and that it also induces hepcidin expression, suggesting a possible mechanistic link between the molecular regulation of metabolism and AI in the elderly.[21]

There is also a substantial connection between the anemia of aging and the anemia of inflammation (AI), formerly known as the anemia of chronic disease. As older patients are more likely to have chronic diseases, it is not surprising that this specific type of anemia is often identified in the aging population. Anemia of inflammation is biochemically characterized by low serum iron and a low iron-binding capacity despite the presence of a normal or elevated serum ferritin, which serves as the distinguishing feature between AI and iron-deficiency anemia. AI is thought to be induced by the protein hepcidin, which is produced by the liver and regulates iron stores by inhibiting absorption of iron from the gastrointestinal tract while also preventing the release of stored iron in macrophage populations. Hepcidin is an acute-phase reactant increased by inflammation, and it is predicted that patients with AI have elevated hepcidin levels. Unlike iron-deficiency anemia, AI is not effectively treated by iron repletion, likely as a result of increased hepcidin levels preventing both the absorption and utilization of stored iron.

It was hypothesized that the availability of hepcidin testing would help establish the diagnosis of AI. However, when hepcidin levels are investigated in cohorts of aging patients, they did not provide clear diagnostic information. Ferrucci et al. evaluated urinary hepcidin levels in conjunction with anemia and measurement of inflammatory cytokines in individuals in the InCHIANTI study. Surprisingly, an elevated excretion of hepcidin was not seen in patients who were anemic with biochemical evidence of AI, although levels did correlate with low plasma iron and elevated IL6.[22] The reason for this remains unclear, but it establishes that single-point-in-time measurements of hepcidin cannot be expected to distinguish AI from other forms of anemia. Further elucidating how and when hepcidin elevation is triggered by inflammatory pathways in aging patients will likely be required in order to most effectively utilize hepcidin levels in the diagnosis or treatment of anemia in the elderly.

Vitamin D deficiency is also known to occur with some frequency in elderly populations. Intriguingly, in a subgroup analysis of the NHANES study population, vitamin D was not only associated with anemia but also demonstrated significant variation based upon anemia subtype.[23] The prevalence of vitamin D deficiency was 56% in study participants with anemia of inflammation, compared to only 33% in the nonanemic population or in those with unexplained anemia.[23] The presence of concurrent vitamin D deficiency and anemia has long been noted in patients suffering from chronic kidney disease, but the suggestion that vitamin D metabolism may play a direct role in mediating the development of anemia raises interesting possibilities for treatment of anemia not only in the elderly but also in other patient populations.

Clinical Connections

The clinical significance of anemia in the elderly patient population can be overlooked because of the relative frequency with which this laboratory abnormality is detected and the often insidious nature of clinical symptoms in patients with mild to moderate anemia. However, an emerging body of literature continues to support the connection between anemia and several clinical conditions with dramatic effects upon quality of life and health care expenditures in the aging population.

Recently published data demonstrates that anemia leads to a statistically significant increase in the likelihood of developing dementia in a large cohort of patients with a median age of 76 years and without dementia at the beginning of an 11-year follow-up period.[24] This association persisted even after correcting for demographics and comorbidities. A study with similar outcomes performed as part of the Women's Health and Aging Study raises the possibility that a better understanding of anemia in this unique population may suggest therapeutic targets for dementia.[25] Beyond the general inflammatory changes associated with aging and certain neurodegenerative processes, it is possible that biological steps uniquely linked to anemia may directly contribute to the pathology of dementia. New data specifically implicates iron deficiency in the elderly with cognitive decline, even in those who had not yet developed clinical anemia as a consequence of iron deficiency.[26] Such findings emphasize the complexity of the connections between the biology of aging and the regulation of erythropoiesis.

The connection between frailty and anemia has long been established. However, it is now becoming clear that not only can anemia itself contribute to the cognitive and physical decline in elderly patients, but it can also function in synergy with other disease processes associated with inflammatory changes to worsen the health status of older adults. Data from the Women's Health and Aging Studies demonstrates that both depression and pulmonary disease act in a synergistic fashion with anemia to worsen overall health status in patients with both disorders when compared to those with only one.[27] What this study does not address is whether the anemia is the driving influence in the cascade of physical decline that leads to frailty or whether it functions as a reflection of another underlying process. Since anemia in the elderly is usually quite mild, the latter seems more likely.

Similarly, accumulating evidence has identified anemia as an important clinical variable in the outcome and disease progression of patients with heart failure, the majority of whom are also elderly. The prospective STAMINA-HFP (Study of Anemia in a Heart Failure Population) found that 34% of patients in a cohort of 1,076 also suffered from anemia.[28] Multiple studies have also demonstrated that heart failure is a state of chronic inflammation, with elevated levels of circulating TNF-α, IL-1, and IL-6, notably the same cytokine profile seen in patients with anemia of inflammation.[29] Furthermore, a subset of heart failure patients is also noted to have iron deficiency anemia.[30] The first randomized, double-blind placebo-controlled trial of iron repletion versus placebo in a small cohort of anemic patients with heart failure led to improvements in hemoglobin as well as NYHA class, 6-minute walk time, and number of hospitalizations.[31] These results were replicated in a larger trial of heart failure patients, and in this larger study, improvement in outcomes in the cohort of patients receiving iron supplementation was seen even in those patients who were not yet clinically anemic.[32]

In an exciting development for possible therapeutic intervention, it has been established that iron deficiency results in a down-regulation of aconitase enzyme pathways in early erythroid progenitors, which subsequently results in decreased erythropoiesis and clinical anemia. There is some suggestion that a similar down-regulation may also occur in response to chronic inflammation. A recent study in animal models suggests that repleting a downstream product of the aconitase pathway can reverse this anemia.[33] Targeting this pathway may thus represent a way to therapeutically address elements of anemia in the elderly caused by both iron deficiency and the inflammatory milieu.

Future Directions

Multiple large-scale and smaller-cohort studies have confirmed that in older patients with anemia, up to one third of study participants will be found to have anemia that is not attributable to classical anemia of inflammation or vitamin deficiencies. The mechanisms behind this unexplained anemia are still being investigated but may ultimately reflect the complexity and intersection of multiple signaling pathways that regulate iron metabolism, inflammatory mediators, and growth factor signaling. Interestingly, while changes in telomere length are considered to be the molecular hallmark of aging, in contrast to other age-related diseases, no association was seen between telomere length and anemia in a large, multicountry population study of adults over age 85.[34] Future studies will be needed to continue to refine not only the overall regulators of erythropoiesis but also the genetic polymorphisms and epigenetic changes that drive the multifactorial biology of anemia in the elderly.

From a practical standpoint, the clinical management of the anemic elderly patient should focus on several things. First, a thorough assessment of nutritional status is critical to identify the estimated third of all elderly anemic patients with deficiencies in iron, folate, B12, or vitamin D, all of which can be effectively treated with supplementation. Second, management of comorbidities, particularly those associated with increased inflammation, is likely to minimize the deleterious effects of anemia associated with inflammation. Finally, appropriate monitoring of overall functional status and ability to perform activities of daily living (ADLs) will continue to help identify frail patients at a stage at which intervention may help prevent the morbidity associated with this condition.

Overall, the etiology of anemia in the aging population is complex and multifactorial. However, it also represents an exciting arena in both clinical patient care and laboratory investigation because of the ever-evolving connections between the common biological pathways and genetic regulation that contribute to a final clinical endpoint of anemia as assessed by hemoglobin measurement. Moving forward, a better understanding of the key features and drivers of anemia in the elderly will allow for improved patient care of this growing vulnerable population. In addition, increased insight into the unique mechanisms of anemia in the elderly may also have wider application in our understanding of other disease processes and the fundamental biology of inflammation.

References

1. Vanasse GJ, Berliner N. Anemia in elderly patients: an emerging problem for the 21st century. *Hematology Am Soc Hematol Educ Program*. 2010; 2010:271–275. PubMed PMID: 21239805. Epub 2011/01/18.

2. Blanc BFC, Hallberg L, et al. Nutritional anaemias. Report of a WHO Scientific Group. *WHO Tech Rep Ser*. 1968; 405:1–40.

3. Guralnik JM, Eisenstaedt RS, Ferrucci L, Klein HG, Woodman RC. Prevalence of anemia in persons 65 years and older in the United States: evidence for a high rate of unexplained anemia. *Blood*. 2004 Oct 15; 104(8):2263–2268. PubMed PMID: 15238427. Epub 2004/07/09.

4. US Census 2010.

5. Moore KL, Boscardin WJ, Steinman MA, Schwartz JB. Age and sex variation in prevalence of chronic medical conditions in older residents of U.S. nursing homes. *J Am Geriatr Soc*. 2012 Apr;60(4):756–764. PubMed PMID: 22463062. Epub 2012/04/03.

6. Patel KV. Epidemiology of anemia in older adults. *Semin Hematol*. 2008 Oct;45(4):210–217. PubMed PMID: 18809090. Epub 2008/09/24.

7. Paller CJ, Shiels MS, Rohrmann S, Menke A, Rifai N, Nelson WG, et al. Association between sex steroid hormones and hematocrit in a nationally representative sample of men. *J Androl*. 2012 Nov–Dec;33 (6):1332–1341. PubMed PMID: 22604627. Epub 2012/05/19.

8. Beutler E, West C. Hematologic differences between African-Americans and whites: the roles of iron deficiency and alpha-thalassemia on hemoglobin levels and mean corpuscular volume. *Blood*. 2005 Jul 15; 106(2):740–745. PubMed PMID: 15790781. Epub 2005/03/26.

9. Thomson CA, Stanaway JD, Neuhouser ML, Snetselaar LG, Stefanick ML, Arendell L, et al. Nutrient intake and anemia risk in the women's health initiative observational study. *J Am Diet Assoc*. 2011 Apr;111(4):532–541. PubMed PMID: 21443985. Epub 2011/ 03/30.

10. Patel KV, Longo DL, Ershler WB, Yu B, Semba RD, Ferrucci L, et al. Haemoglobin concentration and the risk of death in older adults: differences by race/ethnicity in the NHANES III follow-up. *Br J Haematol*. 2009 May;145 (4):514–523. PubMed PMID: 19344387. Epub 2009/04/07.

11. Semba RD, Ricks MO, Ferrucci L, Xue QL, Chaves P, Fried LP, et al. Types of anemia and mortality among older disabled women living in the community: the Women's Health and Aging Study I. *Aging Clin Exp Res*. 2007 Aug;19(4):259–264. PubMed PMID: 17726354. Epub 2007/ 08/30.

12. Woodman R, Ferrucci L, Guralnik J. Anemia in older adults. *Curr Opin Hematol*. 2005 Mar;12(2):123–128. PubMed PMID: 15725902.

13. Kikuchi M, Inagaki T, Shinagawa N. Five-year survival of older people with anemia: variation with hemoglobin concentration. *J Am Geriatr Soc*. 2001 Sep;49(9):1226–1228. PubMed PMID: 11559383.

14. Guralnik JM, Ershler WB, Schrier SL, Picozzi VJ. Anemia in the elderly: a public health crisis in hematology. *Hematology (Am Soc Hematol Educ Program)*. 2005:528–532. PubMed PMID: 16304431.

15. Willems JM, den Elzen WP, Vlasveld LT, Westendorp RG, Gussekloo J, de Craen AJ, et al. No increased mortality risk in older persons with unexplained anaemia. *Age Ageing*. 2012 Jul;41(4): 501–506. PubMed PMID: 22417980. Epub 2012/03/16.

16. Tettamanti M, Lucca U, Gandini F, Recchia A, Mosconi P, Apolone G, et al. Prevalence, incidence and types of mild anemia in the elderly: the "Health and Anemia" population-based study. *Haematologica*. 2010 Nov;95(11): 1849–1856. PubMed PMID: 20534701. PubMed Central PMCID: 2966906. Epub 2010/06/11.

17. Ferrucci L, Corsi A, Lauretani F, Bandinelli S, Bartali B, Taub DD, et al. The origins of age-related proinflammatory state. *Blood*. 2005 Mar 15; 105(6):2294–2299. PubMed PMID: 15572589. Epub 2004/12/02.

18. Furst DE, Kay J, Wasko MC, Keystone E, Kavanaugh A, Deodhar A, et al. The effect of golimumab on haemoglobin levels in patients with rheumatoid arthritis, psoriatic arthritis or ankylosing spondylitis. *Rheumatology (Oxford)*. 2013 Jul 9. PubMed PMID: 23838027. Epub 2013/ 07/11. Eng.

19. Vanasse GJ, Jeong JY, Tate J, Bathulapalli H, Anderson D, Steen H, et al. A polymorphism in the leptin gene promoter is associated with anemia in patients with HIV disease. *Blood*. Nov 17; 118(20):5401–5408. PubMed PMID: 21926355. Epub 2011/09/20.

20. Hubbard RE, Sinead O'Mahony M, Woodhouse KW. Erythropoietin and anemia in aging and frailty. *J Am Geriatr Soc*. 2008 Nov;56 (11):2164–2165. PubMed PMID: 19016962. Epub 2008/11/20.

21. Chung B, Matak P, McKie AT, Sharp P. Leptin increases the expression of the iron regulatory hormone hepcidin in HuH7 human hepatoma cells. *J Nutr*. 2007 Nov;137(11):2366–2370. PubMed PMID: 17951471. Epub 2007/ 10/24.

22. Ferrucci L, Semba RD, Guralnik JM, Ershler WB, Bandinelli S, Patel KV, et al. Proinflammatory state, hepcidin, and anemia in older persons. *Blood*. 2010 May 6; 115(18):3810–3816. PubMed PMID: 20081092. Epub 2010/01/19.

23. Perlstein TS, Pande R, Berliner N, Vanasse GJ. Prevalence of 25-hydroxyvitamin D deficiency in subgroups of elderly persons with anemia: association with anemia of inflammation. *Blood*. Mar 10; 117 (10):2800–2806. PubMed PMID: 21239700. Epub 2011/01/18.

24. Hong CH, Falvey C, Harris TB, Simonsick EM, Satterfield S, Ferrucci L, et al. Anemia and risk of dementia in older adults: Findings from the Health ABC study. *Neurology*. Aug 6; 81(6): 528–533. PubMed PMID: 23902706. Epub 2013/08/02.

25. Deal JA, Carlson MC, Xue QL, Fried LP, Chaves PH. Anemia and 9-year domain-specific cognitive decline in community-dwelling older women: The Women's Health and Aging Study II. *J Am Geriatr Soc*. 2009 Sep;57(9): 1604–1611. PubMed PMID: 19682133. Epub 2009/08/18.

26. Yavuz BB, Cankurtaran M, Haznedaroglu IC, Halil M, Ulger Z, Altun B, et al. Iron deficiency can cause cognitive impairment in geriatric patients. *J Nutr Health Aging*. 2012 Mar;16(3):220–224. PubMed PMID: 22456776. Epub 2012/03/30.

27. Chang SS, Weiss CO, Xue QL, Fried LP. Patterns of comorbid inflammatory diseases in frail older women: the Women's Health and Aging Studies I and II. *J Gerontol A Biol Sci Med Sci*. Apr;65(4):407–413. PubMed PMID: 19933749. Epub 2009/11/26.

28. Adams KF, Jr., Patterson JH, Oren RM, Mehra MR, O'Connor CM, Pina IL, et al. Prospective assessment of the occurrence of anemia in patients with heart failure: results from the Study of Anemia in a Heart Failure Population (STAMINA-HFP) Registry. *Am Heart J*. 2009 May;157(5):926–932. PubMed PMID: 19376323. Epub 2009/04/21.

29. Shah R, Agarwal AK. Anemia associated with chronic heart failure: current concepts. *Clin Interv Aging*. 2013 8:111–122. PubMed PMID: 23403618. Epub 2013/02/14.

30. Nanas JN, Matsouka C, Karageorgopoulos D, Leonti A, Tsolakis E, Drakos SG, et al. Etiology of anemia in patients with advanced heart failure. *J Am Coll Cardiol*. 2006 Dec 19; 48(12):2485–2489. PubMed PMID: 17174186. Epub 2006/12/19.

31. Toblli JE, Lombrana A, Duarte P, Di Gennaro F. Intravenous iron reduces NT-pro-brain natriuretic peptide in anemic patients with chronic heart failure and renal insufficiency. *J Am Coll Cardiol*. 2007 Oct 23; 50(17): 1657–1665. PubMed PMID: 17950147. Epub 2007/10/24.

32. Anker SD, Comin Colet J, Filippatos G, Willenheimer R, Dickstein K, Drexler H, et al. Ferric carboxymaltose in patients with heart failure and iron deficiency. *N Engl J Med*. 2009 Dec 17; 361(25):2436–2448. PubMed PMID: 19920054. Epub 2009/11/19.

33. Richardson CL, Delehanty LL, Bullock GC, Rival CM, Tung KS, Kimpel DL, et al. Isocitrate ameliorates anemia by suppressing the erythroid iron restriction response. *J Clin Invest*. 2013 Aug 1; 123(8):3614–3623. PubMed PMID: 23863711. Epub 2013/07/19.

34. Den Elzen WP, Martin-Ruiz C, von Zglinicki T, Westendorp RG, Kirkwood TB, Gussekloo J. Telomere length and anaemia in old age: results from the Newcastle 85-plus Study and the Leiden 85-plus Study. *Age Ageing*. Jul;40(4): 494–500. PubMed PMID: 21622673. Epub 2011/05/31.

Anemia in Pregnancy

Ariela Marshall, MD, and Jean M. Connors, MD

Epidemiology and Pathophysiology

Anemia is one of the most common physiologic alterations of pregnancy, affecting an estimated 52% of women in nonindustrialized countries and 23% of women in industrialized countries.[1] The Centers for Disease Control and Prevention defines anemia as a hemoglobin less than 11 g/dL during the first and third trimester, or a hemoglobin less than 10.5 g/dL during the second trimester.[2] Alternatively, the World Health Organization has defined anemia as a hemoglobin less than 11 g/dL in any trimester.[3] The prevalence of anemia increases over the course of pregnancy, and by the third trimester, rates are approximately 14–52%, with higher prevalence in women of lower socioeconomic status and living in less developed countries.[4] Of the multiple potential causes of anemia in pregnancy, iron deficiency is by far the most common. We will discuss the specific pathophysiology of each type of anemia in what follows.

Physiologic Anemia

All pregnant women experience dilutional anemia as a consequence of a greater increase in plasma volume relative to the increase in red cell mass. Starting in the sixth week of pregnancy, total plasma volume increases approximately 30–50% above baseline.[5] This is accompanied by a decrease in systemic vascular resistance mediated by rennin, angiotensin, aldosterone, estrogens and progesterone, ADH, and prostacyclin. Total red blood cell mass, however, expands only by about 20–30% starting in the 12th week of pregnancy, leading to a decrease in hemoglobin concentration and hematocrit.[6]

Iron Deficiency Anemia

Iron deficiency is the most prevalent cause of anemia in pregnancy. Iron functions predominantly to transport hemoglobin-bound oxygen from the lungs to tissues and also facilitates both storage in muscle tissue (as myoglobin) and electron transport in cytochromes. Iron is absorbed in the proximal small intestine and released into the bloodstream via ferroportin, then binds to transferrin, whereafter it circulates to the bone marrow and erythrocytes for utilization as well as to the liver and spleen for storage.[7] Intracellular iron is stored inside ferritin, a large 24-subunit protein that can store up to 4,500 iron atoms. Ferritin is an excellent biomarker of iron status.

Due to increased demand from both physiologic anemia and fetal growth as well as to compensate for blood loss at delivery, iron absorption increases from 0.8 mg/day in the first trimester to 7.5 mg /day in the third trimester, averaging 4.4 mg/day throughout gestation.[8] Though intestinal iron absorption increases, dietary intake and existing iron stores are generally inadequate, and iron deficiency anemia develops. While the impact of iron deficiency anemia (IDA) on pregnancy outcomes is controversial, there is at least some evidence that first-trimester IDA is associated with low birth weight and preterm delivery.[9]

Megaloblastic Anemia

Megaloblastic anemia in pregnancy is most commonly due to folate deficiency but can also be a result of vitamin B12 deficiency. Folate is absorbed in the small intestine and transported as 5-methyl-tetrahydrofolate to sites of utilization in a vitamin B12-dependent manner and is stored primarily in the liver. Folate is found in most food sources. The leading cause of deficiency in pregnancy is increased requirement due to high metabolic activity of the fetus and utero-placental unit.[10]

Vitamin B12, which is absorbed in the distal ileum as a complex with intrinsic factor, is stored primarily in the liver as well as the bone marrow. Vitamin B12 deficiency during pregnancy is most often secondary to intestinal malabsorption related to lack of intrinsic factor due to either autoimmune pernicious anemia or to removal of parietal cells as a result of gastrectomy. It can also occur in settings of low oral intake.[10]

Both types of megaloblastic anemia are characterized by defective DNA synthesis in the presence of continued RNA synthesis, resulting in large cells with shortened survival times related to defective membrane architecture.[11]

Hemoglobinopathies

Sickle cell hemoglobinopathies (predominantly hemoglobin SS) are relatively prevalent and can lead to significant complications during pregnancy. Hemoglobin S is due to substitution of glutamic acid with valine in the beta globin gene, whereas hemoglobin C occurs when glutamic acid is substituted by lysine. Deoxygenation leads to agglutination of hydrophobic hemoglobin residues and the formation of tetrameric polypeptides in the erythrocyte. This causes distortion of the erythroid cell membrane, a shortened life span, and a chronic compensated anemia.[12] The increased metabolic demands, hypercoagulable state of pregnancy, and increased venous stasis lead to an increase in vaso-occlusive crises and an overall increase in both maternal and fetal morbidity and mortality, though with modern medical care, outcomes have improved significantly.[13]

Thalassemias occur as a result of decreased synthesis of the α-globin or β-globin chains. α-thalassemia occurs as a consequence of the deletion of variable numbers of α-globin genes. Loss of one is termed the "silent carrier" state, loss of two is called α-thalassemia minor and can occur in either cis (α-thalassemia-1) or trans (α-thalassemia-2) formations, and loss of three is called Hemoglobin H. Loss of all four α-globin genes is incompatible with life. Individuals with α-thalassemia of any type are thought to have normal pregnancy outcomes.[14]

β-thalassemia is a consequence of a variety of point mutations in the β-globin gene. There are two forms, $β^0$ and $β^+$, the former associated with absence of β-globin mRNA and the latter with decreased quantity. Patients with mutations in only one β-globin gene (thalassemia minor) are usually asymptomatic, whereas those with homozygous mutations (β-thalassemia major) are affected by ineffective erythropoiesis, hemolysis, and increased production of fetal hemoglobin.[15] Many female patients with β-thalassemia major are infertile due to iron overload and resultant abnormal pituitary function, and thus pregnancy is rare.[16] However, patients with β-thalassemia minor have unimpaired fertility.

Hemolytic Anemias

Hemolytic anemias are characterized by increased erythrocyte destruction related to either an intrinsic red cell defect or the action of an extrinsic agent. Two of the more common intrinsic defects include hereditary spherocytosis and G6PD deficiency. Hereditary spherocytosis is an autosomal dominant disease characterized by alteration of membrane proteins (most often ankryn), leading to increased fragility, splenic sequestration, and destruction of erythrocytes. G6PD deficiency is an X-linked disorder leading to impaired production of NADPH during aerobic glycolysis, compromising the ability to maintain glutathione in a reduced state and depriving the cell of the capacity to protect from oxidative damage.

Microangiopathic hemolytic anemias are the primary extrinsic hemolytic anemias of pregnancy. They are characterized by intravascular hemolysis and microvascular thrombotic lesions and, in pregnancy, most often present as hemolytic uremic syndrome (HUS) or hemolysis with elevated liver enzymes and low platelets (HELLP). Autoimmune hemolytic anemia (AIHA) is related to production of either a warm (typically IgG) antibody or a cold (IgM) antibody. Warm AIHA can occur in the setting of an underlying autoimmune

disorder or hematologic malignancy, while cold AIHA typically occurs in the postinfectious setting.[17]

Other Anemias

Other notable causes of anemia in pregnancy include infections and aplastic anemia. Infections include predominantly the hemolytic anemia of malarial infection, as well as hookworm, roundworm, and whipworm infection leading to iron deficiency anemia and HIV infection leading to hemolytic and hypoproliferative anemia. Aplastic anemia may be either unmasked by pregnancy or induced through estrogen-mediated inhibition of erythropoiesis. Maternal death, primarily due to hemorrhage or infection, occurs in 20–25% of cases.[6]

Clinical Presentation

Anemia in pregnancy is often asymptomatic and only detected on routine laboratory testing. When symptomatic, anemia manifests in a similar manner regardless of the pathophysiologic basis. The most common symptoms include those of decreased oxygen-carrying capacity, including weakness, dizziness, lightheadedness, and palpitations. Physical findings can include pale skin, tachycardia, and a systolic flow murmur.

Iron deficiency anemia can cause pica, particularly pagophagia (ingestion of ice). Women with megaloblastic anemia due to folate deficiency may present with cheilosis and glossitis, whereas those with B12 deficiency can develop neurologic symptoms such as numbness and paresthesia of the extremities, weakness, ataxia, poor coordination, and changes in mental status – all thought to be related to demyelination.[10]

Women with sickle cell disease may experience an increase in painful crises during pregnancy, as well as an increased rate of infections, preeclampsia, and thromboembolic events.[12] Women with thalassemias generally have few specific complications in pregnancy aside from manifestations of worsening anemia, but there is a high risk of preeclampsia in women carrying a fetus with α-thalassemia related to the large fetal placenta associated with fetal hydrops.

Symptoms of hemolytic anemia vary based on the chronicity of disease. Inherited hemolytic anemias are typically chronic and associated with jaundice, splenomegaly, cholelithiasis, and painful crises, whereas acquired hemolytic anemias present more acutely, often with chills, myalgias, and abdominal pain and vomiting. Microangiopathic hemolytic anemias can present at any time throughout pregnancy, but HUS in particular tends to occur in the peripureum.[17]

Diagnostic Evaluation and Lab Findings

Pregnant women should be evaluated on a regular basis to assess for anemia, defined per CDC or WHO criteria as mentioned. A low serum ferritin reflects iron deficiency.[18] In pregnancy, ferritin <15–30 μg/L is diagnostic and merits iron supplementation.[19,20] Of note, ferritin is generally elevated in pregnancy, as it is an acute-phase reactant, so a normal ferritin does not ensure adequate iron stores. Iron deficiency is also associated with hypochromic microcytosis, decrease in transferrin saturation, and increase in the serum-transferring receptor concentration.[21]

Anemia due to folate or vitamin B12 deficiency is associated with macrocytosis (MCV >100) as well as a low reticulocyte count, macroovalocytes, and hypersegmented neutrophils on peripheral smear and, in more severe cases, leucopenia and thrombocytopenia. Folate deficiency is confirmed with low serum and red blood cell folate levels and normal methylmalonic acid, whereas B12 deficiency is associated with low serum B12 levels and elevation in serum methylmalonic acid and homocysteine.[22] Both types of megaloblastic anemia are associated with hemolysis related to destruction of cells with defective membrane architecture, resulting in elevation in indirect bilirubin and lactic dehydrogenase levels and elevation in serum ferritin and iron levels.[11]

Sickle cell anemia and thalassemia are generally diagnosed via hemoglobin electrohporesis prior to pregnancy. Because of the increased risk of complications in pregnancy, it is recommended that all pregnant women undergo prenatal screening (Rust). Both hemoglobinopathies are generally associated with chronic, hypochromic microcytic anemias. Women with Hemoglobin H will also exhibit moderate hemolysis and reticulocytosis, whereas those with α-thalassemia 1 have only mild anemia and those with α-thalassemia 2 do not have notable laboratory findings. Findings of β-thalassemia major include abnormal erythrocytes with Heinz bodies, nucleated erythrocytes, hyperbilirubinemia (often associated with cholelithiasis), hepato- and spleno-megaly, and extramedullary hematopoiesis with bony malformations. β-thalassemia minor is generally associated with reticulocytosis in addition to hypochromic microcytic erythrocytes.[15]

Hemolytic anemias are characterized by indirect hyperbilirubinemia, elevation of lactate dehydrogenase, low haptoglobin, and often hemoglobinuria. Markers of accelerated compensatory erythropoiesis including reticulocytosis, macrocytosis, leukocytosis, and thrombocytosis develop 5–10 days after an episode of acute hemolysis.[17] Specific tests for each disorder include spherocytes on peripheral smear and increased osmotic fragility in hereditary spherocytosis, Heinz bodies in G6PD deficiency, schistocytes with a negative direct Coomb's test in microangiopathic hemolytic anemias, and positive Coomb's test in autoimmune hemolytic anemia.[17] HELLP syndrome, unique to pregnancy, involves transaminitis and thrombocytopenia in addition to markers of hemolysis.

Treatment

As iron deficiency anemia is so common in pregnancy, some organizations have recommended prophylactic supplementation, either for all women or selectively based on low ferritin level. Supplemental iron increases ferritin, though not necessarily the hemoglobin concentration during pregnancy.[23] However, prophylactic iron is not routinely recommended by all physicians. Iron deficiency may initially be treated with oral iron supplementation of 60–120 mg elemental iron a day divided into three doses, decreased to 30 mg a day after the anemia is corrected (generally within 1–2 weeks given a rise in hemoglobin of approximately 0.2 g/dL per day, though longer for more severe anemia).[24] As high-dose iron supplementation can lead to depletion in zinc, a multivitamin with 15 mg of zinc should be given at a different time of day. If there is no response to oral iron therapy within 4 weeks, other etiologies of anemia should be investigated. If iron deficiency remains the diagnosis, common due to an up to 70% rate of gastrointestinal adverse events with oral supplementation,[25] parenteral iron can be administered. One gram of low-molecular weight iron dextran given over one hour is standard and in some cases is used first-line even without a prior trial of oral iron.[26] Combination of intravenous iron (polymaltose) with oral iron has been demonstrated to lead to significantly higher increases in hemoglobin and ferritin, as well as improvement in quality-of-life parameters, compared to oral iron alone.[27] Recombinant erythropoietin may be efficacious for refractory cases[28] but is not considered standard of care.

Vitamin B12 deficiency is treated with 1,000 ug of cyanocobalamin intramuscularly once weekly for 8 weeks followed by monthly injection; supplementation generally leads to reticulocytosis within 3 days, and anemia typically resolves over 3–4 weeks. Women found to be folate deficient should take 1 mg of oral folate daily, and anemia can be expected to resolve within 4–6 weeks.[10] Vitamin B12 deficiency should be ruled out prior to administration of folic acid, as folic acid may correct many symptoms of B12 deficiency but can lead to worsening of the neurologic sequelae.

Management of pregnant patients with sickle cell disease includes baseline blood work (complete blood count, reticulocyte count, electrophoresis, and serum iron, as well as screening for hepatitis and HIV) and supplementation with 1 mg of folate daily. Patients should have regular obstetric visits with serial ultrasonography for fetal growth and amniotic fluid volume assessments from 24 to 28 weeks monthly through delivery. Vasoocclusive crises are managed as in nonpregnant patients, with intravenous hydration, oxygen therapy, and liberal use of analgesics. The use of prophylactic exchange transfusions is controversial, as it can reduce the risk of vasoocclusive crises during pregnancy but does carry the risks of alloimmunization[29] and is strongly recommended only for women with multiple gestations. Women should be monitored closely in the peurperium, period as risk of infections, painful crises, and thromboembolic disease is high. As women with β-thalassemia major rarely become pregnant and pregnancy is relatively uncomplicated for the less severe variants of both α- and β-thalassemia, obstetric management focuses on first-trimester screening of women (and, if identified, offering the father screening) and subsequently offering counseling and prenatal diagnosis for those couples who are both carriers.

Treatment of the hemolytic anemias in pregnancy is quite varied given the different pathophysiologic basis of each condition. Splenectomy is curative for hereditary spherocytosis. Hemolytic episodes due to G6PD are treated with supportive care. Plasmapheresis is the therapy of choice for microangiopathic hemolytic anemias, and steroids are the initial therapy of choice for warm AIHA.[17] Finally, delivery is the only curative therapy for HELLP syndrome, though supportive measures such as antihypertensives and platelet transfusions in the setting of active bleeding may also be helpful.

References

1. United Nations Children's Fund, University, and WHO. *Iron Deficiency Anaemia. Assessment, Prevention, and Control. A Guide for Programme Managers.* Geneva (Switzerland): World Health Organization; 2001.

2. Centers for Disease Control and Prevention. Recommendations to prevent and control iron deficiency in the united states. *MMWR Recomm Rep.* 1998; 47(RR-3):1–29.

3. World Health Organization. *Nutritional anaemias. Report of a WHO scientific group* 1968. (WHO Technical Report Series, No.405). http://whqlibdoc.who.int/trs/WHO_TRS_405.pdf (Accessed March 13, 2013).

4. Milman N. Prepartum anaemia: prevention and treatment. *Ann Hematol.* 2008; 87(12):949–959.

5. Bernstein IM, Ziegler W, and Badger GJ. Plasma volume expansion in early pregnancy. *Obstet Gynecol* 97(5);669–672.

6. Lee AI, Okam MM. Anemia in pregnancy. *Hematol Oncol Clin N Am.* 2011; 25:241–259.

7. Andrews NC. Forging a field: the golden age of iron biology. *Blood.* 2008; 112(2):219–230.

8. Milman N. Iron and pregnancy – a delicate balance. *Ann Hematol.* 2006; 85 (9):559–565.

9. Scholl TO et al. Anemia vs iron deficiency: increased risk of preterm delivery in a prospective study. *Am J Clin Nutr.* 1992; 55(5):985–988.

10. Cambpell BA. Megaloblastic anemia in pregnancy. *Clin Obstet Gynecol.* 1995; 38(3):455–462.

11. Frenkel EP, Yardley DA. Clinical and laboratory features and sequelae of deficiency of folic acid (folate) and vitamin B12 (cobalamin) in pregnancy and gynecology. *Hematol Oncol Clin N Am.* 2000; 14(5):1079–1100.

12. Rust OA and Perry KG. Pregnancy complicated by sickle hemoglobinopathy. *Clin Obstet Gynecol.* 1995; 38(3):472–484.

13. Rogers DT and Molokie R. Sickle disease in pregnancy. *Obstet Gynecol Clin North Am.* 2010; 37(2):223–237.

14. Fleming AF. Maternal anemia and fetal outcome in pregnancies complicated by thalassemia minor and "stomatocytosis." *Am J Obstet Gynecol.* 1973; 116(3):309–319.

15. Kilpatrick SJ and Laros RK. Thalassemia in pregnancy. *Clin Obstet Gynecol.* 1995; 38(3):485–496.

16. Mordel N et al. Successful full-term pregnancy in homozygous β-thalassemia major: case report and review of the literature. *Obstet Gynecol.* 1989; 73(5):837–840.

17. Leduc L. Hemolytic anemias in pregnancy. *Clin Obstet Gynecol.* 1995; 38(3):463–471.

18. Lipschitz DA, Cook JO, Finch CA. A clinical evaluation of serum ferritin as an index of iron stores. *N Engl J Med.* 1974; 290(22):1213–1216.

19. Breymann C et al. Diagnosis and treatment of iron-deficiency anaemia during pregnancy and postpartum. *Arch Gynecol Obstet.* 2010; 282(5):577–580.

20. Van den Broek NR et al. Iron status in pregnant women: which measurements are valid? *Br J Haematol.* 1998; 103 (3):817–824.

21. Schwartz WJ, Thurnau GR. Iron deficiency anemia in pregnancy. *Clin Obstet Gynecol.* 38(3):443–454.

22. Beck WS. Diagnosis of megaloblastic anemia. *Annu Rev Med.* 1991; 42:311–322.

23. Taylor DJ et al. Effect of iron supplementation on serum ferritin levels during and after pregnancy. *Br J Obstet Gynaecol.* 1982; 89(12):1011–1017.

24. Allen LH. Nutritional supplementation for the pregnant woman. *Clin Obstet Gynecol.* 1994; 37(3):587–595.

25. Reveiz L et al. Treatments for iron-deficiency anaemia in pregnancy. *Cochrane Database Syst Rev.* 2011; 10: CD003094.

26. Auerbach M et al. Safety and efficacy of rapidly administered (one hour) one gram of low molecular weight iron dextran (INFeD) for the treatment of iron deficiency anemia. *Am J Hematol.* 2011; 86(10):860–862.

27. Khalafallah AA et al. Three-year follow-up of a randomized clinical trial of intravenous versus oral iron for anaemia in pregnancy. *BMJ Open.* 2012; 2(5):e000998.

28. Sifakis S et al. Erythropoietin in the treatment of iron deficiency anemia during pregnancy. *Gynecol Obstet Invest.* 2001; 51(3):150–156.

29. Koshy M et al. Prophylactic red-cell transfusions in pregnant patients with sickle cell disease. *N Engl J Med.* 1988; 319(22):1447–1452.

28

Anemias Due to Systemic Diseases

Giada Bianchi, MD, and Ronald P. McCaffrey, MD

Hematologic abnormalities frequently accompany systemic diseases not primarily affecting the bone marrow.

In this chapter, we will review the complex etiology and pathogenesis of the anemias secondary to systemic diseases, represented primarily by Anemia of Chronic Inflammation (ACI), with particularly relevant disease entities considered separately.

Clinical Presentation

The clinical presentation of anemia of chronic inflammation (ACI) is related to the underlying illness causing it. Often, anemia is the first detected abnormality while investigating the etiology of symptoms such as fatigue, decreased stamina, or fever in patients subsequently diagnosed with a systemic inflammatory/infectious condition. Chronic infections, solid and hematologic malignancies, and autoimmune disease are the most frequent causes of ACI.

Chronic cardiac, renal and liver disease, and hypothyroidism are commonly associated with an anemia whose etiology only partially overlap with ACI and will be discussed separately (Table 28.1).

A thorough clinical history and physical examination often provide sufficient data to guide appropriate diagnostic investigations. A history of rash, sinovitis, or arthralgias is often present in patients with rheumatologic diseases, while the presentation of an infectious disease depends on the pathogenic organism, the target organ(s), and the status of the immune system of the host (immunocompetent versus immunodeficient). Generally, fever is present, and a history of compatible exposure can be elicited.

ACI is the second most common form of anemia in the United States (US), after iron deficiency anemia (IDA) and the most prevalent anemia in hospitalized/chronically ill patients.[1] The final, common etio-pathogenic mechanism of ACI is increased inflammatory cytokine production related to activation of T cells and monocytes, resulting in alteration of iron homeostasis via increased hepcidin synthesis; impairment of proliferation and differentiation of erythrocyte precursors; decreased production and response to erythropoietin (EPO); and reduced life span of red cells.[2] In what follows, we will explore this complex pathophysiology in detail.

Table 28.1. Most common systemic diseases accompanied by anemia with the corresponding pathogenesis of anemia

Disease	Pathogenesis of Anemia
Autoimmune Diseases Rheumatoid arthritis Systemic lupus erythematosus Connective tissue diseases Vasculitis Inflammatory bowel diseases Sarcoidosis	ACI
Infectious Diseases Bacterial Viral Fungal Parasitic	ACI
Malignancies Hematologic Solid	ACI; IDA; chemotherapy-related myelosuppression; myelophtisis; folic acid/vitamin B12 deficiency; treatment/cancer-related hemolysis
Chronic Kidney Disease	EPO deficiency; IDA; folic acid deficiency; hyperparathyroidism
Chronic Heart Failure	ACI; IDA; nutritional deficiencies; drug-related myelosuppression
Chronic Liver Disease	ACI; treatment/disease-related myelosuppression or hemolysis; folate/vitamin B12 deficiency
Hypothyroidism	Decreased erythropoietic drive; myelophtisis in advanced mixedema

Abbreviations: ACI: anemia of chronic inflammation; IDA: iron-deficiency anemia

Diagnostic Evaluation and Lab Findings

The main differential diagnosis of ACI is IDA. Diagnostic difficulty can arise because these two conditions can often overlap.

ACI is typically mild to moderate in severity (hemoglobin ≥8 g/dL). The presence of severe anemia usually suggests a different etiology or overlapping diseases. ACI is normochromic/normocytic, albeit mild microcytosis can be present.

Table 28.2. Common laboratory findings in anemia of chronic inflammation (ACI), iron deficiency anemia (IDA), and overlap syndrome (ACI+IDA).

Laboratory Test	ACI	IDA	ACI+IDA
Hemoglobin	Moderately low (typically >8 g/dL)	Moderately/severely low (<8 g/dL)	Moderately/severely low
MCV	Normal/low	Very low	Low
Serum Iron	Low	Low	Low
Transferrin	Normal/low	High	Normal
Transferrin Saturation	Low (~20–25%, rarely <10%)	Very low (typically <10%)	Low
Ferritin	High	Low	Normal
TIBC	Normal/low	High	Normal/high
Serum Hepcidin	High	Normal	Normal/high
Serum Inflammatory Cytokines	High	Normal	Normal/high
TIBC/logFerritin	<1	>1	>1

Abbreviation: TIBC: total iron binding capacity

Iron studies are crucial to the diagnosis. In ACI there is low serum iron, low-to-normal transferrin, normal-to-decreased total iron binding capacity (TIBC), and elevated ferritin. In contrast, IDA is characterized by low serum iron in association with an elevated TIBC, and a low ferritin. If measured, hepcidin and pro-inflammatory cytokines are elevated in ACI but not in IDA (Table 28.2).

The ratio between the concentration of TIBC and the log of ferritin can be helpful in establishing whether IDA is overlapping with ACI. A ratio of less than 1 suggests ACI alone, while a ratio greater than 2 suggests the presence of IDA.

In ACI, the peripheral smear shows normocytic/normochromic erythrocytes. Acanthocytes and anisopoichilo-cytosis are frequent in end-stage liver disease (ESLD), while target cells and macro-ovalocytes are common in early-stage hepatic dysfunction; echynocytes are typical of chronic kidney disease (CKD), while hypothyroidism is associated with macrocytic cells.

Pathophysiology

Anemia of Chronic Inflammation

The hallmark of ACI is functional hyposideremia in face of abundant total-body iron stores. By limiting accessibility to iron, ACI appears to be an anthropologically and evolutionarily preserved defense mechanism against infections by siderophore-carrying bacteria. Hepcidin (liver-expressed antimicrobial peptide 1), the central molecule in ACI, was initially identified as an antimicrobial peptide and acute phase reactant and only subsequently recognized as a master regulator of iron metabolism.[3]

Hepcidin is hepatically synthesized as an 84 amino acid precursor, which is post-translationally cleaved into biologically active 20, 22, and 25 amino acid peptides. Ferroportin is its only recognized ligand and the only known cellular iron exporter, expressed on the reticuloendothelial (RE) system, hepatocytes, and the basolateral membrane of duodenal enterocytes. The binding of hepcidin to ferroportin results in its internalization and lysosomal degradation, causing the inability of iron to be released by these cells.

More than 20 mg of elemental iron are required daily for metabolic functions. Destruction of senescent erythrocytes by the RE system and recycling of iron from the heme group provides the majority of the daily iron need, with diet supplying only 1–1.5 mg/day. Iron is vital to mitochondrial metabolism. It is required for redox reactions during cell respiration, metabolism, and proliferation and for synthesis of oxygen-carrying (hemoglobin) and oxygen-storing (myoglobin) molecules. Excessive iron can result in free-radical formation, oxidative stress, and eventually apoptosis, explaining the need for a tight homeostasis.

Dietary iron is absorbed in its ferrous state by duodenal epithelium via the divalent metal transporter 1 (DMT1). In the enterocyte cytoplasm, it is oxidized to a ferric state that is suitable for export via ferroportin into the portal blood circulation. Iron circulates bound to transferrin, and it is taken up by target cells, in particular hepatocytes, via transferrin receptor 1 and 2 (TfR1 and 2), where it deposits as ferritin. A functional ferroportin is necessary to access this stored iron.

Hepcidin Regulation in Physiologic and Pathologic States

The two major regulators of hepcidin transcription in physiologic states are iron level and bone marrow erythropoiesis.

Elevated intracellular iron induces transcription of bone morphogenic protein 6 (BMP6), a ligand for BMP, a serine-threonine kinase receptor of the transforming growth factor β family expressed on the surface of hepatocytes. The coreceptor hemojuvelin (HJV) enhances the signaling mediated by

BMP6–BMP interaction. HJV is encoded by the hemochromatosis gene 2 (HFE2), the gene mutated in type 2, or juvenile, hemochromatosis. The small mothers against decapentaplegic (SMAD) 1, 5, and 8 are downstream of BMP6-BMP signaling and form a complex with phosphorylated SMAD4. The complex translocates to the nucleus and induces transcription of the hepcidin gene. In a negative feedback loop, hepcidin binds to ferroportin, causing its degradation and thus inhibiting the export of iron from hepatocytes, RE, and duodenum. Erythropoiesis appears to induce hepcidin transcription through the same BMP-SMAD pathway but via different initiator ligands: growth and differentiation factor 15 (GDF15) and twisted gastrulation protein (TWSG1).[4]

In chronic infectious/inflammatory states, activation of monocytes and T lymphocytes causes secretion of pro-inflammatory cytokines: interferon γ (IFN-γ), tumor necrosis factor α (TNF-α), and interleukin 1 and 6 (IL-1 and IL-6).

IL-6 binds to its receptor IL-6R and signals through the Janus Kinase 2 (JAK2) Signal Transducer and Activator of Transcription (STAT3) pathway. JAK2 causes the phosphorylation of STAT3, resulting in its homodimerization and translocation to the nucleus, where it induces expression of hepcidin. Crosstalk exists between the IL-6-JAK2-STAT3 pathway and the BMP6-BMP-SMAD pathway, as liver-specific homozygous deletion of SMAD4 in mice results in decreased hepcidin transcription in response to IL-6, and an intact SMAD-responsive site in the hepcidin promoter is necessary for IL-6-induced hepcidin expression (Figure 28.1).[5]

The Effect of Pro-inflammatory Cytokines on Iron Metabolism and Erythropoiesis

IFN-γ and TNF-α induces expression of DMT1 and downregulates ferroportin, resulting in increased retention of iron in the RE systems and duodenum. IL-1, TNF-α, IFN-α, IFN-β, and especially IFN-γ have a direct inhibitory effect on the erythropoietic precursors, erythroid burst-forming units (BFU-E), and colony-forming units (CFU-E) by causing apoptosis possibly via generation of free-radicals and oxidative stress; inducing erythrophagocytosis; causing decreased expression of EPO receptor; and inhibiting the production of EPO and other erythropoiesis growth factor such as stem-cell factor (Table 28.3).

Anemia of Chronic Renal Disease

The predominant mechanism of anemia in CKD is EPO deficiency. EPO is a glycoprotein hormone mostly (>90%) produced by interstitial fibroblasts bordering the peritubular capillaries of the renal cortex, with perisinusoidal hepatocytes responsible for the remaining production. Hypoxia is the major stimulus for EPO synthesis, which requires an intact renal perfusion. EPO level declines proportionally to loss of creatinine clearance, starting at an eGFR less than 60 ml/min/m^2.[6] EPO deficiency is almost universally present in patients with stage V CKD. EPO is the major erythropoietic hormone, acting on BFU-E, CFU-E, and all the intermediate, developmental stages of red cells until basophilic erythroblasts.

It is unclear whether uremic toxins also contribute to anemia, although it is well accepted that increased blood urea can alter the composition of erythrocyte membranes, causing the characteristic burr cell (echynocyte) appearance.

Excessive parathyroid hormone (PTH) can cause replacement of normal hematopoietic marrow tissue by fibrosis in the process known as osteitis fibrosa cystica, thus inhibiting erythropoiesis. Secondary/tertiary hyperparathyroidism is frequent in CKD, and osteitis fibrosa cystica can occur. Excessive PTH also inhibits production of EPO and blunts EPO response in the bone marrow, as demonstrated by a surge in EPO level and erythropoiesis shortly after parathyroidectomy.[7]

Patients with CKD can also frequently develop folate deficiency, as this is dialyzed off, and iron deficiency either absolute, secondary to blood loss during dialysis, or functional related to the chronic inflammatory state of CKD.

Anemia of Chronic Liver Disease

The pathophysiology of anemia of chronic liver disease is multifactorial. The etiology of liver disease can be causative of anemia, per se. Both ethanol and acetaldehyde suppress erythropoiesis by inducing growth arrest in BFU-E and CFU-E. Folic acid and vitamin B12 deficiencies are also frequently present in alcoholic patients, due to malnutrition, and contribute to produce a macrocytic anemia.

Chronic infection with hepatitis B (HBV) or C virus (HCV) can induce ACI due to the chronic state of inflammation, while acute infection can rarely cause hepatitis-associated aplastic anemia (HAA), a potentially life-threatening condition presenting as pancytopenia. A third of patients with HCV experience anemia while treated with ribavirin, PEG-IFN-α, and protease inhibitor due to direct suppression of erythropoiesis from interferon and hemolytic anemia induced by ribavirin.[8]

In the pediatric population, Wilson disease, an autosomal recessive disorder of copper excretion, is a frequent cause of chronic liver disease. Erythrocytes function as scavenger elements by uptaking copper released after hepatic necrosis. Copper causes free-radical oxidative damage to red cells and intravascular hemolysis. Clinically significant intravascular hemolysis occurs in 20–50% of patients and is the first hint to the diagnosis in 5%.

Regardless of the etiology of liver injury, protracted liver damage results in cirrhosis and portal hypertension, causing splenomegaly and hypersplenism; congestive gastropathy and/or esophageal varices; and chronic, paradoxical activation of the renin-angiotensin system. All these maladaptive phenomena contribute to anemia: extravascular hemolysis from splenic sequestration; chronic or acute iron loss from occult or overt gastrointestinal bleed; and finally hemodilution secondary to plasma volume expansion from salt/water retention.

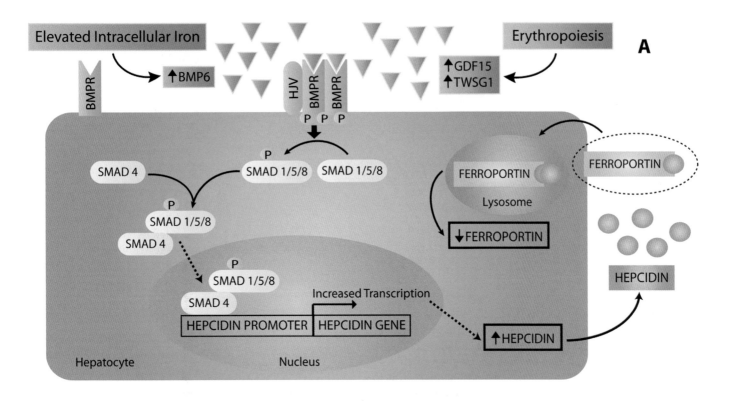

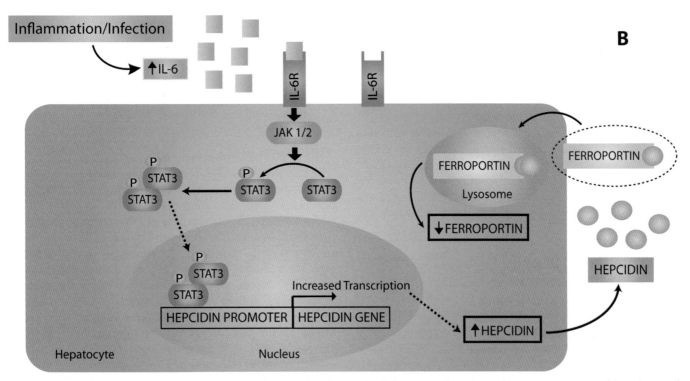

Figure 28.1 Signaling pathway underlying hepcidin upregulation in physiologic and pathologic states. Panel A is a schematic representation of the induction of hepcidin by physiologic stimuli: increased intracellular iron stores and erythropoiesis. Panel B shows the signaling pathway of hepcidin upregulation by IL-6, typical of chronic inflammatory/infectious states.

Abbreviations: BMP6: bone morphogenic protein 6; BMPR: BMP receptor; HJV: hemojuvelin; GDF15: growth and differentiation factor 15; TWSG1: twisted gastrulation protein; SMAD: small mothers against decapentaplegic; IL-6: interleukin 6; IL-6R: Il-6 receptor; JAK: Janus Kinase; STAT: Signal Transducer and Activator of Transcription.

Table 28.3. Molecular mechanisms mediating impaired erythropoiesis and functional hyposideremic state in anemia of chronic inflammation

Target Cell/Organ	Cytokine Mediator	Molecular Mechanism	Biological Effect
RE system	IFN-α, IFN-β, IFN-γ, IL-6 IFN-α, IFN-β, IFN-γ, IL-1, TNF-α, IL-6	Upregulation DMT1 Upregulation hepcidin Downregulation ferroportin Upregulation ferritin	Increased iron uptake Decreased iron export/accessibility Increased iron stores
CFU-E, BFU-E	IFN-α, IFN-β, IFN-γ, IL-1, TNF-α IFN-α, IFN-β, IFN-γ, IL-1, TNF-α IFN-α, IFN-β, IFN-γ, IL-1, TNF-α	Formation free radicals Decreased EPO receptor expression Apoptosis induction	Increased precursor apoptosis Decreased precursor proliferation
Bone Marrow Macrophages	IFN-α, IFN-β, IFN-γ, TNF-α	Induction erythrophagocytosis	
Kidney	IFN-α, IFN-β, IFN-γ, IL-1, TNF-α	Decreased EPO production	
BMSCs	IFN-α, IFN-β, IFN-γ, IL-1, TNF-α	Decreased SCF production	

Abbreviations: RE: reticuloendothelial; IFN: interferon; IL: interleukin; DMT1: divalent membrane transporter 1; TNF: tumor necrosis factor; CFU-E: erythroid colony-forming unit; BFU: burst-forming unit; EPO: erythropoietin; BMSC: bone marrow stromal cells.

The formation of acanthocytes (spur cells) in ESLD is related to aberrant lipoprotein synthesis. The erythrocyte membrane is in constant balance with plasma cholesterol and phospholipids. Advanced hepatic dysfunction causes accumulation of cholesterol without a consensual increase in phospholipids, which causes physical-chemical changes in the erythrocyte membrane typical of acanthocytes. These cells are particularly prone to severe intravascular hemolysis and represent a dismal prognostic sign.[9]

Anemia of Chronic Heart Disease

Anemia is present in 20–35% of patients with chronic heart failure (HF), with a prevalence over 50% in hospitalized patients.[10] Anemia in HF is associated with 1.5-fold excessive mortality, decreased quality of life and exercise tolerance, and increased frequency of hospitalizations.

The etiology of anemia in HF is multifactorial, with IDA and ACI advocated in the majority of the cases. CKD and EPO deficiency, micronutrient deficiency related to cardiac cachexia, and the direct suppressive effect of certain cardiac medications (angiotensin converting enzyme inhibitors and angiotensin receptor blockers) on erythropoiesis are potential contributing factors.[11]

Anemia of Thyroid Disease

As master regulators of metabolism, thyroid hormones stimulate erythropoiesis, directly increasing CFU-E formation and inducing the release of burst-promoting factors from the bone marrow milieu, resulting in increased BFU-E proliferation. Conversely, hypothyroidism is associated with a multifactorial reduction in erythrocyte mass. First, thyroid-hormone-stimulated erythropoiesis is blunted; second, the decreased metabolic requirement exerts a negative feedback loop on erythropoiesis; last, in severe, advanced cases, bone marrow mixedema can be present, causing a significant impairment in normal hematopoiesis.[9]

Anemia of Cancer

Anemia occurs frequently in patients with either hematologic or solid cancer on a multifactorial base. Iron deficiency is often related to tumor bleed, in particular for gastrointestinal malignancies, blood loss from surgeries, nutritional deficiencies, and frequent diagnostic phlebotomies. Certain hematologic tumors, in particular chronic lymphocytic leukemia, and chemotherapies (i.e., gemcitabine) have the potential of causing hemolytic anemia. Malnutrition-related folic and vitamin B12 deficiency, direct myelosuppressive effect of chemotherapy agents, and myelophthisis related to hematopoietic tissue replacement by cancer are major contributors to anemia. Finally, cancer itself is perceived as a chronic inflammatory process and recapitulates the pathophysiology of ACI with relative excess of hepcidin and EPO insufficiency.[12]

Treatment and Prognosis

The presence of anemia during chronic illnesses is associated with worse prognosis and decreased quality of life. The mainstay of treatment is to control or cure the underlying illness, which is often difficult to accomplish. Treatment of anemia has been advocated in order to improve quality of life and possibly prolong survival. A better understanding of the pathophysiologic mechanisms of ACI has led to the development of more targeted therapies, which have largely decreased the need for packed red blood cell (pRBC) transfusion.

The use of recombinant erythropoiesis-stimulating agents (ESA) was the first attempt to correct the pathogenesis of the disease in ESRD patients. Several randomized clinical trials confirmed the effectiveness of ESA in increasing hemoglobin level, resulting in improved quality of life and decreased pRBC requirement. However, significantly increased mortality and cardiovascular events (stroke and cardiac ischemia) were noted when hemoglobin level was above 13 g/dL and in patients requiring higher doses of ESA to achieve the target

Table 28.4. Treatment options for ACI

Target	Treatment	Comments
Anemia	pRBC transfusion	Non–pathogenesis-directed therapy, now declining.
EPO Deficiency	ESAs (epoietin α, darbepoetin)	Target Hb controversial. Overreplacement associated with increased mortality from cardiovascular events in ESRD. Increased mortality in cancer patients under examination.
Increased Hepcidin	Blocking moAb	In preclinical evaluation.
	Anticalins	Protein tetramers with blocking activity. In preclinical evaluation.
	Spiegelmers	In phase IIa clinical trial in cancer patients.
	siRNA	In preclinical evaluation.
	BMP-HJV-SMAD inhibitors	In preclinical evaluation.
	JAK-STAT inhibitors	In preclinical evaluation.
Decreased Ferroportin	MoAb against hepcidin-ferroportin binding site	In preclinical evaluation.

Abbreviations: pRBC: packed red blood cells; EPO: erythropoietin; ESAs: erythropoietin stimulating agents; ESRD: end stage renal disease; Hb: hemoglobin; moAb: monoclonal antibody; siRNA: small interfering RNA; BMP: bone morphogenic protein; HJV: hemojuvelin; SMAD: small mothers against decapentaplegic; JAK: Janus Kinase; STAT: Signal Transducer and Activator of Transcription.

hemoglobin. Currently, guidelines recommend to target a Hb level of 10–11 g/dL, sufficient to improve quality of life, avoid pRBC transfusion, and maintain adequate oxygen delivery.[13]

ESA were FDA-approved for patients with chemotherapy-related anemia in 1989. Their use have been recently debated based on the ESRD data and following a large meta-analysis of randomized trials, which showed increased mortality and decreased overall survival in oncologic patients treated with ESA.[14] However, quality-of-life metrics were improved and requirement for pRBC decreased. Two large prospective, randomized trials are open to specifically address the impact of ESA on mortality in cancer patients. Until those results are available, oncologic and hematologic societies in the US recommend discussing risks and benefits with patients and targeting a hemoglobin less than 11 g/dL if ESAs are used.[15]

Novel therapies targeting the hepcidin-ferroportin axis are under development. RNA interference and antisense oligonucleotides, blocking monoclonal antibodies and proteins, and spiegelmers (single-strand oligonucleotides with inhibitory protein binding properties) were successful at blunting hepcidin transcription, translation, or function, resulting in correction of anemia in murine models of ACI.[16] NOX-H94, an antihepcidin spiegelmers conjugated to PEG, is the most advanced molecule in development, currently being evaluated in a phase IIa, double-blind, randomized trial in patients with cancer-related anemia after proving successful in monkeys.[17]

Alternative strategies to target hepcidin include inhibitors of the BMP6-BMP-HJV-SMAD pathway, IL-6 inhibitors, and inhibitors of the ferroportin-hepcidin interaction site (Table 28.4).

References

1. Cartwright GE. The anemia of chronic disorders. *Seminars in Hematology*. 1966 Oct; 3(4):351–375. PubMed PMID: 5341723.

2. Weiss G, Goodnough LT. Anemia of chronic inflammation. *The New England Journal of Medicine*. 2005 Mar 10; 352(10):1011–1023. PubMed PMID: 15758012.

3. Weinberg ED. Iron withholding: a defense against infection and neoplasia. *Physiological Reviews*. 1984 Jan; 64 (1):65–102. PubMed PMID: 6420813.

4. Means RT, Jr. Hepcidin and iron regulation in health and disease. *The American Journal of the Medical Sciences*. 2013 Jan; 345(1):57–60. PubMed PMID: 22627267. PubMed Central PMCID: 3430792.

5. Gangat N, Wolanskyj AP. Anemia of chronic inflammation. *Seminars in Hematology*. 2013 Jul; 50(3):232–238. PubMed PMID: 23953340.

6. Nurko S. Anemia in chronic kidney disease: causes, diagnosis, treatment. *Cleveland Clinic Journal of Medicine*. 2006 Mar; 73(3):289–297. PubMed PMID: 16548452.

7. Yasunaga C, Matsuo K, Yanagida T, Matsuo S, Nakamoto M, Goya T. Early effects of parathyroidectomy on erythropoietin production in secondary hyperparathyroidism. *American Journal of Surgery*. 2002 Feb; 183(2):199–204. PubMed PMID: 11918889.

8. Romero-Gomez M, Berenguer M, Molina E, Calleja JL. Management of anemia induced by triple therapy in patients with chronic hepatitis C: challenges, opportunities and recommendations. *Journal of Hematology*. 2013 Jul:15. PubMed PMID: 23867320.

9. Handin RI, Lux SE, Stossel TP. *Blood: Principles and Practice of Hematology*. 2nd ed. Philadelphia, PA: Lippincott Williams & Wilkins; 2003:xii, 2304.

10. van Veldhuisen DJ, Anker SD, Ponikowski P, Macdougall IC. Anemia and iron deficiency in heart failure: mechanisms and therapeutic approaches. *Nature Reviews Cardiology*. 2011 Sep; 8(9):485–493. PubMed PMID: 21629210.

11. Groenveld HF, Januzzi JL, Damman K, van Wijngaarden J, Hillege HL, van Veldhuisen DJ, et al. Anemia and mortality in heart failure patients a systematic review and meta-analysis. *Journal of the American College of Cardiology.* 2008 Sep 2; 52(10):818–827. PubMed PMID: 18755344.

12. Dicato M, Plawny L, Diederich M. Anemia in cancer. *Annals of Oncology: Official Journal of the European Society for Medical Oncology/ESMO.* 2010 Oct; 21 Suppl 7:vii, 167–172. PubMed PMID: 20943610.

13. Kliger AS, Foley RN, Goldfarb DS, Goldstein SL, Johansen K, Singh A, et al. KDOQI US Commentary on the 2012 KDIGO Clinical Practice Guideline for Anemia in CKD. *American Journal of Kidney Diseases: The Official Journal of the National Kidney Foundation.* 2013 Jul 25. PubMed PMID: 23891356.

14. Bohlius J, Schmidlin K, Brillant C, Schwarzer G, Trelle S, Seidenfeld J, et al. Recombinant human erythropoiesis-stimulating agents and mortality in patients with cancer: a meta-analysis of randomised trials. *Lancet.* 2009 May 2; 373(9674):1532–1542. PubMed PMID: 19410717.

15. Rizzo JD, Brouwers M, Hurley P, Seidenfeld J, Arcasoy MO, Spivak JL, et al. American Society of Clinical Oncology/American Society of Hematology clinical practice guideline update on the use of epoetin and darbepoetin in adult patients with cancer. *Journal of Clinical Oncology: Official Journal of the American Society of Clinical Oncology.* 2010 Nov 20; 28(33):4996–5010. PubMed PMID: 20975064.

16. Sun CC, Vaja V, Babitt JL, Lin HY. Targeting the hepcidin-ferroportin axis to develop new treatment strategies for anemia of chronic inflammation and anemia of inflammation. *American Journal of Hematology.* 2012 Apr; 87 (4):392–400. PubMed PMID: 22290531. PubMed Central PMCID: 3653431.

17. Schwoebel F, van Eijk LT, Zboralski D, Sell S, Buchner K, Maasch C, et al. The effects of the anti-hepcidin Spiegelmer NOX-H94 on inflammation-induced anemia in cynomolgus monkeys. *Blood.* 2013 Mar 21; 121(12):2311–2315. PubMed PMID: 23349391. PubMed Central PMCID: 3606066.

Transfusion Therapy for Anemia

Joseph D. Sweeney, MD, FACP, FRCPath

Red cell concentrates (RCC) are therapeutic products sourced from prescreened healthy human subjects (blood donors) by either whole-blood donation or using apheresis devices. In developed countries, these donations are plasma depleted by centrifugation, mostly prestorage leukoreduced by filtration, and stored between 1°C and 6°C in specially formulated crystalloid solutions, called additive solutions (AS). In Europe, SAG-M (saline-adenine-glucose-mannitol) is widely used, but in North America, the AS vary slightly in formulation, all containing saline and adenine but differing in the presence of either phosphate or mannitol or the concentration of glucose. The storage container is commonly polyvinylchloride (PVC) plasticized with diethylhexylphalate (DEHP). The maximum duration of liquid storage is 42 days. During this period, the red cells undergo changes collectively referred to as the red cell storage lesion and characterized morphologically by ecchinocytosis.[1] **Surprisingly, this does not appear to have any clinically detectable consequences.**[2] The composition of red cell concentrates is shown in Table 29.1. As is evident, there is considerable variation, and attempts to standardize are generally resisted.[3] Red cell concentrates are more correctly called *red cells, in additive solution* in Europe and *red blood cells* in the U.S., but these terms are rarely used in day-to-day practice.

Epidemiology of Red Cell Transfusion

Red cell concentrates are transfused in two distinct clinical scenarios.[4] First, red cells are transfused to actively bleeding patients with the intent of the restoration of intravascular volume with a fluid capable of oxygen delivery to an acutely oxygen deprived microvasculature. Second, red cell concentrates are transfused to patients with normovolemic anemia, that is, a clinical situation in which there is no active bleeding evident, the patient is not hemodynamically compromised and is isovolemic with the intent of improving oxygen delivery to a microvasculature with subacute or chronic oxygen deprivation. The relative proportion of red cells transfused to either population can vary from institution to institution and depends on the presence of specialized surgical services such as trauma care, cardiac or vascular surgery, solid organ transplantation, and some types of orthopedic surgery. On the medical side, normovolemic red cell transfusion will determine much of the use of red cells, especially in the management of

Table 29.1. Approximate composition of prestorage leukoreduced red cell concentrates in additive solution

	Typical	Range
Total volume (ml)	310	260–420
Volume of red cells (ml)	185	160–255
Hematocrit	55	50–65
Hemoglobin (g)	60	45–80
Additive solution (ml)	100	100 or 110
Carryover (residual) plasma (ml)	25	15–90
Residual leukocytes	5×10^5	10^4–10^6

The actual composition of any one concentrate will depend on the donor hemoglobin, the volume of whole blood collected, the loss of red cells in tubing or filtration, and the centrifugational conditions, which will determine residual (carryover) plasma.

cancer patients and more particularly the hematopoietic malignancies and stem cell reconstitution therapy.

Transfusion incidents rates (TIR) are usually expressed as units RBC/1,000 population/year. In developed countries, this rate can vary greatly. Data for most European countries, with the exception of Denmark, shows TIR between 30 and 45.[5] In the United States, the TIR overall has been decreasing in recent years, although it remains higher than in most European countries, at approximately 40 units/1,000/year.[6] Red cell transfusion within individual hospitals will depend on the complexity and volume of clinical services. Typically, this is expressed as an absolute number of units transfused per year. However, various denominators can be applied such as units RBC/total discharges or units RBC/patient days, which allows for some degree of year-to-year intra-institutional and, to a lesser extent, interinstitutional comparison. Attention needs to be paid to these denominators, however, as a significant number of red cell concentrates are transfused to out-patients, which will distort these ratios, if not removed from the in-patient volume for the calculation.

Dosage of Red Cells

The dose of red cells (# units) in acute major blood loss anemia is determined by the volume of blood loss and the time required to establish hemodynamic stability. By definition, this will vary greatly between patients.

Red cell transfusion in normovolemic anemia is generally less urgent, and the dose of red cells can be determined by defining the target hemoglobin and considering the characteristics of the recipient and the amount of hemoglobin in the RCC. In practice, the latter two aspects are usually unknown. The final hemoglobin posttransfusion can be described as follows; however:

If, Hb^{Final} = Desired post transfusion hemoglobin (g/dL)
$Hb^{initial}$ = Pretransfusion (initial) hemoglobin (g/dL)
BV = Blood volume of recipient (dL)
Product Hb = Product Hb required (g)

$$Hb^{Final} = \frac{\left(Hb^{initial} \times BV\right) + Product\ Hb}{BV}$$

then, $Hb^{Final} \times BV = Hb^{initial} \times BV + Product\ Hb$
$BV\ (Hb^{Final} - Hb^{initial}) = Product\ Hb$
i.e.

$$Increase\ in\ hemoglobin = \frac{Product\ Hb}{Blood\ volume}$$

The increase in hemoglobin is directly proportional to the grams of Hb given and **inversely related to the recipient blood volume**. In general, am RCC containing 50 g hemoglobin will increase the hemoglobin by 1 g/dL in a patient with blood volume of 50 dL, explaining the empirical observation of an approximate increase of 1 g/dL in a recipient, on average, after transfusing a single unit of red cells.[7] However, from Table 29.1, product Hb will vary between units and recipient blood volume even more so: low-blood-volume recipients will respond with a disproportionate increase in hemoglobin and high-blood-volume recipients the reverse. This is well illustrated in Figure 29.1, in which a low blood volume female patient (58′ height; 63 lbs weight) achieved a 4.4 g/dL increase in hemoglobin after the transfusion of two red cell units.

Red Cell Transfusion in Acute Large-Volume Blood Loss Anemia

Acute blood loss anemia can result from spontaneous bleeding, iatrogenic bleeding, or bleeding associated with trauma. In all of these situations, the decision to transfuse red cell concentrates is dependent on the assessment of intravascular volume, visible evidence of the site and amount of bleeding, known or suspected cardiac dysfunction, and the hemoglobin level, if available. In some such instances, a predisposing coagulopathy precipitating the bleeding may need to be addressed with other blood components or derivatives, or a large-volume red cell transfusion may in itself cause a secondary hemodilution coagulopathy, exacerbating any bleeding. Extensive discussion regarding red cell transfusion in this context is beyond the scope of this book: each clinical situation is different, giving rise to considerable variation in practice, especially with regard to the management of trauma.[8] It should be noted, however, that a conservative approach to red cell transfusion is appropriate in some of these scenarios, as shown in a recent randomized control trial.[9]

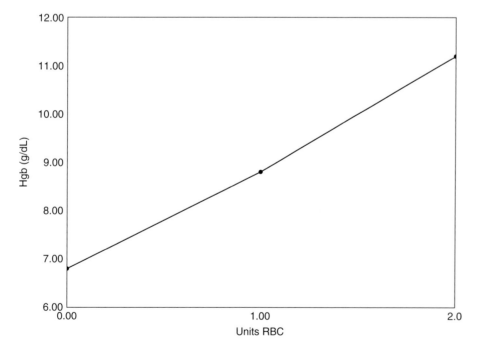

Figure 29.1 Response in hemoglobin to the transfusion of two units of red cells to a low-intravascular-volume recipient.

Red Cell Transfusion in Normovolemic Anemia

Red cell transfusion in normovolemic anemia occurs in two differing clinical scenarios. First, there are patients with normovolemic anemia who will require only one or two episodes of red cell transfusion in the supportive care of their condition during a single hospitalization. Red cell transfusion in this context is dependent on the measured level of hemoglobin and the presence of clinical symptoms of anemia: the dose should be a single unit per prescription (episode) when the pretransfusion hemoglobin is close to the threshold, with reassessment of the post transfusion Hb and any changes in clinical symptoms. The mechanism of anemia in these patients may be multifactorial, with inflammatory disease, renal failure, minor blood loss from the gastrointestinal tract or a recent surgical event, or even diagnostic phlebotomy contributing to the anemia. Many of these patients are in an intensive care unit or a coronary care unit or are recently postoperative from cardiac, vascular, orthopedic or abdominal surgery. Rarely, an acute hemolytic process may be present. There has been considerable attention paid to this population, and some data are available from both observational and randomized controlled trials. The TRICC trial is a landmark RCT which showed no benefit to red cell transfusion if the pretransfusion hemoglobin is 7 g/dL or greater, certainly in the absence of cardiac disease.[10] Various retrospective observation studies[11,12] and one small RCT[13] in patients with acute coronary syndrome or acute myocardial infarction showed a negative effect of red cell transfusion on a clinical outcome in general, especially if the pretransfusion Hb is 8.0 g/dL or more. Similarly, the recent FOCUS RCT showed no benefit of red cell transfusion **in postoperative hip fracture surgery** when the pretransfusion Hb is 8.0 g/dL, even in the presence of cardiac disease.[14] Remarkably, many of these studies show an excess of acute myocardial infarction in the more transfused population, a complication the red cell transfusion is intended to prevent. Recent data on red cell concentrates indicates a potential prothrombotic effect, which may help explain this apparent paradox.[15] Taken together, red cell transfusion in these patients with normovolemic anemia should not be given if the Hb is 7.0 g/dL or more in the absence of cardiac disease and 8.0 g/dL or more in the presence of cardiac disease whether active (acute coronary syndrome or acute myocardial infarction) or otherwise, and the dose should be as a single unit when possible with reassessment posttransfusion.[16]

Second, there are patients with normovolemic anemia who will likely require multiple or chronic red cell transfusion. Patients in this category often have a hypoproliferative anemia from **malignant disease** or the treatment of such, a hereditary anemia, a chronic hemolytic process, recurrent gastrointestinal bleeding from anatomic lesions, or, rarely, recurrent bleeding from a severe bleeding disorder.[4] There are special considerations regarding the transfusion of patients who will undergo chronic red cell transfusion. The anemias described in Sections 3 and 4 encompass many of the clinical situations requiring transfusion in this category.

Special Considerations in Chronic Anemia

a. Phenotype Matching and Red Cell Genotyping:

Patients receiving multiple red cell transfusions are at risk for red cell alloimmunization or the formation of red cell autoantibodies. Routine compatibility testing in the US determines ABO and Rh(D) type and assesses unexpected antibodies using the indirect Coombs test (antibody screen). No further compatibility testing is routinely performed. The lack of routine matching for antigens outside of the ABO or Rh systems sets the stage for alloimmunization to other antigens within the so-called minor blood group systems. The most common antibodies observed in a population of such transfusion recipients is shown in Table 29.2.[17] The two most common antibodies seen are anti-E (RH3) and anti-K (KEL1). Prophylactic matching for these antigens alone would potentially have prevented 60% of the alloantibodies and is a consideration for patients likely to require chronic red cell transfusion, such as patients with hematopoietic malignancies.[18] Prophylactic phenotype matching has been used in other populations, particularly patients with sickle cell syndromes and thalassemias, and has been shown to be effective in reducing alloimmunization but remains controversial.[19,20] This approach is also used in patients with autoimmune hemolytic anemia who can be phenotyped for some but not all minor blood group antigens. The usefulness of this approach in preventing alloimmunization or a hemolytic reaction in this context is unknown.[21]

Red cell genotyping is now available and suitable for implementation in even moderate-size transfusion services.[22] Red cell genotyping is useful for guiding red cell

Table 29.2 One hundred fifty-four red cell alloantibodies identified in 39,431 patients who received 86,750 red cells over a 3-year period. Several other alloantibodies were identified, but only single examples

Antibody	#	%
Anti-E (RH3)	65	38%
Anti-c (RH4)	9	5%
Anti-C (RH2)	7	4%
Anti-KEL1	37	22%
Anti-Jk^a	18	11%
Anti-FY1 (Fy^a)	12	7%
Anti-e (RH5)	3	2%
Anti-C^w (RH8)	3	2%
Total	154	91%

transfusions in recently transfused patients, who have a mixture of autologous and allogeneic red cells and, hence, are difficult to phenotype accurately; patients with autoimmune hemolysis or in patients with either an unidentified high-frequency alloanitbody or multiple alloantibodies.

b. **Red Cell Exchange**: Red cell exchange (RCE) is used as a therapeutic intervention in the sickle cell syndromes,[23] in patients with high-grade parasitemia with babesia or malaria[24] or as a prophylactic intervention to avoid alloimmunization in a mistransfused patient (e.g., Rh(D) red cell given to Rh(D) negative female) or to prevent iron overload in the sickle cell syndromes or thalassemias. Although RCE is an infrequent procedure, the effectiveness of this intervention is largely based on anecdotes and small case series, and it will require more years to determine the effectiveness of RCE versus simple transfusion with iron chelation therapy in the sickle cell/thalassemia population.

c. **Leukoreduction**: The standard whole-blood donation contains approximately 2×10^9 white cells at the time of collection. High-efficiency leukoreduction filters can decrease this white cell yield to approximately 5×10^5 or a 4-$\log_{10}$ reduction. Such a reduction can successfully reduce the frequency of febrile nonhemolytic reactions, the transfusion of some herpes viruses such as cytomegalovirus, and avoid primary HLA alloimmunization to Class I HLA antigens. This latter effect is most beneficial for chronically transfused patients, especially patients with hemolytic malignancies who will require platelet transfusions or undergo bone marrow transplantation. Most red cells transfused in the United States and Europe are prestorage leukoreduced, although universal leukodepletion remains controversial.[25]

d. **Irradiation**: an irradiated blood product is a product exposed to electromagnetic radiation of high-energy either gamma photons or, less commonly, X-rays. Blood can be irradiated using the same devices as are used in radiation therapy departments or in special devices called blood irradiators. These blood irradiators contain a radioactive isotope, either cesium (Cs[137]) or cobalt (Co[60]), which emits gamma radiation from nuclear decay. X-ray generating devices capable of delivering a high-energy dose are also available. Irradiation takes 2–8 minutes, depending on the age of the source and the "dose" used. Dose is expressed as "absorbed radioactive dose" and measured in units called *"rads"* or *"grays"* (100 rads = 1 Gy). Typically, irradiated blood is exposed to 2500 rads (25 Gy). Irradiated blood is used to prevent a rare complication of blood transfusion known as transfusion-associated-graft-versus-host-disease,[26] and the indications for the use of irradiated cells are shown in Table 29.3. Note that recipients of solid organ transplants (unless alemtuzumab is used as immunosuppressant),

Table 29.3. Suggested indications for irradiated red cells

1. Potential or actual nonmarrow transplant patients. Allogeneic patients should receive irradiated products upon the start of conditioning and indefinitely after transplantation; autologous patients at least 10 days prior to any harvest of stem cells and on conditioning until 3–6 months posttransplantation.

2. Patients with a diagnosis of Hodgkin's disease regardless of stage.

3. Patients with aplastic anemia receiving immunosuppressive therapy with rabbit ATG, which is more immunosuppressant than horse ATG, or immunosuppressive therapy with alemtuzumab.

4. Patients with other hematopoietic malignancies or severe T-Cell immune defects considered at risk for TAGVHD. Routine irradiation for acute leukemia is controversial and not recommended.

5. Pediatric patients with a diagnosis of malignancy.

6. Patients who are receiving purine analogues (fludarabine, claradibine, bendamustine deoxycoformycin, clofarabine) who have taken purine analogues within the past 2 years or use of alemtuzumab (anti-CD52, CAMPATH).

7. Fetus and Neonates: All intrauterine transfusions; all exchange transfusions (ET) when the *neonate received an IUT*; other ETs, irradiation is recommended but not mandatory. All "Top up" transfusions when the *neonate received an IUT*; evidence of or known immunodeficiency of the T cell system.

8. Certain products:
   a. Directed donations from genetically related family members
   b. All HLA matched platelets
   c. All granulocyte concentrates

patients with HIV, and neutropenic patients are NOT considered as subpopulations of transfusion recipients who should routinely receive irradiated cellular products. It is preferable to irradiate red cells immediately prior to transfusion,[27] but continued liquid storage is possible, but only to 28 days. Stored irradiated red cells show an exacerbation of the storage lesion, and supernatant potassium concentrates may increase to high levels (50–100 mEq/L), which could be a concern if multiple units are transfused to a recipient with renal compromise.

e. **Washed Red Cells**: A washed red cell product is a liquid stored or thawed cellular product that has been washed in saline or ACD-saline and finally suspended in saline. Red cells suspended in additive solutions with carryover plasma may contain soluble substances or particulate matter, which cause metabolic, allergic, or immunologic reactions. Washing removes most of these contaminants but is performed infrequently, mostly in the context of a history of severe allergic reactions to red cells.[28]

Table 29.4. Red cell transfusion in neonates

	Transfusion Threshold
Cardiovascular disease: requiring oxygen administration and ventilator support	Hct 30–45 depending on severity
Symptomatic anemia: poor weight gain; tachycardia; dyspnea; weak suck; lethargy	Hct < 20

Red Cell Transfusion in Neonates and Children

The neonatal period is arbitrarily deferred to as the first 4 months of life, and red cell transfusion is not uncommon in this population, particularly for premature neonates.[29] The risk of transfusion is inversely related to weight at birth. Some suggested indications and threshold for transfusion are shown in Table 29.4, but universal agreement is lacking as to these thresholds and the indications. Neonatal transfusions can be divided into whole-blood exchange transfusion and simple (top-up) transfusion. Whole-blood exchange transfusions are performed manually with fresh red cell (<5 days of liquid storage) reconstituted with plasma. Irradiation may be indicated under certain circumstances (Table 29.3). Whole-blood exchange typically occurs with hemolytic disease of the newborn. Simple top-up transfusions are given at a dose of 15–20 ml/kg of red cell concentrates. Historically, fresh red cells suspended in anticoagulated plasma (CPD-red cells) were the preferred product, but in recent years, red cells in AS have been used and transfused to the end of the liquid storage period (42 days). This practice allows the transfusion service to "dedicate" a single red cell unit to a predetermined neonate and, thus, minimize donor exposure.[30] Many transfusion services choose to transfuse only Group O, Rh(D) compatible red cells to neonates and no compatibility testing is routinely performed: non-O red cells are most commonly transfused in the context of directed donation, a practice that should be discouraged. Some blood centers manufacture Group O red cells with four attached satellite bags, allowing for four separate doses. It is preferable, however, to use a sterile connecting device to remove a predetermined volume from the red cell unit, especially when very small volumes are transfused to low-birth-weight premature infants. Red cell transfusion in older infants and children is closer to adult practice: the dose of RCC prescribed needs to take the intravascular volume into account, especially in infants and younger children.[31]

Case Study

A 60-year-old male resident of Central Rhode Island presented to the emergency room with a 1-week history of drenching sweats, chills, headache and fatigue and a fever of 104°F. He had been diagnosed 1 week previously with Lyme disease

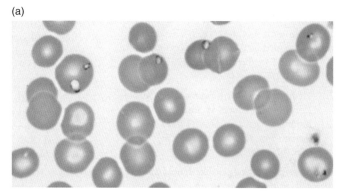

Figure 29.2a Pre–red cell exchange. Dense red cell parasitemia (6.2%) with babesia is present.

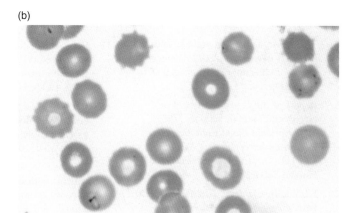

Figure 29.2b Immediate post–red cell exchange. Parasitemia is reduced (1.1%), and several ecchinocytes are evident representative of in vitro storage changes in the transfused allogeneic red cell.

after a target lesion was observed on his right thigh and had been started on doxycycline. His vital signs showed a heart rate of 95/min, BP 136/74, RR 18, and temperature 97.5°F. Oxygen saturation on room air was 96%. Relevant laboratory results showed a hemoglobin 10.1 g/dL, MCV 90 fL, platelet count 93 × 10⁹/L, MPV 11.6 fL, white cell count 6.3 × 10⁹/L, LDH 963 1U/L (N: 50–175), total bilirubin 1.3 mg/dL, creatinine 2.8 mg/dL. A blood smear showed intra-erythrocytic red cell inclusions identified as *M. bancroti* and enumerated as parasitemia of 6.2% of red cells. The smear is shown in Figure 29.2a. The patient typed as Group A, Rh(D) positive, antibody screen negative. Direct Coombs test negative. The patient was commenced on intravenous clindamycin and oral quinine sulphate. On account of the high degree of parasitemia and the elevated creatinine, a red cell exchange was performed with 2,950 mls of allogeneic Group A red cells, a total of 9 units. The procedure was tolerated well. A post–RCE hemoglobin was 9.1 g/dL, platelet count 58 × 10⁹/L, and level of parasitemia decreased to 1.1% (82% decrease). The post RCE smear is shown in Figure 29.2b. The patient was discharged 6 days later, symptomatically improved and afebrile, with <0.01% red cell parasitemia.

References

1. Tinmouth A, Chin-Yee, I. The clinical consequences of the red cell storage lesion. *Transfus Med Rev.* 2001; **15**:91–107.

2. Heddle NM, Cook RJ, Arnold DM. et al. Effect of short-term vs. long-term blood storage on mortality after transfusion. *N Eng J Med.* 2016; **375**:1937–1945.

3. Sweeney JD. Standardization of the red cell product. *Transfusion and Apheresis Science.* 2006; **34**:213–218.

4. Wallis JP, Wells AW, Chapman CE. Changing indications for red cell transfusion from 2000 to 2004 in the North of England. *Transfus Med.* 2006; **16**:411–417.

5. The collection, testing and use of blood products in Europe (2007), Council of Europe Publishing, Strasbourg, 2007, www.edqm.eu.

6. Report of the U.S. Department of Health and Human Services. *The 2011 National Blood Collection and Utilization Survey Report.* Washington, DC: U.S. Department of Health and Human Services, 2011.

7. Elizalde JI, Clemente JL, Marin J, et al. Early changes in hemoglobin and hematocrit levels after packed red cells transfusion in patients with acute anemia. *Transfusion.* 1997; **37**:573–576.

8. Hess JR, Dutton RBH, Holcomb JB Scalea TM. Giving plasma at a 1:1 ratio with red cells in resuscitation: Who might benefit? *Transfusion.* 2008; **48**:1763–1765.

9. Villanueva C, Colomo A, Bosch A, et al. Transfusion strategies for acute upper gastrointestinal bleeding. *N Eng J Med.* 2013; **368**:11–21.

10. Hebert PC, Wells G, Blajchmann MA, et al. A multicenter, randomized, controlled clinical trial of transfusion requirements in critical care. *N Eng J Med.* 1999; **340**:409–417.

11. Rao SV, Jollis JG, Harrington RA, et al. Relationship of blood transfusion and clinical outcomes in patients with acute coronary syndromes. *JAMA.* 2004;**292**:1555–1562.

12. Chatterjee S, Wetterslev J, Sharma A, et al. Association of blood transfusion in increase mortality in myocardial infarction: meta-analysis and diversity adjusted study sequential analysis. *JAMA Intern Med.* 2013; **173**:132–139.

13. Cooper HA, Rao SV, Greenberg MD, et al. Conservative versus liberal red cell transfusion in acute myocardial infarction. *Am J Cardiol.* 2011; **108**:1108–1111.

14. Carson JL, Liberal or restrictive transfusion in high risk patients after hip surgery. *N Eng J Med.* 2011; **1**:1–10.

15. Sweeney JD, Kouttab N, Kurtis JD. Stored red cell supernatant facilitates thrombin generation. *Transfusion.* 2009; **49**:1569–1579.

16. Carson JL, Grossman BJ, Kleinman S, et al. Red blood transfusion: A clinical practice guideline from the AABB. *Ann Intern Med.* 2012; **157**:49–58.

17. LeGolvan M, Pilz J, Sweeney JD. Should patients with malignancies receive phenotyped matched red cells? *Transfusion.* 2005 ;**45**:132A.

18. Sanz C, Nomdedeu M, Belkaid M, et al. Red blood cell alloimmunization in transfused patients with myelodysplastic syndrome or chronic myelomonocytic leukemia. *Transfusion.* 2013; **53**:710–715.

19. Tahhan HR, Holbrook CT, Braddy LR, et al. Antigen-matched donor blood in the transfusion management of patients with sickle cell disease. *Transfusion.* 1994; **34**(7):562–569.

20. Chou ST, Jackson T, Vege S, et al. High prevalence of red blood cell alloimmunization in sickle cell disease despite transfusion from Rh-matched minority donors. *Blood.* 2013; DOI:10.1182/Blood-2013-03-490623.

21. Ziman A, Cohn C, Carey PM et al. Warm-reactive (immunoglobulin G) autoantibodies and laboratory testing best practices: review of the literature and survey of current practice. *Transfusion.* 2017; **57**:463–477.

22. Anstee D. Red cell genotyping and the future of pretransfusion testing. *Blood.* 2009; **114**:248–256.

23. Miller ST. How I treat acute chest syndrome in children with sickle cell disease. *Blood.* 2011; **117**:5297–5305.

24. Spaete JE, Rich J, Sweeney JD. Red cell exchange for babesiosis in Rhode Island. *J Clin Apheresis.* 2009; **24**:97–105.

25. Sweeney JD. Universal leukoreduction of cellular blood components in 2001? *Yes. Am J Clin Pathol.* 2001; **115**:666–673.

26. Treleaven J, Gennery A, Marsh J, et al. Guidelines for the use of irradiated blood components prepared by the British Committee for Standards in Haematology blood transfusion task force. *Br J Haem.* 2010; **152**:35–51.

27. Moroff G, Holme S, AuBuchon JP, et al. Viability and in vitro properties of gamma irradiated AS-1 red blood cell. *Transfusion.* 1999; **39**:128–134.

28. Goldfinger D, Lowe C. Prevention of adverse reactions to blood transfusion by the administration of saline-washed red blood cells. *Transfusion.* 1981; **21**:277–280.

29. Luban NLC. Neonatal red cell transfusion. *Vox Sang.* 2004; **87**: S184–188.

30. Luban NLC, Strauss RG, Hume HA. Commentary on the safety of red cells preserved in extended-storage media for neonatal transfusions. *Transfusion.* 1991; **31**:229–235.

31. Lacroix J, Hebert PC, Hutchinson JS, et al. Transfusion strategies for patients in pediatric intensive care units. *N Eng J Med.* 2007; **356**:1609–1619.

Chapter

30

Transfusion Reactions

Alex Ryder, MD, PhD, Edward Snyder, MD, and David Unold, MD

General Principles

Patients who are anemic may need transfusion of blood products. Regardless of how many times a patient has been successfully transfused, every transfusion of human blood products poses a risk of a transfusion reaction. Accordingly, it is imperative for clinicians to be aware of and know how to treat the types of transfusion reactions that may occur.

Transfusion reactions may be categorized as hemolytic or nonhemolytic, acute or delayed, and immune-mediated or non–immune-mediated.[1] Transfusion reactions can result in significant morbidity and mortality, and the types of reactions differ with regard to pathophysiology, presentation, prevention, treatment, and laboratory workup. While these differences can be complex, there are general principles that can be followed to ensure that any reaction is recognized and treated properly. Table 30.1 depicts the recognized transfusion reaction categories that will be detailed in this chapter.

Proper transfusion practice requires monitoring a patient's vital signs and his/her signs and symptoms. A patient's vital signs should be monitored immediately prior to transfusion, 5–15 minutes after the infusion begins, and then periodically, or as per institutional policy.[2] The patient thus should be assessed for the signs and symptoms of a transfusion reaction including fever, chills, rigors, respiratory distress, hypertension, hypotension, flank pain, rash, infusion site pain, hives, pruritis, angioedema, jaundice, hemoglobinuria, nausea, vomiting, coagulopathy, and anuria.[1] Changes in vital signs, presentation of new signs and symptoms, or worsening of preexisting signs and symptoms should prompt the clinical staff to evaluate the patient and consider ordering a transfusion reaction workup (see Table 30.2).

Suspected transfusion reactions should never be ignored or presumed to be benign until the appropriate workup and evaluation has been completed. In general, for any patient who is suspected of having a transfusion reaction, the transfusion should be stopped, vital signs recorded, and the volume infused noted.[1] The patient should be assessed by a physician or trained health care professional, and the blood bank should be notified that a possible transfusion reaction has occurred. Once stopped, for most reactions, the transfusion should not be restarted, but for a mild allergic reaction (e.g., a few hives), restarting a transfusion is acceptable. Never restart a transfusion if fever or chills have occurred.

Table 30.1. Classification of transfusion reactions

1. Hemolytic Transfusion Reactions
   a. Immune Mediated
      i. Acute Hemolytic Transfusion Reactions
         1. Extravascular hemolysis
         2. Intravascular hemolysis
      ii. Delayed Hemolytic Transfusion Reactions
         1. Extravascular hemolysis
         2. Intravascular hemolysis
   b. Non–Immune-Mediated
      i. Physical damage during storage or infusion
         1. Mechanical
         2. Thermal
         3. Age-related

2. Allergic
   a. Anaphylactic
   b. Minor Allergic Reactions

3. Transfusion–Related Acute Lung Injury (TRALI)

4. Transfusion-Associated Circulatory Overload (TACO)

5. Transfusion-Associated Graft-Versus-Host Disease (TA-GVHD)

6. Septic Transfusion Reactions
   a. Bacterial
   b. Vital
   c. Fungal
   d. Protozoal

7. Transfusion Associated Dyspnea

8. Post Transfusion Purpura

9. Hypothermia

10. Metabolic Derangements of Transfusion
    a. Iron Overload
    b. Citrate Toxicity/Hypocalcemia
    c. Hypokalemia/hyperkalemia

The patient's clinical team should initiate appropriate treatment, and the blood bank should be consulted for guidance regarding disposition of the product(s) implicated in the reaction as well as the patient samples that are needed to complete a transfusion reaction workup. The blood bank will notify a transfusion medicine physician about the reaction, and this physician can assess the suspected reaction and help guide the

Table 30.2 Acute clinical signs/symptoms that might prompt a transfusion reaction workup

- Notable changes in vital signs
  - Fever
  - Hypothermia
  - Hypertension/hypotension
  - Tachycardia/bradycardia
  - Oxygen desaturation
- Chills/Rigors
- Respiratory distress
- Angioedema
- Pruritis
- Urticaria
- Pain at the IV site
- Back or flank pain
- Oliguria/Anuria
- Hematuria
- Epistaxis/Oozing at IV site
- Nausea
- Feeling of 'impending doom'
- Any notable change in clinical status potentially explainable by transfusion

workup and treatment of the patient as necessary. Product bags and patient samples, as applicable, should be promptly sent to the laboratory. If multiple products were given to a patient before a reaction is noted, any one of the products could be the sentinel unit (or units) responsible, as the reaction may be delayed. Thus, the workup should include, if possible, all recently infused blood products.

Transfusion reaction prevention depends on the type of reaction to be prevented as well as the patient's history of prior reactions to transfusion. The best way to prevent a transfusion reaction is to avoid transfusion entirely. That said, the choice of blood product to be transfused, premedication, and specific infusion parameters can all be tailored to minimize, albeit never completely eliminate, the risk of a transfusion reaction. It is notable that pretransfusion medication prophylaxis such as with acetaminophen or diphenhydramine is recommended by some[1] but is controversial and is increasingly being discouraged by others.[3]

Hemolytic Transfusion Reactions

Hemolytic transfusion reactions can cause significant morbidity and represent a substantial proportion of transfusion-related mortality. Between 2011 and 2015, there were 37 fatalities associated with hemolytic transfusion reactions reported to the FDA. This comprises 21.5% of all transfusion-associated fatalities.[4]

Most hemolytic transfusion reactions are a result of recipient immune responses that lead to the destruction of transfused donor RBCs. However, it is also possible that transfusing products containing large amounts of donor RBC antibody can cause hemolysis of recipient RBCs. Specifically, there are reports of hemolytic transfusion reactions resulting from transfusion of donor type O plasma containing high-titer anti-A or anti-B antibodies.[5,6] Additionally, there are nonimmune causes for hemolysis during transfusion.

The severity of hemolytic transfusion reactions can range from mild, with subclinical signs and symptoms, to life-threatening reactions requiring prompt recognition and intervention. If there are clinical and/or laboratory findings suggestive of any type of hemolytic transfusion reaction, rapidly instituting appropriate interventions is essential to minimize morbidity and mortality. Interventions generally involve stopping the cause of hemolysis when possible (e.g., stopping transfusion of an implicated blood product) and initiating a transfusion reaction workup. Once the etiology of the reaction is identified, the management of the patient can be tailored to the cause of hemolysis. The patient should be treated for anemia and the effects, if any, of hemoglobinemia, such as renal failure.

Evaluating the presence and cause of a hemolytic transfusion reaction based on clinical symptoms alone is inadequate, and laboratory investigation is critical. Laboratory investigation for hemolysis should include: (a) a CBC to identify an insufficient increment in hemoglobin and hematocrit in response to the transfusion or any acute decreases in hemoglobin and hematocrit; (b) micro- and macroscopic urinalysis including urine urobilinogen; (c) peripheral blood smear to check for abnormal RBC morphology; (d) lactate dehydrogenase; (e) bilirubin (total and direct); (f) direct antiglobulin test; (g) haptoglobin; and (h) visual inspection of the patient's plasma for hemolysis. While a sample with a plasma hemoglobin of greater than 20 mg/dL will appear pink when inspected visually, automated methods for determining hemolysis are more sensitive and specific indicators.[7] When a suspected hemolytic reaction is reported in a transfusion recipient, if a donor specimen is still available, a repeat type and screen and a repeat crossmatch is indicated.

Different types of hemolytic transfusion reactions are distinguished by the timing and location of hemolysis, and determining the mechanism of hemolysis has implications for patient management. Such reactions can be characterized by the temporal relationship between the reaction and the transfusion (e.g., acute versus delayed) as well as the fluid compartment in which the hemolysis occurs (e.g., intravascular or extravascular). Immune-mediated hemolysis, whether acute or delayed, can be identified by a positive DAT and/or eluate, provided that the targeted red blood cells have not been cleared by the immune response.

Acute Hemolytic Transfusion Reactions

Within 24 hours of a transfusion, a patient having an acute hemolytic transfusion reaction may experience signs/symptoms such as back pain, flank pain, chills, rigors, disseminated intravascular coagulation (DIC), epistaxis, fever, hematuria, hypotension, oliguria, anuria, pain at the IV site, oozing at the IV site, and renal failure.[8] While acute hemolytic transfusion reactions may occur anytime within 24 hours of transfusion, signs and symptoms of an acute hemolytic reaction generally develop more rapidly and often manifest sooner. Reactions may occur during the inciting transfusion; however, as explained previously, the transfusion of multiple blood products may confound identification of the sentinel unit, as an acute hemolytic transfusion reaction may take place several hours after transfusion.

Laboratory studies may demonstrate hypofibrinogenemia, decreased haptoglobin levels, bilirubinemia, elevated lactate dehydrogenase, hemoglobinemia, hemoglobinuria, hemolysis evident upon visual inspection of the patient's plasma, and spherocytes on peripheral blood smear.[8]

Acute hemolytic transfusion reactions are commonly caused by preformed recipient antibodies against antigens on infused donor red blood cells.[1] These reactions may result in either extravascular or intravascular hemolysis with the most severe reactions, as seen in ABO mismatch events, being intravascular.

Treatment of intravascular hemolysis should include at least 24 hours of aggressive hydration with crystalloid products and concurrent diuresis in order to preserve renal function. Close monitoring of vital signs and laboratory studies of renal, hepatic, and hemostatic function during this period of time is important to detect signs of organ dysfunction. Advanced supportive care, including support of airway and blood pressure, may be necessary in some patients. Treatment of extravascular hemolysis is typically less aggressive. Vital signs should still be monitored for signs of hemodynamic compromise, and patients should be hydrated as tolerated. In general, extravascular hemolysis poses less of a clinical risk than does intravascular hemolysis.

Intravascular and Extravascular Hemolysis

Intravascular hemolysis is associated with complement-mediated RBC lysis in the vascular space, whereas extravascular hemolysis is most often due to the removal of antibody- or complement-coated RBCs by phagocytic cells in the reticuloendothelial system. Predicting the severity of a hemolytic transfusion reaction can be challenging. However, due to extensive fixation of complement, intravascular hemolysis, as is seen in acute reactions due to ABO mismatch, is usually associated with more severe reactions than is extravascular hemolysis. In general, reactions increase in severity as the amount of the transfused incompatible product increases.

Intravascular RBC hemolysis arises from activation of the classical complement pathway, initiated by antigen-antibody complexes.[9] Transfused donor RBCs that display nonrecipient antigens may serve as a focal point for recipient alloantibody development. Alternatively, hemolysis can arise from preexisting RBC antibodies in the recipient, specifically anti-A and anti-B, that arise naturally. When recipients are transfused with donor allogeneic RBCs that display antigens to which

the recipients have antibodies, these antibodies complex with the donor red cell antigens, and the Fc portion of the antibody can bind C1q, initiating the classical complement cascade. This cascade can stall after the addition of C3b, and while these complement-coated cells are highly opsonized for uptake by the reticuloendothelial system, they do not lyse intravascularly. If the terminal complement cascade is activated through C9, however, the membrane attack complex (C5b–C9) can directly lyse cells, leading to intravascular hemolysis. Intravascular hemolysis typically occurs acutely because induction of the complement membrane attack complex is rapid.

Immunoglobulins vary widely in their ability to fix complement. Pentameric IgM antibodies are the most potent at fixing complement. IgG antibody subclasses range widely in their complement-fixing ability: IgG1 and IgG3 are relatively efficient at fixing complement, while IgG2 is intermediate and IgG4 actually inhibits complement fixation.[10] It follows that intravascular hemolysis is most often associated with IgM-type RBC antibodies; however, complement-fixing IgG subclasses of antibodies are also capable of initiating the complement cascade that leads to acute intravascular hemolysis. More commonly, however, preformed IgG class antibodies do not fix complement to C9 and instead stop at C3b or fail to bind complement at all, thus leading to an acute extravascular hemolytic reaction as coated RBCs are removed while circulating through the liver and spleen.

Delayed Hemolytic Transfusion Reactions

A delayed hemolytic transfusion reaction (DHTR) takes place greater than 24 hours after transfusion, typically within days to weeks of the implicated transfusion. The signs and symptoms of a delayed hemolytic transfusion reaction may be very non-specific (fever, malaise, and anemia) and often are subclinical. Evidence for a DHTR in an asymptomatic patient may only be detectable by laboratory studies (positive DAT, positive eluate, indirect hyperbilirubinemia, new alloantibody on antibody screen, increased lactate dehydrogenase, and spherocytes on peripheral smear).[8]

DHTRs do not typically occur during the primary immune response (e.g., when a patient is exposed to red blood cell antigens and creates an antibody against a red blood cell antigen for the first time).[1] Rather, they occur after the titer of a previously preformed antibody has fallen below the level of detection. In this situation, the pretransfusion antibody screen may initially appear to be negative, and crossmatch of donor RBCs and recipient serum may therefore appear to be compatible. Reexposure to the inciting antigen as occurs with subsequent transfusions results in an anamnestic immune response. The fall of antibody levels over time (also known as antibody evanescence) is common.[11] In fact, up to 64% of newly formed blood group alloantibodies have been shown to become undetectable over a period of 5 years.[11] Clinicians should always take a careful transfusion history and notify the blood bank of patients who have had transfusions at other institutions in order to help identify evanescent antibodies and potentially prevent DHTRs.

If clinically significant hemolysis results, this reaction is known as a DHTR. If there is no clinical evidence of hemolysis, and the antibody is identified by serology alone, the reaction is called a delayed serologic transfusion reaction (DSTR). Delayed type transfusion reactions, either hemolytic or serologic, are identified in approximately 1 in 1,300 transfused blood components, with DSTRs being more common than DHTRs.[12]

In patients with evidence for a DHTR, treatment depends on whether the reaction is intravascular or extravascular, as described previously for acute hemolytic transfusion reactions.

Hemolytic Transfusion Reactions in Sickle Cell Disease

Patients with sickle cell disease represent a unique population with regard to hemolytic transfusion reactions. These patients have extensive exposure to multiple blood products, and this largely ethnically African patient population has red blood cell antigen phenotypes that may differ from the predominantly Caucasian blood donor population.[13] Thus, sickle cell disease patients frequently form RBC alloantibodies (including evanescent alloantibodies) and are at risk for immune-mediated hemolytic transfusion reactions.[13] Additionally, patients with sickle cell disease may experience hyperhemolytic reactions in relation to RBC transfusion.[14] These reactions are characterized by the immune destruction of both transfused donor RBCs and the patient's own RBCs (commonly known as "bystander" hemolysis), leading to a posttransfusion hemoglobin/hematocrit level lower than the pretransfusion levels and occasionally producing severe, life-threatening anemia. The mechanism(s) for hyperhemolytic reactions are not completely understood but may involve complement or antigen–antibody complexes binding to the patient's own cells. Strategies for managing transfusions in patients with a history of hyperhemolysis include use of intravenous corticosteroids, IVIG, rituximab, and plasma exchange with red blood cell replacement.[14] As a general rule, sickle cell patients who experience hyperhemolysis should not be transfused unless absolutely necessary, as this can exacerbate the hemolysis. The advantages and disadvantages of transfusion in some patients must be carefully assessed for each individual case.

Non–Immune-Mediated Hemolytic Transfusion Reactions

Nonimmune hemolytic transfusion reactions also occur and are typically related to physical properties of the transfused blood. Causes include use of improper storage conditions and exposure to temperature extremes, damage to a blood component during transit, and physical shearing of transfused red blood cells passing through large-bore IVs.[15] Additionally, prosthetic heart valves have had a recognized association with hemolysis, although severe hemolysis is rare in valve patents today, as modern valves are less likely to induce hemolysis.[16]

Depending on the degree of hemolysis, the manifestations of nonimmune hemolytic transfusion reactions may share similarities with immune-mediated hemolytic transfusion reactions, leading to confusion as to the etiology of the reaction.

Febrile Nonhemolytic Reactions

Although their incidence has decreased with the widespread use of leukocyte-reduced red blood cell and platelet products, febrile nonhemolytic transfusion reactions (FNHTRs) are still common.[17] They are defined as a temperature greater than or equal to 38°C and a change in temperature of at least 1°C during, or as many as 4 hours after, a transfusion.[8] In addition, chills or rigors are recognized as surrogates for fever and temperature changes.[8] The temperature changes seen in FNHTRs are thought to be due, at least in part, to antibodies in the recipient against white cells in the donor unit, or cytokines transfused from the donor unit to the recipient.[18]

Temperature changes in a transfused patient with a recent history of febrile illness or sepsis should *not* be ignored or presumed to be only a manifestation of the patient's underlying disease. Temperature changes may also be a sign of hemolytic transfusion reaction, septic transfusion reaction, transfusion-related acute lung injury (TRALI), and even transfusion-associated circulatory overload (TACO).[19] If an FNHTR is suspected, the transfusion should be stopped, and a full transfusion reaction workup should be performed. Never restart the same unit of blood if an FNHTR is suspected, since inadvertent reinfusion of an ABO-incompatible unit of blood or a septic unit of blood or platelets could be fatal.

Febrile nonhemolytic reactions can often be prevented by modification of the product and/or use of premedication strategies. Use of prestorage leukoreduced red blood cell or platelet units has been demonstrated to decrease the incidence of FNHTRs.[20] The use of premedication (e.g., acetaminophen or diphenhydramine directly preceding transfusion) is controversial, and it has been argued that there is little evidence to support such practice (see section regarding Allergic Reactions).[3]

When a FNHTR is suspected, the transfusion should be stopped, an open intravenous line should be maintained to allow for hydration should the reaction prove to be a hemolytic transfusion reaction with or without hypotension, and acetaminophen should be administered as clinically tolerated and as practical. There are no data supporting the use of diphenhydramine for treatment of FNHTRs. Patients experiencing chills and rigors can be supported using warm blankets. As with most other suspected transfusion reactions, further transfusions are typically avoided until the blood bank workup is completed. The standard blood bank work up is designed to rule out an ABO/Rh incompatibility not detected during the initial crossmatch and ensure that the patient has not developed new alloantibodies to red blood cell antigens. Transfusion reaction evaluations in the blood bank do not specifically determine a reaction to be a FNHTR (or, similarly, an allergic reaction) but instead rule out hemolytic transfusion reactions so that the diagnosis of other types of reactions, such as an FNHTR, may be entertained.

Transfusion-Related Acute Lung Injury

As agreed upon by a working group of the National Heart, Lung, and Blood Institute (NHLBI), TRALI is defined as "new acute lung injury (ALI) occurring during or within 6 hours after a transfusion" and "that develops with a clear temporal relationship to transfusion, in patients without or with risk factors for ALI other than transfusion."[21] The following signs of ALI have become important diagnostic criteria for both clinicians and transfusion medicine specialists: the development of bilateral lung infiltrates imaged by chest radiograph with concurrent hypoxemia (oxygen saturation $\leq$90% on room air).[21] Other findings that may be seen in TRALI include dyspnea, cyanosis, tachycardia, hypotension, hypertension, fever, and transient leukopenia.[21]

The pathophysiology of acute lung injury is complex but is thought to be due primarily to antineutrophil antigen antibodies (anti-HNA) and anti-HLA antibodies. There are two prevailing hypotheses about the specific mechanism of injury by these antibodies. The first posits that these antibodies directly cause lung injury (donor antibody hypothesis[22]). The second posits an initial insult, generally an inflammation-inducing event such as infection or recent surgery, that results in endothelial damage and leukocyte accumulation in pulmonary capillaries, followed by transfusion of products containing antibodies that result in activation of these leukocytes to cause injury ("two-hit model"[23]). The donor population group at most risk of developing these anti-WBC antibodies is multiparous females, and the components that contain the greatest burden of anti-HNA and anti-HLA antibodies are plasma-rich products, including fresh frozen plasma and platelets. Surveillance data has shown that female donors of plasma-rich products, specifically those who have anti-HNA or anti-HLA antibodies, are significantly more likely to provide blood products that are associated with TRALI.[24]

As of 2015, TRALI was the leading cause of FDA-reported transfusion-associated deaths; however, as reflected by FDA-reported transfusion-associated fatalities and prospective surveillance studies, the incidence of TRALI has decreased significantly since the implementation of TRALI mitigation strategies.[4,25] While previous strategies restricted high plasma-volume component donations to male donors, recent revisions have allowed for female donors with low risk of HLA or HNA alloimmunization, including nulliparous females and females who have delivered and subsequently tested negative for HLA antibodies, to again donate high plasma-volume products.[26]

Transfusion-Associated Circulatory Overload

Transfusion-associated circulatory overload (TACO) has been shown to increase mortality and prolong inpatient lengths of stay.[27] Additionally, according to the FDA, between fiscal years 2011 and 2015, TACO represented the second-highest cause of reported transfusion-related fatalities.[4]

TACO is characterized by signs and symptoms that include: acute respiratory distress, elevated central venous pressure, elevated brain natriuretic peptide, left heart failure, positive fluid balance, and cardiogenic pulmonary edema (as evidenced by radiology findings).[8] Other signs may include hypertension, tachycardia, and elevated pulmonary wedge pressure.[28] These findings typically occur 6 hours or less after a transfusion.[8] Patients with congestive heart failure or chronic kidney disease are at greater risk for TACO, likely because of an inability to tolerate increases in blood volume.[27]

TACO may be prevented by slowing the infusion rate, transfusing only single (or split) units at any one time, and administering diuretics such as furosemide prior to transfusion.[29] Certainly, avoidance of transfusion is the best way to prevent TACO. For anemic patients, however, clinicians should be sensitive to individuals at-risk for TACO (as described earlier) when ordering blood transfusions. It has been suggested that nursing staff should not only monitor patients for signs and symptoms of TACO during transfusion but also advocate against unnecessary transfusion in patients who are at greater risk for TACO by working more closely with the patient's ordering physician.[29]

TACO and TRALI are typically both part of the differential diagnosis for a transfused patient with acute respiratory distress, hypoxia, and pulmonary edema.[30] The edema in TACO is due to increased capillary hydrostatic pressures and due to cardiac/vascular insufficiency, while the edema in TRALI is related to permeability reflecting an allergic capillary leak syndrome.[30,31] The two entities can be difficult to differentiate, but some features in TACO that are not typically present in TRALI include hypertension, transudative pulmonary edema fluid, and response to diuresis.[32] The utility of elevated brain natriuretic peptide (BNP) and N-terminal pro-brain natriuretic peptide (NT-pro-BNP) levels to differentiate TACO from TRALI is favored by some investigators but not by others.[33,34] The two entities are important to differentiate, as diuretics are central to the treatment of TACO but considered to be contraindicated for most patients with TRALI.[31] This is because diuretics can induce hypovolemia in patients with TRALI who are euvolemic, thus precipitating hypotension.[31,35]

When respiratory distress occurs within 24 hours of a transfusion and TACO, TRALI, and an allergic reaction (discussed in what follows) are ruled out, the reaction may be called transfusion-associated dyspnea (TAD).[8]

Allergic Reactions

Allergic reactions vary in their presentation. They range from mild and benign (e.g., pruritus) to severe and life-threatening (e.g., anaphylaxis).[1,18] These reactions may be self-limited, may respond well to simple medication, or may necessitate aggressive treatment to maintain vital functions and prevent death.

Allergic reactions can occur during the administration of any form of human blood product, but human plasma in any product is often implicated as the cause of allergic transfusion reactions.[36,37] Recipients may develop a response to allergens (e.g., plasma proteins) contained within the plasma of donated products.[1,37] This is manifest as a Type I hypersensitivity reaction resulting from IgE, allergen, mast cell, and basophil interactions.[36] It has been suggested that previous exposure to plasma in human blood products increases the risk of allergic transfusion reactions.[36] Anaphylactic reactions due to IgG antibodies against IgA may be seen in individuals with IgA deficiency (true total lack of IgA); however, most anaphylactic reactions are not due to anti-IgA antibodies.[38] The cause of most reactions may be antibodies to substances and allergens other than IgA.[1,38]

The clinical signs and symptoms of an allergic reaction include the following: conjunctival edema; edema of lips, tongue, and uvula; erythema and edema of the periorbital area; generalized flushing; hypotension; localized angioedema; maculopapular rash; pruritis (itching); respiratory distress; bronchospasm; and urticaria (hives).[8] Isolated pruritis and hives are typically a benign manifestation of allergic reactions. Anaphylactic reactions, however, may be life threatening and present as respiratory distress (dyspnea, wheezing, and stridor) with hypotension, hypotonia, and/or syncope.[1,8]

Allergic transfusion reactions may be prevented or ameliorated by washing red blood cells or platelets prior to administration.[36] This practice shortens the shelf life of the product because component processing must be performed in an open system. Further, washing may shorten the survival time of platelets and may reduce the number of platelets transfused.[36] Patients with known anti-IgA antibodies who have a history of anaphylactoid reactions to blood product administration should receive plasma from IgA-deficient donors or have red blood cells and platelets washed prior to transfusion.[1]

Patients who have had previous allergic reactions may be premedicated with an antihistamine such as diphenhydramine or a corticosteroid such as solumedrol prior to transfusion.[1] The premedication of all patients receiving a transfusion is controversial, however. Some transfusion medicine specialists insist that there is not enough evidence to support premedication as an effective means of preventing transfusion reactions.[3] A 2010 Cochrane Review of three randomized control trials studying transfusion premedication concluded that premedication did not prevent nonhemolytic transfusion reactions, including allergic transfusion reactions.[17]

Treatment of mild allergic reactions includes merely pausing the transfusion. If the reaction resolves and there are no other signs and symptoms suggestive of a febrile or hemolytic transfusion reaction (e.g., fever, chills, flank pain, etc.), transfusion may be continued following mild allergic reactions. Administration of additional volumes of the implicated product in the initial absence of anaphylaxis is not likely to lead to anaphylaxis but, perhaps, a recurrence of the mild symptoms originally seen (e.g., hives). In patients with more severe reactions, diphenhydramine and solumedrol may be administered to help alleviate symptoms. More advanced supportive care (including airway management) as well as administration of intramuscular or subcutaneous epinephrine may be necessary in patients who develop anaphylaxis.[37] Additionally, those patients who develop anaphylaxis should be checked for a true deficiency of IgA as well as the presence of anti-IgA antibodies.

Septic Transfusion Reactions

Despite various measures to ensure that donated blood products are safe and free of viral, fungal, bacterial, and protozoal agents, microbial contamination remains a rare but serious risk of transfusion. Between 2011 and 2015, there were 18 microbial infection-related deaths reported to the FDA.[4] This represents 10% of total FDA-reported transfusion-associated deaths. Interestingly, 16.7% of all microbial infection-related deaths during this time period were attributed to *Babesia microti*, an intraerythrocytic parasite that is most commonly spread by tick bites.[4] Currently, there is no routine screening of donated products for babesia species, although this is a topic of intense discussion, especially in regions where this parasite is common. Results of laboratory-based blood donor screening pilot programs in New England are already being published and will likely continue to gain momentum as babesiosis is recognized as a significant transfusion-associated health risk.[39]

Although deaths due to septic transfusion reactions are rare, as many as 1 in 3,000 transfused platelet products may contain some level of bacterial contamination. However, most of these do not result in clinical sepsis.[40] Platelets, which are stored at room temperature, have the highest rate of septic transfusion reactions among blood components, with approximately 1 in 20,000 platelet transfusions resulting in clinical sepsis.[40] Bacterial species reported in fatal septic reactions due to platelet transfusion include *S. aureus, S. Marcescens, S. epidermidis,* and *coagulase-negative staphylococci.*[4] Apheresis platelets, which are collected from a single donor, are generally considered to have a lower risk of microbial contamination than do pooled platelets, although recent data demonstrate that both products carry risk.[4] RBC units are stored in the cold at 1 to 6°C, limiting the ability of most bacteria to replicate to significant levels. Although the prevalence of bacterial contamination of RBC products is 2.6 per 100,000 units, clinically significant septic transfusions due to RBC units are estimated to be 1 in 250,000 transfusions,[40] with *Y. enterocolitica, Pseudomonas* species and *S. liquefaciens* being the gram-negative organisms most capable of replication at cold temperature.[41]

Prevention of septic transfusion reactions is a priority for the transfusion medicine community. Targeting the preparation and processing of blood components can limit the risk of postcollection contamination and minimize some of the processing steps that contribute to contamination. For example, collection practices that utilize diversion pouches on the donor collection bags can prevent skin plugs from contaminating a blood product. Additionally, culturing blood products in close proximity to the time of collection can detect bacterial contamination in advance of transfusion of a product. There is published evidence, however, that culturing platelet products multiple days after their collection leads to increased sensitivity of detection of bacterial contamination, presumably by allowing bacteria to enter a log phase of growth.[42]

Pathogen Reduction

Possible methods to reduce bacterial contamination, especially given the relative insensitivity of bacterial detection at the time of collection of platelet products, could include reculture of products at a later date or rapid point-of-issue bacterial or pathogen reduction techniques. Pathogen reduction is an attractive solution to microbial contamination of blood products because it may be effective against not just bacteria but also viruses and parasites.[43] There are multiple pathogen reduction methods for different blood components (i.e., methods differ for whole blood, platelets, and plasma components). Pathogen reduction can be accomplished either by interfering with pathogen nucleic acids pathways, or by dissolving pathogen membranes.[43a,43b] Solvent detergents may be effective at disturbing pathogen membranes in plasma products.[43a,43b] Methylene blue combined with UV-A irradiation may be useful for pathogen reduction through interfering with pathogen nucleic acids in plasma products.[43a,43b] Psoralen, a natural product derivative, combined with UV-A irradiation, interferes with nucleic acids and has been used for plasma and platelet products.[43a,43b] Riboflavin combined with UV-A irradiation may be effective at interfering with pathogen nucleic acids in whole blood, plasma, platelets, and RBC components.[43a,43b] Although European countries have made extensive use of pathogen reduction techniques, especially for platelet products, for more than a decade, they have been only slowly adopted in the United States.[44] Since the December 2014 FDA approval of a commercial platform for pathogen inactivation of plasma and platelet products, utilization of such technology in the United States is starting to increase. The use of pathogen reduction methods for RBC products is currently investigational; however, it is an area of intense interest to combat RBC intracellular parasites, such as babesiosis.[43a,43b,44]

Transfusion-Associated Graft-Versus-Host Disease

Transfusion-associated graft-versus-host disease (TA-GVHD) is an uncommon but potentially fatal complication of blood transfusion that occurs in selected at-risk populations of transfused patients. It occurs when donor T-lymphocytes contained within a transfused product engraft in a susceptible host. Due to either host immune compromise or a close match between donor and recipient HLA types, the donor lymphocytes cannot be effectively cleared and instead proliferate in the recipient, eventually attacking the recipient's tissue and, most importantly, host bone marrow elements, inducing bone marrow aplasia.

When a donor is homozygous for an HLA type, and the recipient is heterozygous for this same type, the donor T-lymphocytes can evade immune detection by the recipient yet still attack recipient cells bearing the unrecognized HLA antigens.[45] This can occur in immunocompetent hosts who receive either directed donations from relatives or HLA-matched transfusions. The level of immune compromise that renders a recipient susceptible to TA-GVHD can vary. It can occur, for example, in patients receiving high-dose chemotherapy, including cyclophosphamide and fludarabine, patients with congenital immunodeficiencies, stem cell transplant recipients, and patients with acute leukemia and Hodgkin's disease. It can also occur in infants with hemolytic disease of the fetus and newborn (HDFN) and in recipients of intrauterine transfusions.[45] TA-GVHD is not a significant concern in patients with HIV/AIDS, possibly due in part to the ability of unaffected recipient CD8+ T-cells to eliminate donor T-cells, and, in part, to the virus itself eliminating susceptible donor and recipient T-cells.[46]

Patients who develop TA-GVHD may experience fever, rash, gastrointestinal tract involvement, often manifesting as diarrhea, and, characteristically, pancytopenia. The pancytopenia is unrelenting and can be fatal. Supportive measures are the only treatment option for patients who have developed TA-GVHD. Mortality approaches 90%.[45] Transfusion medicine services can eliminate risk of TA-GVHD by gamma irradiating blood products intended for susceptible patients. This process stops donor lymphocytes from proliferating and is thus protective against TA-GVHD.

A dose of 2,500 cGy is adequate to eliminate the risk of TA-GVHD from donor T-cells contained within a transfused blood product. Although RBC units resuspended in approved additive solutions have a shelf life of 42 days, once an RBC unit has been irradiated, it must be transfused within 28 days, due to an increase in RBC breakdown products (primarily potassium) in the supernatant of irradiated units. Irradiation of platelet products does not alter the shelf life, and the importance of irradiation of HLA-matched platelet units, specifically, cannot be overlooked. These products are often transfused to a patient population already at risk for TA-GVHD due to immune compromise, and transfusion of products with a close HLA match between donor and recipient presents an additional risk factor for TA-GVHD.

Metabolic Derangements Due to Transfusion

While transfusion can help a patient achieve normalization of anemia, thrombocytopenia, or a coagulopathy, it may also result in changes to the patient's chemistry. This is because blood products contain more than just the cells or proteins of interest that are transfused. They contain endogenous and exogenous substances including anticoagulants and preservatives that may also affect the recipient.

Transfusion of a unit of red blood cells results in administration of 200–250 mg of iron.[1,47] Accumulation of iron in the chronically transfused patient, notably patients with thalassemia major or sickle cell disease, may result in end organ damage particularly to the liver, heart, and endocrine organs.[47] Chronically transfused patients should have ferritin levels followed and iron chelation therapy initiated to treat iron overload. In patients with sickle cell disease, red cell exchange as an alternative to chronic simple transfusion may slow the acquisition of iron overload.

The use of citrate in blood products may cause hypocalcemia in massively transfused patients. Patients with liver disease are particularly sensitive to this complication because of an impaired ability to metabolize citrate to bicarbonate. "Citrate toxicity" causing hypocalcemia may result in perioral and peripheral tingling, nausea, muscle spasms or cramps, hyperventilation, and cardiac dysfunction.[1] Additionally, patients with liver failure who cannot metabolize citrate to bicarbonate (and incidentally cannot metabolize lactate) may develop a metabolic acidosis after large-volume transfusion.[48] Calcium supplementation may be necessary to treat the effects of hypocalcemia due to citrate toxicity.

Storage of red blood cells results in release of intracellular potassium. The amount of potassium ranges from 0.5 mEq to 7 mEq depending on the age of the unit.[1] Furthermore, a portion of transfused red blood cells may lyse after infusion, and irradiation increases the release of potassium from red blood cells. The amount of potassium transfused is unlikely to cause problems in most adult patients, but patients with renal disease and small pediatric patients, especially those given large amounts of blood products, may be susceptible to hyperkalemia with resultant cardiac dysfunction.[1,48] Units may be washed to remove potassium in the supernatant prior to transfusion to sensitive patients.[48]

Hypokalemia due to transfusion is more common than hyperkalemia.[1] Transfused red cells can absorb the patient's circulating potassium.[1] Aldosterone, antidiuretic hormone, catecholamines, and administration of potassium-poor solutions during resuscitation also contribute to hypokalemia.[48] In massive transfusion, the citrate in blood products is metabolized to bicarbonate, resulting in a metabolic alkalosis.[48] To compensate, H+ is released from red blood cells and potassium is absorbed to normalize the ionic balance of the red cell; this can potentiate hypokalemia. Potassium levels should be monitored in massively transfused patients, and potassium should be judiciously supplemented as needed.[48]

Hypothermia

Administration of a large volume of blood products without a blood warmer may result in hypothermia, as these products are, at best, administered at room temperature (platelets) and, at worst, administered immediately after refrigeration between 1°C and 6°C (red cells). Hypothermia as a complication of massive transfusion setting may result in coagulopathy.[48] Use of a monitored blood warmer can help prevent hypothermia in the transfused patient, and patients can also be supported with the use of warm blankets or a warming apparatus. Never use a standard microwave or hot tap water to warm a unit of blood.[2] This practice may result in hemolysis that may be harmful or fatal to the recipient.

Posttransfusion Purpura

A diagnosis of post transfusion purpura (PTP) may be considered in a patient with thrombocytopenia who has been recently transfused. The diagnosis can be made when anti-HPA (or other) alloantibodies against platelet-specific antigens are detected, typically in a patient with newfound thrombocytopenia presenting between 5 to 12 days after transfusion.[8] The anti-HPA (usually anti-HPA-1a) alloantibodies develop after previous pregnancy or transfusion, and these alloantibodies may actually crossreact with antigen-negative platelets in the recipient.[1] The differential diagnosis includes heparin induced thrombocytopenia (which can have a similar time course), idiopathic thrombocytopenic purpura, thrombotic thrombocytopenic purpura, disseminated intravascular coagulation, drug-induced thrombocytopenia, and bone marrow suppression.[1,49] Although typically self-limited, PTP may last for up to a month and can be treated with immunosuppressive therapy such as IVIG.[1,49,50] Therapeutic plasma exchange may be considered for profoundly thrombocytopenic and bleeding patients refractory to IVIG.[50] PTP uncommonly recurs, but transfusion of autologous or antigen-negative units is recommended to prevent recurrence.[1] Leukoreduction appears to have a role in reducing the incidence of PTP.[1]

Concluding Thoughts

The field of transfusion medicine is constantly evolving to identify and eliminate risks for adverse reactions to blood products. Clinicians can take an active role in this process by familiarizing themselves with the basic principles of transfusion medicine, including an awareness of these adverse reactions. Medical practitioners should know not only how adverse reactions to transfusion can be recognized and reported but also how these risks can be minimized. Adhering to evidence-based transfusion practices is an important part of this process. Understanding that there are risks and benefits associated with blood component transfusion can substantially improve patient outcomes.

References

1. Mazzei CA, Popovski MA, Kopko PM. Noninfectious complications of blood transfusion. In: Roback JD, Grossman BJ, Harris T, Hillyer CD, eds. *Technical Manual.* 17 ed. Bethesda: AABB; 2011; 727–762.

2. Sink BLS. Administration of blood components. In: Roback JD, Grossman BJ, Harris T, Hillyer CD, eds. *Technical Manual.* 17 ed. Bethesda: AABB; 2011; 617–629.

3. Tobian AA, King KE, Ness PM. Transfusion premedications: a growing practice not based on evidence. *Transfusion.* 2007 Jun; 47(6):1089–1096.

4. Fatalities reported to FDA following blood collection and transfusion: annual summary for fiscal year 2015 [electronic document]. United States Food and Drug Administration Web Site. Available at: www.fda.gov/downloads/BiologicsBloodVaccines/SafetyAvailability/ReportaProblem/TransfusionDonationFatalities/UCM518148.pdf. Accessed May 21, 2017.

5. Lozano M, Cid J. The clinical implications of platelet transfusions associated with ABO or Rh(D) incompatibility. *Transfusion Medicine Reviews.* 2003 Jan; 17(1):57–68.

6. Valbonesi M, De Luigi MC, Lercari G, et al. Acute intravascular hemolysis in two patients transfused with dry-platelet units obtained from the same ABO incompatible donor. *The International Journal of Artificial Organs.* 2000 Sep; 23(9):642–646.

7. Hawkins R. Discrepancy between visual and spectrophotometric assessment of sample haemolysis. *Annals of Clinical Biochemistry.* 2002 Sep; 39(Pt 5):521–522.

8. National Healthcare Safety Network Biovigilance Component Hemovigilance Module Surveillance Protocol Version 2.4 [electronic document]. 2017 January. In: CDC Web Site. Available at: www.cdc.gov/nhsn/PDFs/Biovigilance/BV-HV-protocol-current.pdf. Accessed May 21, 2017.

9. Giles CM. The role of complement in immunohematology. *Transfusion.* 1989 Nov–Dec; 29(9):803–811.

10. Tao MH, Canfield SM, Morrison SL. The differential ability of human IgG1 and IgG4 to activate complement is determined by the COOH-terminal sequence of the CH2 domain. *The Journal of Experimental Medicine.* 1991 Apr 1; 173(4):1025–1028.

11. Tormey CA, Stack G. The persistence and evanescence of blood group alloantibodies in men. *Transfusion.* 2009 Mar; 49(3):505–512.

12. Pineda AA, Vamvakas EC, Gorden LD, Winters JL, Moore SB. Trends in the incidence of delayed hemolytic and delayed serologic transfusion reactions. *Transfusion.* 1999 Oct; 39(10): 1097–1103.

13. Vichinsky EP, Earles A, Johnson RA, Hoag MS, Williams A, Lubin B. Alloimmunization in sickle cell anemia and transfusion of racially unmatched blood. *New England Journal of Medicine.* 1990; 322(23):1617–1621.

14. Uhlmann EJ, Shenoy S, Goodnough LT. Successful treatment of recurrent hyperhemolysis syndrome with immunosuppression and plasma-to-red blood cell exchange transfusion. *Transfusion.* 2013 May 21. [Epub ahead of print].

15. Sowemimo-Coker SO. Red blood cell hemolysis during processing. *Transfusion Medicine Reviews.* 2002 Jan; 16(1):46–60.

16. Shapira Y, Vaturi M, Sagie A. Hemolysis associated with prosthetic heart valves: a review. *Cardiology in Review.* 2009 May–Jun; 17(3):121–124.

17. Marti-Carvajal AJ, Sola I, Gonzalez LE, Leon de Gonzalez G, Rodriguez-Malagon N. Pharmacological interventions for the prevention of allergic and febrile non-haemolytic transfusion reactions. *The Cochrane Database of Systematic Reviews.* 2010(6):CD007539.

18. Circular of Information: for the Use of Human Blood and Blood Components [electronic document]. Revised November 2013. In: AABB Web Site. Available at: www.aabb.org/tm/coi/Documents/coi1113.pdf. Accessed May 21, 2017.

19. Andrzejewski C, Jr., Popovsky MA, Stec TC, et al. Hemotherapy bedside biovigilance involving vital sign values and characteristics of patients with suspected transfusion reactions associated with fluid challenges: can some cases of transfusion-associated circulatory overload have proinflammatory aspects? *Transfusion.* 2012 Nov; 52(11):2310–2320.

20. King KE, Shirey RS, Thoman SK, Bensen-Kennedy D, Tanz WS, Ness PM. Universal leukoreduction decreases the incidence of febrile nonhemolytic transfusion reactions to RBCs. *Transfusion.* 2004 Jan; 44(1):25–29.

21. Toy P, Popovsky MA, Abraham E, et al. Transfusion-related acute lung injury: definition and review. *Crit Care Med.* 2005; 33(4):721–726.

22. Popovsky MA, Abel MD, Moore SB. Transfusion-related acute lung injury associated with passive transfer of antileukocyte antibodies. *The American Review of Respiratory Disease.* 1983 Jul; 128(1):185–189.

23. Silliman CC, Ambruso DR, Boshkov LK. Transfusion-related acute lung injury. *Blood.* 2005 Mar 15; 105(6): 2266–2273.

24. Eder AF, Herron R, Strupp A, et al. Transfusion-related acute lung injury surveillance (2003–2005) and the potential impact of the selective use of plasma from male donors in the American Red Cross. *Transfusion.* 2007 Apr; 47(4):599–607.

25. Toy P, Gajic O, Bacchetti P, et al. Transfusion-related acute lung injury: incidence and risk factors. *Blood.* 2012 Feb 16; 119(7):1757–1767.

26. AABB Revises and Clarifies TRALI Risk Reduction Requirements. *AABB Weekly Report* [serial online]. 2013 Sept 27. Available at: www.aabb.org/resources/publications/weeklyreport/2013/Pages/wr130927.aspx. Accessed February 4, 2014.

27. Murphy EL, Kwaan N, Looney MR, et al. Risk factors and outcomes in transfusion-associated circulatory overload. *The American Journal of Medicine.* 2013 Apr; 126(4):357 e329–e338.

28. Popovsky MA. Pulmonary consequences of transfusion: TRALI and TACO. *Transfusion and Apheresis Science: Official Journal of the World Apheresis Association: Official Journal of the European Society for Haemapheresis.* 2006 Jun; 34(3):243–244.

29. Alam A, Lin Y, Lima A, Hansen M, Callum JL. The prevention of transfusion-associated circulatory overload. *Transfusion Medicine Reviews.* 2013 Apr; 27(2):105–112.

30. Pandey S, Vyas GN. Adverse effects of plasma transfusion. *Transfusion.* 2012 May; 52 Suppl 1:65S–79S.

31. Kopko PM, Holland PV. Transfusion-related acute lung injury. *British Journal of Haematology.* 1999 May; 105(2): 322–329.

32. Skeate RC, Eastlund T. Distinguishing between transfusion related acute lung injury and transfusion associated circulatory overload. *Current Opinion in Hematology.* 2007 Nov; 14(6): 682–687.

33. Li G, Daniels CE, Kojicic M, et al. The accuracy of natriuretic peptides (brain natriuretic peptide and N-terminal pro-brain natriuretic) in the differentiation between transfusion-related acute lung injury and transfusion-related circulatory overload in the critically ill. *Transfusion.* 2009 Jan; 49(1):13–20.

34. Tobian AA, Sokoll LJ, Tisch DJ, Ness PM, Shan H. N-terminal pro-brain natriuretic peptide is a useful diagnostic marker for transfusion-associated circulatory overload. *Transfusion.* 2008 Jun; 48(6):1143–1150.

35. Levy GJ, Shabot MM, Hart ME, Mya WW, Goldfinger D. Transfusion-associated noncardiogenic pulmonary edema. Report of a case and a warning regarding treatment. *Transfusion.* 1986 May–Jun; 26(3):278–281.

36. Tobian AA, Savage WJ, Tisch DJ, Thoman S, King KE, Ness PM. Prevention of allergic transfusion reactions to platelets and red blood cells through plasma reduction. *Transfusion.* 2011 Aug; 51(8):1676–1683.

37. Hirayama F. Current understanding of allergic transfusion reactions: incidence, pathogenesis, laboratory tests, prevention and treatment. *British Journal of Haematology.* 2013 Feb; 160(4):434–444.

38. Gilstad CW. Anaphylactic transfusion reactions. *Current Opinion in Hematology.* 2003 Nov; 10(6):419–423.

39. Young C, Chawla A, Berardi V, et al. Preventing transfusion-transmitted babesiosis: preliminary experience of the first laboratory-based blood donor screening program. *Transfusion.* 2012 Jul; 52(7):1523–1529.

40. Hillyer CD, Josephson CD, Blajchman MA, Vostal JG, Epstein JS, Goodman JL. Bacterial contamination of blood components: risks, strategies, and regulation: joint ASH and AABB educational session in transfusion medicine. *Hematology/the Education Program of the American Society of Hematology. American Society of Hematology. Education Program.* 2003:575–589.

41. Brecher ME, Means N, Jere CS, Heath D, Rothenberg S, Stutzman LC. Evaluation of an automated culture system for detecting bacterial contamination of platelets: an analysis with 15 contaminating organisms. *Transfusion.* 2001 Apr; 41(4):477–482.

42. Murphy WG, Foley M, Doherty C, et al. Screening platelet concentrates for bacterial contamination: low numbers of bacteria and slow growth in contaminated units mandate an alternative approach to product safety. *Vox Sanguinis.* 2008 Jul; 95(1):13–19.

43a. Pelletier JP, Transue S, Snyder EL. Pathogen inactivation techniques. Best practice & research. *Clinical Haematology.* 2006; 19(1):205–242.

43b. Snyder EL, Stramer S, Benjamin R. Safety of the blood supply – time to raise the bar. *The New England Journal of Medicine.* 2015; 372(20):1882–1885.

44. Seltsam A, Muller TH. Update on the use of pathogen-reduced human plasma and platelet concentrates. *British Journal of Haematology.* 2013 Aug; 162(4):442–454.

45. Anderson KC, Weinstein HJ. Transfusion-associated graft-versus-host disease. *The New England Journal of Medicine.* 1990 Aug 2; 323(5): 315–321.

46. Fast LD. Developments in the prevention of transfusion-associated graft-versus-host disease. *British Journal of Haematology.* 2012 Sep; 158(5):563–568.

47. Thuret I. Post-transfusional iron overload in the haemoglobinopathies. *Comptes Rendus Biologies.* 2013 Mar; 336(3):164–172.

48. Sihler KC, Napolitano LM. Complications of massive transfusion. *Chest.* 2010 Jan; 137(1):209–220.

49. Padhi P, Parihar GS, Stepp J, Kaplan R. Post-transfusion purpura: a rare and life-threatening aetiology of thrombocytopenia. *BMJ Case Reports.* May 24, 2013. [published online].

50. Schwartz J, Winters JL, Padmanabhan A, et al. Guidelines on the use of therapeutic apheresis in clinical practice-evidence-based approach from the Writing Committee of the American Society for Apheresis: the sixth special issue. *Journal of Clinical Apheresis.* 2013 Jul; 28(3):145–284.

Chapter

31

Pharmacologic Therapy of Anemia

Nicholas Short, MD, and Elisabeth M. Battinelli, MD, PhD

In anemic patients who are hemodynamically stable and lack an urgent need for allogeneic blood transfusion, anemia is generally treated with specific therapies targeting its underlying etiology (nutritional deficiencies, hemolysis, ongoing blood loss, etc.). Iron deficiency anemia is the most common cause of anemia worldwide, and therefore hematologists must be especially familiar with the nuances of iron repletion. This chapter provides an in-depth discussion of the dosing, safety, and clinical indications of oral and intravenous (IV) iron formulations. In contrast, erythropoiesis-stimulating agents (ESAs) are indicated for the treatment of hypoproliferative anemias due to a broad spectrum of clinical conditions. This chapter will also discuss the pharmacology of the various ESAs as well as their safety, efficacy, and clinical indications. Details of therapy with cyanocobalamin and folic acid for megaloblastic anemias and androgens for aplastic states are discussed in Chapters 14 and 18, respectively.

Iron Repletion

Oral Iron Therapy

In asymptomatic patients with iron deficiency anemia, oral iron therapy is often adequate to reverse anemia and replete iron stores. Daily oral intake of 150–300 mg of elemental iron is advised, which results in absorption of up to 50 mg of iron per day in most patients without underlying malabsorption. Gastrointestinal absorption of oral iron is indirectly related to overall body iron content (i.e., plasma ferritin concentration) and decreases as iron stores are repleted.[1] Available iron preparations differ in their elemental iron content (Table 31.1), and as long as equivalent daily doses of elemental iron are provided, there is no evidence that any oral iron formulation is superior for replacing iron stores and raising hemoglobin. Various dietary and drug interactions can impair the absorption of oral iron (Table 31.2). Conversely, iron absorption may be augmented with the addition of ascorbic acid, which increases the acidity of the gastric environment and reduces ferric (Fe^{+++}) iron to the more easily absorbed ferrous (Fe^{++}) form.[2]

Gastrointestinal side effects are common and occur in almost 50% of patients treated with some oral iron formulations, leading to discontinuation of therapy in up to 15% of patients.[3–4] Oral iron supplements can cause nausea,

abdominal pain, constipation, and (less commonly) diarrhea. The frequencies of gastrointestinal side effects are directly related to the elemental iron content of the preparation.[5] Enteric-coated and sustained-release iron formulas cause fewer gastrointestinal side effects than other oral iron preparations but have significantly lower absorption because they bypass the

Table 31.1 Elemental iron content of common oral iron preparations

Oral Iron Preparation	Approximate Elemental Iron Concentration (mg/g)	Strength (Elemental Iron Content), mg[1]	Route
Ferrous gluconate	110	240 (27)	Tablet
		325 (36)	Tablet
Ferrous sulfate	200	195 (39)	Tablet
		325 (65)	Tablet
		220 (44)	Solution
		300 (60)	Solution
Ferrous fumarate	330	325 (108)	Tablet
Polysaccharide–iron complex	1,000	150 (150)	Tablet
		50 (50)	Tablet

[1] Strengths for all iron solutions are based on a 5 ml dose.

Table 31.2 Dietary and drug interactions with oral iron

Dietary Interactions
- Dairy products
- Phytates (e.g., bran, oats and rye fiber)
- Polyphenols (e.g., coffee, tea, and some fruits and vegetables)
- Tannins (e.g., tea and wine)

Drug Interactions[1]
- Antisecretory agents (e.g., H2RAs and PPIs)
- Aluminum-containing phosphate binders
- Calcium supplements and calcium salt-containing antacids
- Pancreatic enzyme replacement (pancrelipase)
- Phosphate supplements
- Tetracyclines

H2RA histamine 2 receptor antagonists, *PPI* proton pump inhibitor.
[1] Interactions only apply for orally administered medications or supplements.

duodenum and proximal jejunum. For patients who are intolerant of oral preparations, a reduced dose of iron supplement can be attempted with slow up-titration.

The typical response to oral iron repletion is a reticulocytosis that peaks in approximately 7–10 days, an increase in hemoglobin by 2 g/dL within 3 weeks, and a normalization of hemoglobin within 6–8 weeks. Despite correction of the anemia, oral iron therapy should be continued for at least 6 months in patients with severe iron deficiency anemia if full repletion of iron stores is desired.

Intravenous Iron Therapy

IV iron therapy offers a number of potential advantages over oral iron repletion in patients with iron deficiency anemia. Unlike oral iron therapy, some formulations of IV iron can provide enough iron to reverse anemia and replace iron stores with only one infusion. IV iron is particularly advantageous in patients who cannot tolerate oral iron preparations or who are otherwise nonadherent or refractory to oral iron repletion.

IV Iron Dosing

A number of IV iron formulations are currently available (Table 31.3). These preparations primarily differ in their concentration of elemental iron and their approved maximum daily dose.[6] When treating a patient with IV iron, the following formula should be used to calculate a patient's iron deficit, which is used to estimate the necessary dose of IV iron:

Table 31.3 Intravenous iron preparations

Iron Preparation	Maximum Daily Dose of Elemental Iron (mg)	Concentration of Elemental Iron (mg/ml)	Test Dose Required[1]
HMW iron dextran[2]	1,000[3]	50	Yes
LMW iron dextran	1,000[3]	50	Yes
Ferric gluconate	125	12.5	No
Iron sucrose	300	20	No
Ferumoxytol	510	30	No
Ferric carboxymaltose	1,500	50	No

HMW high molecular weight, *LMW* low molecular weight.
[1] The test dose should be given as 25 mg of elemental iron infused over 5 minutes. The rest of the dose may be given 30 minutes later if the test dose is tolerated.
[2] Due to its relatively high adverse event rate, the use of HMW iron dextran is not recommended.
[3] Manufacturer's labeling recommends 100 mg maximum dose, although 1,000 mg doses have been safely given.

$$\text{Total iron deficit (mg)} = \text{Body weight (kg)} \times 2.3 \times \left(14 - \text{patient's hemoglobin, g/dL}\right)$$

If repletion of iron stores is also desired, an additional 500 mg to 1,000 mg of iron should be provided. To calculate the volume of IV iron required to replete the iron deficit and/or iron stores, the desired dose of iron should be divided by the concentration of the particular iron formulation being administered. Up to 1,000 mg of low-molecular-weight (LMW) iron dextran and 1,500 mg of ferric carboxymaltose can be administered in one infusion. When the full dose of iron cannot be given in one administration, repeat doses can be given on a weekly basis.

Safety of IV Iron

Historically, IV iron has been avoided because of concerns of serious adverse events. However, newer and safer preparations have been developed, lowering the threshold of many clinicians to consider IV therapy for the treatment of iron-deficient patients. Life-threatening adverse events (e.g., anaphylaxis) occur in approximately 11.3 per million patients treated with high-molecular-weight (HMW) iron dextran, a rate significantly higher than with other IV iron formulations [7]. Self-limiting fever, arthralgias, and myalgias can occur with any IV iron preparation, generally resolve within 24 hours, and often respond to non-steroidal anti-inflammatory drugs. Other non–life-threatening adverse events occurring in <5% of patients include pruritus, nausea, dyspepsia, dyspnea, and chest pain.

Indications for IV Iron

Indications for IV iron therapy are summarized in Table 31.4. IV iron repletion should be considered in the iron-deficient patient who is intolerant or nonadherent or who does not respond to oral iron therapy. Gastrointestinal malabsorption is a common cause of failure of oral iron therapy.[8] Patients with achlorhydria, either from an underlying disease (e.g., autoimmune or atrophic gastritis) or iatrogenic causes (e.g., gastric bypass or gastric resection), often have diminished iron absorption. Pathologies affecting intestinal transport of nutrients in the duodenum and proximal jejunum particularly impair iron absorption.

In patients with chronic blood loss (e.g., gastrointestinal or uterine bleeding), IV iron repletion is often required due to the inability of oral iron administration to surpass the rate of iron loss from bleeding. In patients with a rate of blood loss greater than 100 ml per day, oral iron therapy alone is insufficient to achieve positive iron balance (assuming maximum oral elemental iron absorption of 50 mg per day). In patients with lower rates of chronic blood loss, oral iron therapy may take a prohibitively long time to reverse anemia and replete iron stores.

IV iron is preferred to oral iron therapy for many patients receiving concomitant treatment with ESAs. In cancer patients receiving ESAs, IV iron has been shown to synergize with ESAs to increase hemoglobin response and also decrease transfusion requirement.[9] Data are mixed, however, regarding the relative efficacy of IV iron compared to oral iron in cancer patients.[10–11] Thus, the route of iron delivery in these patients should be individualized. In contrast, in chronic kidney disease (CKD) patients on hemodialysis (HD), IV iron has been consistently shown to increase hemoglobin response and decrease ESA requirements compared to oral iron.[12] These benefits are seen whether or not the patient is receiving concomitant ESA therapy. IV iron therapy is preferred in all CKD patients with overt iron deficiency, as oral iron is frequently inadequate to keep up with iron loss from HD and frequent blood draws.

Table 31.4 Indications for intravenous iron therapy

Indication	Comments
Idiopathic nonresponders to oral iron	
Intolerance of oral iron	Gastrointestinal side effects occur in almost 50% of patients on some oral iron preparations and cause discontinuation in up to 15%.
Nonadherence to oral iron therapy	Common reasons include gastrointestinal side effects and three-times-a-day dosing.
Acute need for iron repletion	Oral iron therapy requires up to 6 months to fully replete iron stores, whereas IV iron can replace iron stores within weeks (and sometimes after one dose).
Chronic iron and/or blood loss	Oral iron therapy cannot cause a positive iron balance if blood loss exceeds 100 ml per day (i.e., approximately 50 mg of elemental iron per day).
Gastrointestinal malabsorption	E.g., bacterial overgrowth, celiac disease, autoimmune gastritis, *H. pylori* gastritis, inflammatory bowel disease, gastric bypass, partial or total gastric resection
Active malignancy	Compared to oral iron therapy, data is mixed regarding the superiority of IV iron in cancer patients concomitantly receiving ESAs.
ESRD	Compared to oral iron therapy, IV iron increases hematopoietic response and decreases ESA requirements in CKD patients concomitantly receiving ESAs. Benefit is seen in patients with overt or "functional" iron deficiency.

IV intravenous, *ESA* erythropoiesis-stimulating agent, *CKD* chronic kidney disease.

Erythropoiesis-Stimulation Agents (ESAs)

ESAs are effective at raising hemoglobin levels and reversing anemia in a variety of hypoproliferative anemias. ESA therapy avoids some potential complications of blood transfusions, including iron overload, transfusion reactions, infection, and the development of alloantibodies to blood products. Treatment with ESAs is also useful in patients who refuse blood transfusion for religious or other reasons. However, significant improvement of hemoglobin and anemia-related symptoms with ESA treatment often takes weeks to months. Thus, for the symptomatic patient, blood transfusion is still often required due to its rapid reversal of symptoms and hemodynamics.

Epoetin Alfa and Darbepoetin Alfa

Epoetin alfa and darbepoetin alfa are the two most commonly prescribed ESA formulations. Both agents are 165 amino acid glycoproteins that share the identical primary structure of endogenous erythropoietin (EPO).[13] These agents can be given either IV or subcutaneously (SC) and exhibit dose-dependent erythropoietic effects (Table 31.5). Darbepoetin alfa contains five N-linked oligosaccharide chains (compared to three chains in epoetin alfa), which results in a three-fold longer half-life of IV darbepoetin and two-fold longer half-life of SC darbepoetin compared to IV and SC epoetin alfa, respectively. The half-life of each ESA is longer with the SC route than the IV route. This difference is more notable with epoetin alfa than with darbepoetin alfa. In patients treated with ESAs, deficient iron stores should be repleted prior to ESA therapy in order to obtain optimal hematopoietic effects from the ESAs.

Safety of ESAs

Epoetin alfa and darbepoetin alfa share a similar side effect profile. Common mild side effects include injection site pain,

Table 31.5 Dose conversion between epoetin alfa and darbepoetin alfa

Epoetin Alfa Dose (units per week)[1]	Darbepoetin Alfa Dose (mcg per week)
<2,500	6.25
2,500–4,999	12.5
5,000–10,999	25
11,000–17,999	40
18,000–33,999	60
34,000–89,999	100
≥90,000	200

[1] Epoetin alfa dosing 2–3 times per week is equivalent to darbepoetin alfa weekly dosing. Epoetin alfa weekly dosing is equivalent to darbepoetin alfa dosing every 2 weeks. The darbepoetin alfa dose to be administered every 2 weeks is derived by using the total epoetin alfa dose over a two-week period for conversion.

flu-like syndrome, and headache. ESAs can also cause or worsen hypertension, which is most common in patients with CKD and can be severe and life-threatening. Blood pressure should be monitored carefully when initiating ESAs and titrating doses. The risk of hypertension due to ESAs can be mitigated with slower correction of anemia and lower hemoglobin targets. Adverse cardiovascular events including myocardial infarction, stroke, and death are associated with higher hemoglobin targets in patients treated with ESAs.[14] In patients with heart failure, ESAs are associated with significantly increased risk of venous thromboembolism (VTE) and a trend toward increased mortality (without clinically significant benefits).[15] Because of these safety concerns, ESAs are not recommended in heart failure patients. Pure red cell aplasia due to the development of anti-EPO antibodies is an extremely rare consequence of ESA therapy, most often seen with SC treatment in patients with CKD.

Indications for ESAs

Anemia of Chronic Kidney Disease

ESAs are commonly used in anemic patients with CKD, including predialysis patients and those receiving peritoneal dialysis (PD) or hemodialysis (HD). In CKD patients, ESAs raise hemoglobin levels, decrease blood transfusions, and alleviate anemia-related symptoms.[16] Treatment with an ESA should be considered when the hemoglobin level falls below 10 g/dL, especially if symptoms attributable to anemia are present. In most CKD patients, hemoglobin levels between 10 g/dL and 11.5 g/dL should be targeted, as the risk for serious cardiovascular events, stroke, and mortality is increased in CKD patients when hemoglobin levels are maintained >13 g/dL with ESA therapy.[14] However, the hemoglobin goal should be individualized for each patient, weighing the symptomatic benefit from the treatment of anemia with the patient's estimated risk for adverse events. Nearly all CKD patients (especially those on dialysis) will require iron maintenance to ensure adequate hematopoietic response to ESA therapy.

Common initial doses of epoetin alfa and darbepoetin alfa in predialysis, PD, and HD patients are shown in Table 31.6. For both ESAs, dose increases should be made no more frequently than every 4 weeks, though dose decreases can be made more frequently if necessary. If hemoglobin levels fail to increase by $\geq$1 g/dL over a 4-week period, the ESA dose should be increased by 25%. Conversely, if hemoglobin levels increase by >1 g/dL over any 2-week period, the ESA dose should be reduced by at least 25% to prevent adverse cardiovascular events, which are associated with rapid increase in hemoglobin due to ESA therapy.[17]

Chemotherapy-Associated Anemia

Chemotherapy-associated anemia is a major cause of morbidity in cancer patients. ESAs are effective at increasing hemoglobin and decreasing blood transfusions in patients with anemia due to myelosuppressive chemotherapy, although they

Table 31.6 Common initial doses of epoetin alfa and darbepoetin alfa in CKD patients

Agent	CKD Population	
	Predialysis and Peritoneal Dialysis[1]	Hemodialysis[2]
Epoetin alfa	50–100 U/kg SC weekly	50 U/kg IV three times a week
Darbepoetin alfa	0.45 mcg/kg SC weekly or 60 mcg SC every 2 weeks	0.45 mcg/kg IV weekly or 0.75 mcg/kg IV every 2 weeks

CKD chronic kidney disease, *SC* subcutaneously, *IV* intravenously.
[1] SC route of administration is usually preferred in patients with CKD but not on hemodialysis due to increased convenience compared to IV administration.
[2] IV route of administration is usually preferred in patients on hemodialysis to the ease of administration of IV medications during dialysis sessions.

have not been consistently shown to significantly improve quality of life or anemia-related symptoms.[18] Patients with anemia due to malignant involvement of the bone marrow or anemia of chronic disease are less likely to respond to ESA therapy than are those with chemotherapy-associated anemia.

Patients with active malignancy who are treated with an ESA develop venous thromboembolism (VTE) at higher rates than do cancer patients not receiving ESA therapy.[18] Risk factors for ESA-associated VTE have not yet been fully elucidated, although VTE events do not appear to be strongly influenced by either baseline hemoglobin or target hemoglobin levels. Treatment with ESAs is associated with inferior survival in patients not receiving chemotherapy.[18–19] Survival is also decreased when an ESA is initiated in patients with baseline hemoglobin levels >12 g/dL.

In light of these adverse outcomes, ESAs are not recommended for cancer patients whose anemia is not due to myelosuppressive chemotherapy (except in patients with low-risk myelodysplastic syndrome in whom data suggest that ESA therapy is safe and effective). Patients with significant risk factors for VTE events (e.g., history of VTE, planned surgery, or treatment with chemotherapy regimens associated with increased VTE risk) should avoid ESAs. While controversial, some guidelines recommend against ESA use in patients receiving chemotherapy with the intent of cure.[20]

Epoetin alfa and darbepoetin alfa appear to have similar safety and efficacy in patients with chemotherapy-associated anemia. SC darbepoetin is most commonly used because of its longer half-life and ease of administration. Starting doses and titration guidelines for epoetin alfa and darbepoetin alfa in patients with anemia due to myelosuppressive chemotherapy are summarized in Table 31.7. ESAs should be discontinued if, after 8 weeks of therapy, there is no significant increase in hemoglobin levels or if blood transfusions are still required. ESAs should also be stopped when the patient is no longer receiving chemotherapy.

Table 31.7 Initial doses and dose titration guidelines for epoetin alfa and darbepoetin alfa in patients with chemotherapy-associated anemia

	Epoetin Alfa	Darbepoetin Alfa
Initial Dose	**150 U/kg SC Three Times a Week** or **40,000 U SC Weekly**	**2.25 mcg/kg SC Weekly** or **500 mcg SC Every 3 Weeks**
Reduce dose if:	Hemoglobin reaches level needed to avoid blood transfusion *or* increases by >1 g/dL in any 2-week period	
Recommended dose reduction	25%	40%
Withhold dose if:	Hemoglobin exceeds level needed to avoid blood transfusion[1]	
Increase dose if:	After the initial 4 weeks of therapy, increase in hemoglobin is insufficient to avoid blood transfusion *and* hemoglobin does not increase by ≥1 g/dL	After the initial 6 weeks of therapy, increase in hemoglobin is insufficient to avoid blood transfusion *and* hemoglobin does not increase by ≥1 g/dL[2]
Recommended dose increase	300 U/kg SC three times a week or 60,000 U SC weekly	4.5 mcg/kg SC weekly[2]

SC subcutaneously.

[1] The drug should be resumed when the hemoglobin approaches a level when blood transfusion may be required. When the drug is resumed, epoetin alfa dose should be decreased by 25% and darbepoetin alfa dose should be decreased by 40%.

[2] Further dose adjustment of darbepoetin alfa in patients receiving the drug every three weeks is not recommended.

Patients Who Refuse Blood Transfusions

Patients who refuse blood transfusions should be considered for ESA therapy. In acutely ill patients with significant anemia, ESAs can be combined with IV iron in order to increase the rate of erythropoiesis. However, even with adequate nutritional stores (e.g., iron, folate, and vitamin B12), reticulocytosis does not begin until 3–4 days after initiation, limiting the use of ESAs in the acute setting. For patients with plans for surgery in whom there is concern for significant perioperative blood loss, ESAs can be initiated as early as 3 weeks prior to surgery, either with or without plans for autologous blood transfusion.[21]

Conclusions

Iron and ESAs are among the most common agents used to treat anemia. While in many iron-deficient patients oral iron repletion is adequate to reverse anemia and replace iron stores, IV iron is often necessary in patients with poor tolerance of oral iron preparations, chronic blood loss, gastrointestinal malabsorption, chemotherapy-associated anemia, or CKD. Historically clinicians have been hesitant to use IV iron due to serious adverse events with HMW iron dextran. However, newer formulations of IV iron are significantly safer and better tolerated, challenging the paradigm that IV iron should be used only if oral iron repletion fails.

In patients with anemia due to CKD or myelosuppressive chemotherapy, as well as in anemic patients who refuse allogeneic blood transfusion, epoetin alfa and darbepoetin alfa are effective at increasing hemoglobin levels and decreasing blood transfusion requirements. Repletion of iron stores is required to ensure sufficient ESA-mediated hematopoiesis, and therefore iron is often administered concomitantly with ESAs. Due to the potential risk for serious cardiovascular and VTE events with ESA therapy, the lowest ESA dose required to prevent the need for blood transfusion and alleviate anemia-related symptoms should generally be used.

References

1. Bothwell TH. Overview and mechanisms of iron regulation. *Nutr Rev.* 1995; **53**:237–245.

2. Teucher B, Olivares M, Cori H. Enhancers of iron absorption: ascorbic acid and other organic acids. *Int J Vitam Nutr Res.* 2004; **74**:403–419.

3. Cancelo-Hidalgo MJ, Castelo-Branco C, Palacios S, et al. Tolerability of different oral iron supplements: a systematic review. *Curr Med Res Opin.* 2013; **29**:291–303.

4. Melamed N, Ben-Haroush A, Kaplan B, et al. Iron supplementation in pregnancy—does the preparation matter? *Arch Gynecol Obstet.* 2007; **276**:601–604.

5. Rimon E, Kagansky N, Kagansky M, et al. Are we giving too much iron? Low-dose iron therapy is effective in octogenarians. *Am J Med.* 2005; **118**:1142–1147.

6. Auerbach M, Ballard H. Clinical use of intravenous iron: administration, efficacy, and safety. *Hematol Am Soc Hematol Educ Program.* 2010; **2010**:338–347.

7. Chertow GM, Mason PD, Vaage-Nilsen O, et al. Update on adverse drug events associated with parenteral iron. *Nephrol Dial Transplant.* 2006; **21**:378–382.

8. Fernández-Bañares F, Monzón H, Forné M. A short review of malabsorption and anemia. *World J Gastroenterol.* 2009; **15**:4644–4652.

9. Gafter-Gvili A, Rozen-Zvi B, Vidal L. Intravenous iron supplementation for the treatment of chemotherapy-induced anaemia – systematic review and meta-analysis of randomised controlled trials. *Acta Oncol.* 2013; **52**:18–29.

10. Steensma DP, Sloan JA, Dakhil SR, et al. Phase III, randomized study of the effects of parenteral iron, oral iron, or no iron supplementation on the erythropoietic response to darbepoetin alfa for patients with chemotherapy-associated anemia. *J Clin Oncol.* 2011; **29**:97–105.

11. Henry DH, Dahl NV, Auerbach M, et al. Intravenous ferric gluconate significantly improves response to epoetin alfa versus oral iron or no iron in anemic patients with cancer receiving chemotherapy. *Oncologist.* 2007; **12**:231–242.

12. Albaramki J, Hodson EM, Craig JC, et al. Parenteral versus oral iron therapy for adults and children with chronic kidney disease. *Cochrane Database Syst Rev.* 2012; **1**:CD007857.

13. Macdougall IC, Padhi D, Jang G. Pharmacology of darbepoetin alfa. *Nephrol Dial Transplant.* 2007; **22 Suppl** 4:iv2–iv9.

14. Palmer SC, Navaneethan SD, Craig JC, et al. Meta-analysis: erythropoiesis-stimulating agents in patients with chronic kidney disease. *Ann Intern Med.* 2010; **153**:23–33.

15. Kansagara D, Dyer E, Englander H, et al. Treatment of anemia in patients with heart disease: a systematic review. *Ann Intern Med.* 2013; **159**:746–757.

16. Cody J, Daly C, Campbell M, et al. Recombinant human erythropoietin for chronic renal failure anaemia in pre-dialysis patients. *Cochrane Database Syst Rev.* 2005; **3**:CD003266.

17. Lau JH, Gangji AS, Rabbat CG, et al. Impact of haemoglobin and erythropoietin dose changes on mortality: a secondary analysis of results from a randomized anaemia management trial. *Nephrol Dial Transplant.* 2010; **25**:4002–4009.

18. Tonia T, Mettler A, Robert N, et al. Erythropoietin or darbepoetin for patients with cancer. *Cochrane Database Syst Rev.* 2012; **12**:CD003407.

19. Smith Jr. RE, Aapro MS, Ludwig H, et al. Darbepoetin alpha for the treatment of anemia in patients with active cancer not receiving chemotherapy or radiotherapy: results of a phase III, multicenter, randomized, double-blind, placebo-controlled study. *J Clin Oncol.* 2008; **26**:1040–1050.

20. National Comprehensive Cancer Network Clinical Practice Guidelines in Oncology: Cancer- and Chemotherapy-Induced Anemia (V.2.2014). Available at www.nccn.org/professionals/physician_gls/pdf/anemia.pdf (Accessed December 11, 2013).

21. Goodnough LT, Monk TG, Andriole GL. Erythropoietin therapy. *N Engl J Med.* 1997; **27**:933–938.

Splenectomy
Indications and Consequences

Sophia Fircanis Rizk, MD, Andrew Brunner, MD, and Fred J. Schiffman, MD, MACP

Introduction

For most causes of anemia, there are therapeutic modalities that will improve the patient's clinical status or even cure the underlying illness. However, there are some conditions in which the spleen is the primary cause or the site of red blood cell sequestration or destruction; in select instances, surgical removal of the spleen is warranted as treatment of the anemia.

Selected Hematologic Indications for Splenectomy

Hereditary Spherocytosis (HS)

Splenectomy for HS is frequently considered in patients with severe anemia or with symptomatic splenomegaly related to disease. It can also be considered in patients to help reverse growth failure or skeletal changes related to extramedullary hematopoiesis. Removal of the spleen stops the hemolysis associated with HS and in fact was historically considered a first-line treatment for the disease. More recently, data suggest that although splenectomy does help arrest the hemolytic process, it is also associated with a higher incidence of delayed adverse vascular events,[1,2] including venous thromboembolic events and pulmonary hypertension.[3,4]

Particularly among children with HS, there may be a role for partial rather than total splenectomy. Several series report that both total and partial splenectomy are effective in halting hemolysis; although slightly less effective, partial splenectomy results in sustained, improved hemoglobin levels.[5] These patients also retain splenic immune function.[6] Durable hematologic responses have been reported with partial splenectomy; in one case series, less than 5% of children subsequently required total splenectomy for recurrent anemia or abdominal pain.[5]

Autoimmune Hemolytic Anemia

Splenectomy has been utilized as a second-line treatment for patients who have limited or no response to treatment of autoimmune hemolytic anemia (AIHA) with continuous corticosteroids or other immune-modulating medications.[7] Splenectomy has been employed in patients with ITP and Coombs' positive AIHA, as well as more rare conditions such as Evans' syndrome.[8] The spleen is not only the major site of destruction for antibody- or complement-coated erythrocytes, but it also plays a role in antibody synthesis.

There are not well-defined criteria for moving to second-line therapy in AIHA; proposed criteria include patients who have not responded to continuous corticosteroid therapy, those who have had multiple relapses, or those who require persistent dosing of prednisone above 15 mg/day. When second-line therapy is being considered, it is critical to confirm the diagnosis of AIHA. Documented cases of corticosteroid nonresponders have later been shown to have hemolytic anemia, related to occult malignancy or other causes, where splenectomy would not be beneficial or could even harm the patient.[9]

Approximately 50% of patients who undergo splenectomy for AIHA have an initial beneficial response; however, it is not uncommon to have a postsplenectomy relapse, and the overall cure rate from splenectomy may be closer to 20%.[7] Nonetheless, 40–80% of patients will experience either a partial or complete remission postsplenectomy.[10] A significant challenge is patient selection, since there is no standardized or predictable response to splenectomy for AIHA. Ideally, splenectomy would be reserved for those patients most likely to respond.

Thalassemias

Patients with beta thalassemia have also been noted to have progressive overactivity of the spleen, which is thought to relate to chronic hemolysis.[11] This leads to splenomegaly (work hypertrophy) and hypersplenism in some patients with severe disease, particularly beta thalassemia major.

Splenectomy may be indicated in patients with thalassemia major, as well as some patients with thalassemia intermedia, particularly among younger patients, in order to avoid growth retardation, reduce cytopenias, and decrease the degree of extramedullary hematopoiesis, which itself can cause hypersplenism. Splenectomy improves hemoglobin levels and similarly reduces the need for transfusion, which may protect patients from the complications of iron overload. One strategy for consideration of splenectomy is based upon annual transfusion requirements. When transfusion exceeds approximately 1 unit of packed red blood cells per kilogram body weight per year, there may be benefit to considering splenectomy as a way of decreasing transfusion requirements in order to limit iron overload.[12] A long-term retrospective study assessing the effects of splenectomy on iron balance in patients with thalassemia demonstrated that transfusion dependence was decreased in splenectomized patients; however, markers of iron overload, such as serum ferritin, decreased much more slowly. It is still unclear how splenectomy affects systemic iron balance, and there may be a role for MRI imaging to further assess end-organ iron deposition.[13] Moreover, a recent analysis found that patients treated with splenectomy appear to have higher complication rates, including rates of thrombosis, pulmonary hypertension, and heart failure, compared to those who did not, underscoring the importance of balancing the risks of splenectomy with its potential benefits;[14] this is particularly relevant since the advent of new iron chelation therapies may decrease the morbidity and mortality of continued transfusion.

Felty Syndrome (FS)

Felty syndrome is the triad of rheumatoid arthritis (RA), neutropenia, and splenomegaly. Although anemia is not necessarily a part of the diagnosis, it is not uncommon to see anemia among patients with Felty syndrome. Anemia may relate to chronic inflammation, similar to other patients with RA, or may be present as a hemolytic anemia related to the underlying autoimmune process.

Splenectomy may be considered in patients with FS who have persistent neutropenia and associated recurrent infections. Neutropenia may improve in approximately 80% of patients undergoing splenectomy.[15] Splenic embolization may also be an effective therapy.

A condition that may mimic or be coexistent with Felty syndrome is large granular lymphocyte leukemia (LGL leukemia). LGL leukemia is also commonly associated with RA and may result in cytopenias and splenomegaly due to infiltration of the red pulp cords and sinusoids with lymphoid cells. Specifically in LGL leukemia there is a clonal expansion of lymphoid cells. However, in clinical practice, this distinction between FS and LGL is not always clear, and in fact the diseases may be more closely related than previously suspected. Splenectomy for LGL leukemia appears less successful in improving cytopenias or symptomatic splenomegaly compared to Felty syndrome and may even worsen disease.[16] The role of splenectomy in Felty syndrome may also be reconsidered as newer immunosuppressive agents and disease-modifying antirheumatic drugs play an increasing role in the treatment of a variety of rheumatic diseases.

Myelofibrosis

Splenomegaly is present in nearly all patients with myelofibrosis (MF) and can be severe, often resulting in symptoms related to the size of the spleen itself. Abdominal discomfort and recurrent splenic infarction are the most common

indications for splenectomy, but patients with persistent thrombocytopenia or portal hypertension related to splenomegaly, or high transfusion requirements, may also be considered for surgery. In a review of 316 patients who underwent splenectomy for one of these indications at a single institution, 76% received palliative benefit.[17] However, this benefit lasted for a median of 12 months (1- to 96-month range), and complications of splenectomy were more common in patients with presplenectomy thrombocytopenia related to their disease. Postsplenectomy thrombocytosis was seen in approximately 30% of patients and was associated with higher perisplenectomy complications. Survival was not affected by splenectomy, and indications were typically palliative in nature. Other therapies for splenomegaly in myelofibrosis, including hydroxyurea, palliative radiation, and more recently JAK2 inhibitors, also have a place in the treatment algorithm.[18]

Approach to Splenectomy

Historically, open splenectomy has been performed for removal of the spleen and is usually done via a midline or subcostal incision. Due to the vascular nature of the organ, hemorrhage is a frequent complication associated with surgery. Recently, laparoscopic splenectomy has become more commonly used;[19] this may have the benefit of decreasing surgical trauma. Complications are associated with both of these techniques.

Complications of Splenectomy

In general, splenectomy is a well-tolerated surgery. Compared to open splenectomy, laparoscopic splenectomy may have a lower rate of complications overall, although portal vein thrombosis is a concern that should be considered,[20,21] particularly among patients with underlying myeloproliferative neoplasms. One meta-analysis of laparoscopic splenectomy, encompassing 51 published series and containing a total of 2,940 patients, showed that laparoscopic splenectomy was associated with significantly shorter hospital stays compared to open splenectomy.[22] Laparoscopic splenectomy was associated with significantly fewer pulmonary, wound, and infectious complications but had an increase in hemorrhagic complications and thrombotic complications such as splenic and portal vein thrombosis.

Some common surgical complications of splenectomy include pulmonary embolism (PE), deep venous thrombosis, myocardial infarction, and infection.[22] These are not seen at any higher rate than with other intermediate-risk abdominal surgeries.[23] One retrospective review identified 60 patients who underwent splenectomy as treatment for immune thrombocytopenic purpura (ITP) or AIHA over a 15-year period at a single institution and reported that the most common short-term complications were PE, urinary tract infection, and pneumonia. There were no splenectomy-related deaths within the first 30 days.[24]

A concern in splenectomy is the risk of perioperative bleeding; although laparoscopic approaches minimize surgical trauma, they have also been associated with an increase in hemorrhagic complications.[20] Due to the vascular nature of the spleen, as well as technical concerns related to preoperative magnitude of splenomegaly, laceration of the spleen and parenchymal damage remain concerns. In addition, proper isolation and visualization of the splenic vascular supply is critical and may be technically more difficult with laparoscopic splenectomy. Medical correction of any coexisting coagulopathy may help minimize bleeding risk. Preoperative splenic artery embolization may be considered to help minimize bleeding risks but is not routinely performed.[25]

The most common long-term complications of splenectomy are not related to the surgery itself but rather relate to the loss of the spleen. A cohort study of the U.S. veteran population evaluated the long-term medical effects of splenectomy. This study included 8,149 patients, all of whom underwent splenectomy for various indications, including trauma and splenic injury. After trauma, hematologic disorders were the most common reason for splenectomy. This cohort was followed for at least 27 years, and the rates of postsplenectomy complications were measured.[26] The rate of infections including pneumonia (RR 2.06), meningitis (RR 2.44), and septicemia (RR 3.38) were higher in asplenic patients. These patients were also more likely to die as a result of their infection compared to patients with spleens. The risk of infection appears to be highest immediately following splenectomy,[27] but infectious complications persist, even after 10 years following spleen removal.[26]

Patients who underwent splenectomy also had higher incidences of cancers, both solid tumor (esophageal, liver, colon, pancreas, lung) and hematologic conditions such as non-Hodgkin's lymphoma, Hodgkin's lymphoma, chronic myelocytic leukemia, and other leukemias. Although interpretations of this finding are limited by the retrospective nature of this analysis, the authors propose that the spleen's role in immune function may facilitate cancer immune surveillance, and therefore splenectomy may potentially increase the risk of malignancy via the loss of this immune surveillance mechanism.[26]

Postoperative thrombosis of the splenic and/or portal vein is not uncommon in patients undergoing splenectomy. Splenic vein thrombosis is more frequently seen compared to portal vein thrombosis, occurring in up to between 2 and 20% of patients[25,28–29] and is felt to be slightly more common in patients undergoing laparoscopic splenectomy due to the technical approach of the laparoscopic process itself. Some evidence suggests that insufflation of the abdomen and prolonged Trendelenberg positioning may increase the risk of thrombosis.[30] Other data suggest that the incidence of splenic vein thrombosis relates to the preoperative splenic vein diameter, and thrombosis is higher in those with splenic vein diameter greater than 8 mm.[31] Although thrombosis may relate to the surgical procedure, other potential causes should be considered, including hematologic conditions that may relate to the splenomegaly and indication for splenectomy. This includes conditions such as essential thrombocytosis or paroxysmal nocturnal hemoglobinuria,[33] as well as other non-hematologic conditions such as chronic pancreatitis.

Splenic vein thrombosis, which may be asymptomatic, may be associated with vague abdominal discomfort or, in severe cases, may be associated with ascites. Routine screening for splenic vein thrombosis is not typically performed; however, in one study of 40 patients screened for the presence of thrombus, 52.5% of patients were found to have either splenic or portal vein thrombus postoperatively. Although many of these events are asymptomatic, progression of the thrombus could cause concern for compromise of the mesenteric circulation.[31,32] Treatment with anticoagulation is effective in resolving the clot;[23] the use of perioperative, systemic anticoagulation in high-risk patients as a preventative measure remains under investigation.[29]

Another complication following splenectomy is thromboembolism. There is an increased risk of DVT and PE in patients after splenectomy.[26] In addition, there is an increased risk of developing pulmonary arterial hypertension, which may relate to chronic thromboembolism.[3,4] Other associations with thrombotic risk may be disease specific; for instance, adults with HS may have relative protection against thrombosis prior to splenectomy, as well as an increased risk of atherothrombosis following splenectomy, possibly related to altered lipid profiles.[35]

Postsplenectomy Care
Fever and Antibiotics

Fever in the postsplenectomy patient should always be taken seriously, especially in patients with other risk factors for significant infection, including older age, immune compromise, and comorbid conditions. Postsplenectomy sepsis is a life-threatening condition and requires prompt identification and treatment. Previously, daily prophylaxis with penicillins was the standard of care; however, this practice is currently not routinely advised for patients due to concern for antibiotic resistance and patient compliance.[36]

Any fever in an asplenic patient should prompt immediate medical evaluation. In addition, current guidelines recommend initiating treatment of any febrile illness empirically at home, as soon as possible. Although no prospective trials have been performed to evaluate the efficacy of this method, current expert opinion states the use of any of the following regimens immediately upon fever development is appropriate until additional medical care can be provided:[37,38]

- Amoxicillin-clavulanate 875 mg / 125 mg twice daily
- Cefuroxime 500 mg twice daily
- Levofloxacin 750 mg daily or moxifloxacin 400 mg daily or gemfloxacin 320 mg daily

After taking the antibiotics, patients should report to the emergency room for further evaluation.[37]

Since antibiotic and vaccination recommendations change periodically, up to date information should always be sought from the Centers for Disease Control or other authoritative agencies. Also, recommendations for adults and children may be different.

Vaccinations

The spleen is an essential component of the immune system. It is a major site of synthesis of IgM antibodies and plays a critical role in the clearance of opsonized-encapsulated bacteria. This is underscored by the post splenectomy increased risk of infection with encapsulated bacterial organisms, commonly resulting in pneumonia and meningitis.[26] It is therefore critical to provide immunization against infections from *S. pneumoniae*, *N. meningitides*, and *H. influenzae* type b. This can largely be accomplished via appropriate and timely vaccination.

Vaccination should be considered in the presplenectomy period for elective procedures in order to optimize antibody response. If this is not possible due to urgent or emergent surgical indications, then approximately 2 weeks should elapse postsplenectomy so that vaccination results in the best immune response possible, since there is relative immune suppression in the immediate perioperative period.[38]

Appropriate vaccinations include:

- Pneumococcal vaccines (13-valent followed by 23-valent vaccine recommended in adults, spaced apart by 8 weeks, with reimmunization every 5 years).[39]

- *Haemophilus influenzae b* vaccine – single dose after splenectomy, particularly if not previously vaccinated

- Meningococcal vaccine – two doses given 8 weeks apart, repeated every 5 years. The meningococcal quadrivalent conjugate vaccine is recommended for individuals between 2 and 55 years.[40]

- Influenza vaccine – while asplenic patients are not at higher risk for influenza itself, being infected with influenza puts patients at higher risk for secondary infection with encapsulated organisms, and so routine influenza vaccination is recommended,[39,40]

There is no known contraindication to live, attenuated vaccine administration in asplenic individuals.

Summary

In summary, splenectomy is indicated for selected patients with anemia in whom more conservative treatments have failed. Techniques and consequences of splenectomy should be well understood by caregivers managing patients who are being considered for or who have undergone splenectomy.

References

1. Schilling RF. Risks and benefits of splenectomy versus no splenectomy for hereditary spherocytosis – a personal view. *Br J Hematol.* 2009; 145:728–732.

2. Schilling RF, Gangnon RE, Traver MI. Delayed adverse vascular events after splenectomy in hereditary spherocytosis. *J Thromb Haemost.* 2008; 6:1289–1295.

3. Jaïs X, Ioos V, Jardim C, et al. Splenectomy and chronic thromboembolic pulmonary hypertension. *Thorax.* 2005; 60:1031–1034.

4. Hoeper MM, Neidermeyer J, Hoffmeyer F, et al. Pulmonary hypertension after splenectomy? *Ann Intern Med.* 1999; 130:506–509.

5. Buesing KL et al. Partial splenectomy for hereditary spherocytosis: a multi-institutional review. *J Pediatric Surg.* 2011;46(1):178–183.

6. Seims AD et al. Partial versus total splenectomy in children with hereditary spherocytosis. *Surgery.* 2013; 154 (4):849–855.

7. Lechner K, Jager U. How I treat autoimmune hemolytic anemias in adults. *Blood.* 2010; 116(11):1831–1838.

8. Li Y et al. Splenectomy in the management of Evans syndrome in adult: Long-term follow-up of 32 patients. *Surgical Practice.* 2014; 18 (1):15–22.

9. Jaime-Perez JC, Rodriguez-Martiniez M, Gomez-de-Leon A, Tarin-Arzaga L, Gomez-Almaguer D. Current approaches for the treatment of autoimmune hemolytic anemia. *Arch Immunol Ther Exp.* 2013; 61:385–395.

10. Akpek G, McAneny D, Weintraub L. Comparative response to splenectomy in Coombs-positive autoimmune hemolytic anemia with or without associated disease. *Am J Hematol.* 1999; 61:98–102.

11. Rachmilewitz E, Giardina P. How I treat thalassemia. *Blood.* 2011; 118:3479–3488.

12. Graziano JH, Piomelli S, Hilgartner M, et al. Chelation therapy in beta thalassemia major: the role of splenectomy in achieving iron balance. *J Pediatriacs.* 1981; 99(5):695–699.

13. Casale M, Cinque P, Ricchi P, Constantini S, Spasiano A, Prossomariti L, Minelli S, Frega V, Filosa A. Effect of splenectomy on iron balance in patients with B-thalassemia major: a long term follow-up. *Eur Hematol.* 2013; 91(69–73):__.

14. Taher AT, Mussallam KM, Karimi M, et al. Overview on practices in thalassemia intermedia management aiming for lowering complication rates across a region of endemicity: the OPTIMAL CARE study. *Blood.* 2010; 115(10):1886–1892.

15. Rashba, EJ, Rowe, JM, Packman, CH. Treatment of the neutropenia of Felty Syndrome. *Blood Rev.* 1996; 10:177–184.

16. Lamy T, Loughran T. How I treat LGL leukemia. *Blood.* 2011; 117:2764–2774.

17. Mesa RA, Nagorney DS, Schwager S, Allred J, Tefferi A. Palliative goals, patient selection, and perioperative platelet management; outcomes and lessons from 3 decades of splenectomy for myelofibrosis with myeloid metaplasia at the Mayo Clinic. *Cancer.* 2006; 107(2):361–370.

18. Cervantes F. How I treat splenomegaly in myelofibrosis. *Blood Cancer J.* 2011; 1 (10):e37.

19. Bell RL et al. A ten-year, single institution experience with laparoscopic splenectomy. *JSLS.* 2005 Apr–Jun; 9 (2):163–168.

20. Harris W, Marcaccio M. Incidence of portal vein thrombosis after laparoscopic splenectomy. *Can J Surg.* 2005 Oct; 48(5):352–354.

21. Krauth MT et al. The postoperative splenic/portal vein thrombosis after splenectomy and its prevention–an unresolved issue. *Haematologica.* 2008; 93(8):1227–1232.

22. Winslow ER, Brunt LM. Perioperative outcomes of laparoscopic versus open splenectomy: A meta-analysis with an emphasis on complications. *Surgery.* 2003; 134(4):647–653.

23. Dindo D et al. Classification of surgical complications: a new proposal with evaluation in a cohort of 6336 patients and results of a survey. *Ann Surg.* 2004 August; 240(2):205–213.

24. Patel NY et al. Outcomes and complications after splenectomy for hematologic disorders. *Am J Surg.* 2012; 204(6):1014–1020.

25. Bhandharkar DS, Katara AN, Mittal, G, Shah, R, Udwadia, TE. Prevention and management of complications of laparoscopic splenectomy. *Ind J Surg.* 2011;73(5):324–330.

26. Kristenssen SY et al. Long-term risks after splenectomy among 8,149 cancer-free U.S. veterans: a cohort study with up to 27 years follow-up. *Haematologica.* 2014;99:392–398.

27. Thomsen R, Schoonen M, Farkas DK, Rils A, Jacobsen J, Fryzek J, Sorensen HT. Risk of hospital contact with infection in patients with splenectomy: a population based cohort study. *Ann Intern Med.* 2009; 151(8):546–556.

28. Svensson M, Wiren M, Kimby E, Hagglund H. Portal vein thrombosis is a common complication following splenectomy in patients with malignant haematological disease. *Eur J Haematol.* 2006; 77(3):203–209.

29. Vecchio R, Cacciola E, Cacciola RR, Marchese S, Intagliata E. Portal vein thrombosis after laparoscopic and open splenectomy. *J Laparoendosc Advanc Surg Techniq.* 2011; 21(1):71–75.

30. James AW, Rabl C, Westphalen A, Fogarty P, Posselt A, Campos G. Portomesenteric venous thrombosis after laparoscopic surgery; a systematic literature review. *JAMA Surg.* 2009; 144 (6):520–526.

31. Danno K et al. Splanchnic vein thrombosis: new risk factors and management. *Surgery.* 2009; 145 (5):457–464.

32. Crary SE, Buchanan GR. Vascular complications after splenectomy for hematologic disorders. *Blood.* 2009; 114 (14):2861–2868.

33. Donadini MP et al. Splanchnic vein thrombosis: new risk factors and management. *Thromb Res.* 2012; 129 (1):S93–S96.

34. Hayag-Barin JE, Smith R, Tucker FC, Jr. Hereditary spherocytosis, thrombocytosis, and chronic pulmonary emboli: a case report and review of the literature. *Am J Hematol.* 1998; 57:82–84.

35. Troendle SB, Adix L, Crary SE, et al. Laboratory markers of thrombosis risk in children with hereditary spherocytosis. *Pediatr Blood Cancer.* 2007; 49:781–785.

36. Keenan RD, Boswell T, Milligan DW. Do post-splenectomy patients take prophylactic penicillin? *Br J Haematol.* 1999; 105:509–510.

37. Grohskopf LA, Sokolow LZ, Broder KR, et al. Prevention and control of seasonal influenza with vaccines: recommendations of the Advisory Committee on Immunization Practices – United States, 2017–18 Influenza Season. *MMWR Recomm Rep.* 2017;66(No. RR-2):1–20. DOI: 10.15585/mmwr.rr6602a1

38. Rubin LG, Schaffner W. Care of the asplenic patient. *N Engl J Med.* 2014; 371:349–356.

39. Centers for Disease Control and Prevention. Use of the 13-valent pneumococcal conjugate vaccine and the 23-valent pneumococcal polysaccharide vaccine for adults with immunocompromising conditions: recommendations of the Advisory Committee on Immunization Practices (ACIP). *MMWR Morb Mortality Weekly Report.* 2012:61(40):816.

40. Cohn AC, MacNeil JR, Clark TA, Ortega-Sanchez IR, Briere EZ, Meissner HC, Baker CJ, Messonnier NE. Prevention and control of the meningococcal disease: recommendations of the Advisory Committee on Immunization Practices (ACIP). *MMWR Recomm Rep.* 2013:62(RR-2):1.

Anemias
Summary, Conclusions, and Future Prospects

Edward J. Benz, Jr., MD

Anemias arise from many etiologies that impair the production of erythrocytes, reduce their longevity in the circulation, or both. Fortunately, these diverse etiologies converge on a few final common pathways that disrupt red cell homeostasis. These pathways can be readily detected by careful evaluation of the patient and her or his basic hematologic parameters. As outlined in the preceding chapters, characterization of these abnormalities permits one to develop a rational approach to identifying the underlying etiology. In about 70–80% of patients, these basic stratagems will provide a sufficiently precise diagnosis to guide the best available clinical management. While many more elaborate tools are available to measure a variety of characteristics of the red cell and its progenitors in the bone marrow, these invariably provide only confirmatory information or refinements of the basic diagnosis. Absent the first basic steps advocated in this text, efforts to deal with anemia in the individual patient will inevitably result in overtesting and frustration at one's failure to pinpoint the processes driving anemia in that patient. It is our hope that this book has provided the reader with a straightforward approach to the initial evaluation of anemia and guidance on when to escalate the work-up in a focused and rational way that avoids excessive and unnecessary testing.

As outlined in the volume, some anemias arise from primary abnormalities in bone marrow function, in the structure and function of hemoglobin, in essential enzymes required for heme synthesis or red cell metabolism, or in the components needed for stability of the red cell membrane. However, in a substantial majority of patients with anemia, the underlying etiology is lodged in extrinsic factors such as infections, drug toxicities, or allergies or reflects disruption of the function of other organ systems such as is encountered in chronic renal failure, protein-calorie malnutrition, or chronic gastrointestinal or genitourinary blood loss. The best clinical approach to the diagnosis and treatment of anemias, therefore, must be thoroughly and well grounded in an excellent understanding and mastery of general medicine, the performance of a thorough multisystem history and physical examination, and the judicious use of the clinical laboratory and imaging facility to pursue disease states that could lead to anemia as a secondary complication. By employing this approach, it should be possible to reach an accurate diagnosis of the nature of the anemia

and its underlying causes most of the time. Well-informed decisions about therapy and clinical management of the patient's overall condition can then follow.

There is almost certainly no other cell type that has been more thoroughly investigated and understood at the molecular and cellular level than the red cell and its progenitors. Similarly, no protein or its encoding gene, genomic and epigenomic structure, and structure function relationships is better understood than hemoglobin, the major component of the red cell. Yet it is not possible to characterize anemia precisely in as many as 20–30% of patients, even in the most sophisticated centers. Despite exquisitely precise understanding of the underlying molecular and cellular pathophysiology of many red cell disorders, definitive treatments targeting correction of those basic abnormalities remains elusive for all too many patients. Thus, for example, the precise molecular defect responsible for sickle-cell anemia was delineated in the late 1940s, yet hydroxyurea remains the only therapy targeting the homeostasis of hemoglobins in a sickle cell patient that has provided meaningful therapeutic efficacy. Even in this case, the therapy does not achieve correction of the underlying molecular abnormality. Rather, it causes a shift in hemoglobin gene expression that partially reduces the production of sickle hemoglobin in favor of fetal hemoglobin. Similarly, despite extraordinarily detailed knowledge about the molecular and cellular dynamics leading pluripotent stem cells to commit to and execute the process of erythropoiesis, we are all too often unable to utilize this information to correct the disrupted dynamics leading to hypoproliferative anemias. The "diagnosis" of two increasingly common forms of anemia, the anemia of aging and the anemia of chronic inflammation, are in fact only descriptions of common features of anemias occurring in a particular setting. They are likely to be a heterogeneous collection of marrow and red cell abnormalities occurring in response to inflammation and the aging process. The seemingly idiosyncratic response or nonresponse of these patients to therapeutic efforts probably reflects the heterogeneity of mechanisms underlying the anemia. In this regard, research in the field of anemia serves as a cautionary paradigm for those believing that molecular and cellular insights into a cell or tissue or physiologic phenomenon lead in a straightforward or predictable way to definitive cures.

The care of patients with anemia has benefitted from the judicious application of progress in general medical care. As a result, we have achieved an increased survival and improved quality of life for many patients afflicted with disorders like sickle cell anemia, inherited enzyme and membrane disorders, and bone marrow failure syndromes despite the absence of definitive therapies addressing the underlying etiology. Thus, development of iron chelating agents, better blood typing and cross-matching techniques, and screening for blood-borne pathogens has made chronic red cell transfusion support compatible with longer survival and reduced morbidity in patients requiring lifelong chronic transfusion support. Supportive care has aided patients with myelodysplasia. These facts once again emphasize that one can be a good hematologist only by being a good general physician. Every approach to the anemic patient must be embedded in a solid grounding across the broader areas of general medicine and nursing care.

Anemias are among the most common afflictions in the world, causing morbidity and mortality for millions of people in all areas of the globe. While some of these may arise from primary hematologic etiologies such as hemoglobinopathies in the "malaria belt," the vast majority of patients for whom anemia is a significant clinical issue develop anemia as a consequence of other conditions, often infectious, that derange red cell homeostasis. Examples include the hemolysis of malaria and other bacterial or parasitic infections, iron deficiency and/or folate deficiency resulting from helminthic infections or starvation, or bone marrow suppression due to exposure to toxins. Even in the developed world, anemias become a frequent and inevitable accompaniment to the process of aging or of other chronic diseases increasingly common in economically advanced societies. Prime examples include the anemia of chronic inflammation, the anemia of the aged, and myelodysplasia. High-technology approaches leading to novel therapeutics would help important subsets of these patients. However, for the foreseeable future, these are likely to be expensive, confined to major medical centers, and applicable to relatively small groups of patients. The overwhelming need is for better access to basic medical services and appropriately prepared medical personnel. Much morbidity and mortality could be averted simply by treatment or prevention of the relevant infections and better utilization of extremely inexpensive and relatively nontoxic (when used appropriately) therapeutics such as folic acid, vitamin B12, iron, and blood transfusion services.

Decades of research focused on the pathobiology of the red cell and anemias has benefited broader fields of biomedicine, because the regulated production of red cells, the mechanisms contributing to prolonged red cell survival in the circulation, and the tightly controlled processes by which aged red cells are removed are more amenable to detailed analysis than many other systems. Many advanced tools of medical science and technology have their origins in the study of red blood cells. Application of these tools to human physiology and illness has offered critical insights into other conditions that have led to improved methods for early detection, management, and life-changing therapies. Examples include the application of erythropoietin for the management of chronic renal failure, the discovery of hemoglobin A1C, and recognition of its utility for improved longitudinal monitoring of blood glucose control in diabetes. These two advances alone have facilitated the development of better strategies and therapeutics for chronic disease control. Similarly, the founding of the science of transfusion medicine and then of stem-cell transplantation had its origins in the field of red cell transfusion support. One can argue that clinical immunology arose in large measure from the study of red cell antigens that in turn arose from the need to identify safe donor–recipient pairs for transfusion. Continued progress in the entire field of biomedicine thus needs a robust community of investigators who continue to focus on this paradigm-setting cell. Fortunately, after two to three decades of declining interest in red cell research, enthusiasm for the study of the erythron and engagement by talented investigators appears to be on the rise again.

Future Considerations

At the present time, most patients with anemia can be offered a reasonably accurate diagnosis and either definitive therapy or sufficient supportive care to mitigate the impact of the anemia on their lives. For all too many, however, anemia continues to be the major factor interfering with quality of life or reducing survival. It is thus appropriate for us to conclude this book with a few thoughts about the future prospects for better control of anemia as a worldwide health issue:

First, recent research is making it increasingly clear that the erythrocyte is a far more complicated cell than had been previously appreciated. Red cells, while much simpler in composition than most cells, do not simply float in the circulation for the sole purpose of procuring and delivering oxygen and buffering blood pH via CO_2 exchange. Rather, red cells are far more interactive with the vasculature and other blood cells than previously thought. For example, red cells serve as major reservoirs and governors of the supply of critical nitrate- or nitrite-containing compounds that influence vascular tone and hemodynamics. The utilization of this information for clinical purposes has yet to be realized, but several attempts are underway.

Similarly, red cells play a more important role in hemostasis, thrombosis, and inflammation than previously appreciated. Conversely, the interactions among red cells, the vascular wall, and a multiplicity of cytokines, chemokines, procoagulant and anticoagulant molecules, and the surfaces on which they reside are proving to be important factors in driving previously underappreciated aspects of the pathophysiology of major hematologic conditions like sickle cell anemia, hemolytic-uremic syndrome, and others. Red cells also support somewhat limited but important signal transduction functions, and these govern some of the interactions among red cells, platelets, leukocytes, and the vascular wall which influence basic hemostatic, inflammatory, hemodynamic, and immune activities. Following from these discoveries is the identification of many potential targets for potential diagnostic and therapeutic application. The importance of these processes for conditions such as sickle cell crisis, TTP, and DIC is currently under intense investigation. Clinical trials for the use of agents such as selectin inhibitors to interdict these complex interactions are underway.

The relevance of red cells to immunity and inflammatory process is also becoming evident as increasingly potent agents are being introduced into clinical trials and clinical practice, especially in oncology. One example includes the potential toxicity of agents that enhance monocytes/macrophage uptake of tumor cells bearing neo-antigens in patients with cancer. These can provoke profound hemolytic anemia by blocking previously underrecognized signals on the red cell (in this case, CD47), that inform the reticuloendothelial system not to phagocytose nonaged red cells.

Taken together, these recent insights suggest that red cells can impact a wide array of physiologic functions well beyond their classical role as transporters of oxygen and modulators of blood pH. Even quantitatively minute biochemical phenomena occurring within an individual red cell can exert substantial impact when multiplied by the trillions of cells circulating in intimate contact with the vasculature, platelets, leukocytes, and plasma proteins. As technology allows increasingly more sensitive measurements of biochemical phenomena in individual cells, it can be anticipated that additional features of erythrocyte behavior will be uncovered and that at least some of these will influence physiology and pathophysiology because of the sheer bulk of circulating red cells. Identification of these mechanisms should lead to a more sophisticated and precise understanding of the pathophysiology of anemias and the impact of the erythron on numerous physiological and pathological processes. These insight should in turn generate therapeutic targets for better management of anemia.

As of this writing, our understanding of the physiologic consequences of anemia is almost completely bounded by the notion that anemia causes inadequate oxygen delivery to tissues. The progress just summarized suggests that other functions served by the normal circulating red cell mass may also aggravate the symptomatology of anemia. This may be especially true for lifelong chronic anemia and could also complicate the morbidity of conditions associated with anemia. For example, anemia has been identified as a negative prognostic feature of cancer and HIV/AIDS, but the mechanism is not known.

Second, recent progress in the areas of cell, tissue, and genetic engineering should influence our approach to the clinical management of major red cell disorders. It is ironic that these approaches have not yet yielded more substantive therapeutic applications to life-threatening anemias even though red cells and hemoglobin have invariably been at the forefront of discovery bioscience. Indeed, study of globin genes and the molecular pathology of hemoglobinopathies literally opened the door to the incursion of molecular biology and 'omics into medical science and medical practice. Yet applications of these technologies to achieve beneficial clinical outcomes has perhaps been more extensive and profound in other areas than it has in the management of red cell diseases like congenital hypoplastic anemias and hemoglobinopathies. This is due at least in part to the fact that many of the features that made red cell pathobiology so suitable and attractive for application of the early primitive techniques of molecular genetics five decades ago also render the therapeutic manipulation of red cell homeostasis among the most difficult challenges for the practical use of genetic engineering strategies in the treatment of life-threatening anemias.

Red cell differentiation occurs in a very tightly regulated limited time frame of 2–3 weeks, during which a small subset of genes such as the globin genes and the genes for the red cell membrane cytoskeleton are expressed at high rates; in the case of globin genes, expression is induced at almost the most extraordinarily high rate encountered in nature. Many of these genes are expressed in no other cell type and at no other time. The mature red cell, the product of this process, thus contains large amounts of highly purified proteins that were readily isolated and characterized. Moreover, the reticulocyte, readily accessible in the circulation, contains polyribosomes on which the resident messenger RNA is comprised of more than 90% globin and a few other mRNAs coding for these specialized proteins. Even before gene cloning was available, it was possible to isolate these and to gain insight into the molecular mechanisms governing these diseases at the level of their immediate genes and gene products. Thus, the globin genes were the first human genes to be isolated and characterized by recombinant DNA technology and the first to be expressed in heterologous host cells by gene transfer techniques that are the forbearer of today's efforts in gene therapy. Hemoglobinopathies were the first human disorders to be understood at the fundamental level of their DNA sequence mutations. Unfortunately, these very same parameters make the application of gene transfer and gene engineering daunting in practical terms. Any gene therapy strategy for hemoglobinopathies, for example, must be able to promote extremely high levels of gene expression in a very tightly and precisely controlled manner in only one cell type for only a very limited period of time. Experimentally and clinically, these are very hard goals to achieve. Indeed, they have been achieved only within the last 10–15 years in animal models.

Recent advances in gene transfer technology are providing viral vectors that provide safer and more precise platforms by which one can insert the desired gene(s) and surrounding regulatory elements into the genomes of appropriate stem cells from the patient. These can then be reintroduced by autologous bone marrow transplantation. Advances in the purification and characterization of hematopoietic stem cells is in turn providing safer and more robust hosts for the transferred genes. Among the most advanced examples of gene therapy for anemias are multiple studies in which engineering of globin gene constructs has achieved tightly regulated yet highly abundant production of the desired globin chains. Early-phase human trials for sickle cell anemia and thalassemia are in progress, with some preliminary promising results.

Equally exciting is the development of CRISPR technology, which allows, in principle, precise "editing" of genes bearing deleterious mutations, potentially at the level of single nucleotide corrections. While many formidable technical challenges remain to be addressed, technological progress is rapid, and many investigators and biotechnology firms are engaged in this expanding area of applied research. It is reasonable to anticipate that clinical trials utilizing this technology for the treatment of disorders of hemoglobin, red cell metabolic enzymes, membrane cytoskeletal components, and growth factor receptors will be underway within the next few years.

Third, the field of stem cell and bone marrow transplantation continues to make steady progress. Many of the red cell disorders described in this text can be, and in several cases have been, treated effectively by this modality. Replacement of the patient's own hematopoietic stem cells with those from a healthy donor should clearly be curative when the anemia is due to intrinsic defects of the red cell or its progenitors. The most common indications include hemoglobinopathies, bone marrow failure syndrome such as aplastic anemia and paroxysmal nocturnal hemoglobinuria, Fanconi anemia, Diamond Blackfan syndrome, and so forth. In addition, occasional patients with severe autoimmune hemolytic anemias refractory to immunomodulating therapies have also benefitted from replacement of their erythroid cells by those of a donor not expressing the antigen(s) targeted by the disease. The widespread utilization of stem cell transplantation in these settings is, of course, severely limited by the well-known short- and long-term consequences attendant to this modality. For patients destined to survive for a decade or more with a chronic anemia, it is often difficult to justify exposure to the toxicities of regimens used to ablate or create transplantable niches in the marrow, the risks of significant immunosuppression, and graft-versus-host disease. Moreover, the pool of well-matched related or unrelated donors remains a severely limiting factor. This is especially true among some underserved minority populations in whom the relevant disorders are especially common.

Fortunately, progress is being made in all these areas. We can anticipate that the management of complications and the expansion of the donor pool will make this approach feasible for larger percentages of patients with relevant disorders. The base of suitable donors is being expanded by using a variety of techniques to prevent or mitigate graft-versus-host disease from donors who are unrelated and/or carry one or more mismatched tissue compatibility antigens. These advances should also make the procedure more tolerable for broader groups of patients who could be treated under the present donor–recipient matching algorithms. The widespread use of electronic media to raise awareness of the critical need for donors, the safety and low invasiveness of circulating stem cell donations, and the beneficial impact on recipients should, strategically used, increase both the breadth and depth of the donor pool. Given the increasing ethnic heterogeneity of societies that have the capacity to provide stem cell transplantation, globalization of registries will be necessary. Finally, as described in more detail in what follows, the same techniques that are advancing the fields of gene therapy, stem cell medicine, and clinical immunology are raising the promise of creating "manufactured" universal donor or immunologically customized stem cells. These could presumably be safe for any recipient and allow for transplantation without the need for extreme immune suppression or the consequent specter of graft-versus-host disease (GVHD).

Management and support of patients during the vulnerable periods of the acute transplant episode is also improving. The recent introduction of agents that reduce the risks of posttransplant vaso-occlusive disease is but one example. Similarly, multiple strategies are under investigation in clinical trials that utilize both better drug prophylaxis and refined removal or deliberate infusion of immunocytes that promote or suppress GVHD, respectively.

Bone marrow and stem cell transplantation have clearly yielded the desired outcomes in patients who have been able to weather the intercurrent toxicities of the procedure and avoid excessive issues with chronic immunosuppression GVHD. A major unmet need is a means to identify which patients have prognoses that make exposure to the risks of transplantation (or gene therapy) justifiable, on the one hand, and which donor–recipient pairs pose the least risk for significant GVHD, on the other. Predictive biomarkers are needed to address both questions. Presently the best predictive models rely largely on clinical features of the patient's underlying condition and the progression of the illness. This area of research is somewhat limited presently and needs to be expanded.

Progress in this area suggests that one can anticipate a continually expanded use of stem cell transplantation as a therapy of curative intent for those more severely affected by the conditions mentioned earlier. Even as gene therapy and gene editing are being evaluated as more definitive forms of therapy, the modality of "classical" stem cell replacement will become more feasible for a broader group of patients. Indeed, it will remain as the best curative option for those conditions in which correction of a single genetic lesion is not adequate as a therapy because the underlying cause of the illness is not a targetable gene.

Fourth, future patients with anemia are likely to benefit from the application of gene and stem cell engineering methods to the manufacture of stem cell and blood cell products. The benefits of having "universal donor" stem cell products have been mentioned already. The potential that now exists for manufacturing "universal donor" red cells that are free of blood-borne pathogens, longer lived in the circulation, inexpensively storable, and easily transportable merits equal attention. Achieving the monumental scale of manufacturing needed to provide literally trillions of red cells to the large numbers of patients requiring either short-term or chronic transfusion support is a formidable challenge. Yet, several significant efforts to produce bulk amounts of red cells by "stem cell farming" strategies are already underway. Belief that the basic technological capabilities are in place is evident from the formation of a number of start-up companies hoping to manufacture red cells, white cells, and platelets for transfusion into humans. This would offer substantial benefits for patients in developed areas of the world. It would be a paradigm-changing advance for patients in areas of the world where the infrastructure for blood donor centers, appropriate typing and cross-matching, and the like are not widely available. In principle, engineering "universal donor" red cells capable of being reliably produced in large numbers is feasible. Actually achieving a manufacturing scale sufficient to impact the public health challenge and developing a cost-effective product that can be safely stored and disseminated will be more a far more difficult but ultimately attainable goal.

Finally, the future should hold greater promise for the substantial reduction of morbidity and mortality from anemia on a global basis, but an open question is whether it will. A great deal of progress could be made in this regard simply by broadening and deepening the access of patients in many areas of the developing world to basic hematologic care and therapeutic capabilities that are simple and inexpensive. Examples include access to educated providers, basic laboratory testing, iron, folate, B12, hydroxyurea, and iron chelating compounds and basic transfusion services. In this regard, hematologists will need to become more active in the emerging field of global medicine. Pioneers in this new discipline are innovating rapidly to exploit the power of technologies, informatics, electronics, nanotechnology and materials science, and system engineering. These efforts are certain to create better mechanisms for disseminating essential health care capabilities to previously unserved areas. As part of this effort, there needs to be an explicit focus on how these approaches can be applied to the recognition, characterization, and treatment of anemias. In particular, basic management of helminthic infections, malaria, and other zoonoses would eliminate a great deal of anemia due to iron deficiency secondary to GI bleeding, hemolysis due to microbe infestation, and so on. In other cases, access to basic nutritional supplementation with iron, folates, vitamin B12 would address the most common causes of anemia and mitigate anemia during otherwise normal pregnancies. In still other situations, far more accessible "low-tech" methods for identifying patients who have hemoglobinopathies, enzymopathies, and membrane disorders are desperately needed. These conditions are especially prevalent in the equatorial areas of the world that are in developing countries where resources for care are limited and must be prioritized for those in most urgent need.

Despite remarkable advances, anemias continue to be among the most common causes of morbidity and mortality across the globe. Fortunately, an appropriate diagnosis that provides a rational basis for therapy of these conditions can be achieved in most cases using relatively simple approaches outlined in the preceding chapters. A thorough history and physical examination, careful examination of the complete blood count, differential and reticulocyte counts and peripheral blood smear, and a few basic laboratory tests that assess markers for hemolysis, iron, and vitamin status continue to provide the most successful strategy for proper diagnosis and characterization of the anemia and any underlying causes. More sophisticated and complex testing usually provides confirmatory information or refinement of the diagnosis. However, much remains to be learned if we are to be able to treat all anemias effectively and to decipher at a far more precise level the diagnosis occurring in 20–30% of patients in whom even the most expert hematologists are unable to pinpoint the exact nature of the anemia. It is thus fortunate that research into the production, circulating lifespan, and destruction of red cells should continue to be at the forefront of biomedical science. One can expect that these efforts will continue to generate insights leading to novel therapies, particularly for those patients with red cell disorders originating in intrinsic derangements of the erythron. The editors and authors of this book hope that the approaches and information provided in this text will be useful to those who, prior to reading this material, were less conversant with the present state of this area of medicine and to those more expert who might have supplemented their knowledge of the many causes of anemia and the ways by which a few thoughtful approaches can simplify our efforts to offer our patients the appropriate diagnosis, therapy, and individualized care of anemia.

References

1. *Marks PW*. Approach to Anemia in the Adult and Child, 2013. In: Hoffman R, Benz EJ Jr., Silberstein LE, Heslop HE, Weitz JI, Anastasi J, eds. *Hematology: Principles and Practice*, 6th edn. Philadelphia: Elsevier: 418–426.

2. Zhang D, Xu C, Manwani D, Frenette PS. Neutrophils, platelets and inflammatory pathways at the nexus of sickle cell disease. *Blood.* 2016; 127:801–809.

3. Hoban MD, Orkin SH, Bauer DE. Genetic treatment of a molecular disorder: gene therapy approaches to sickle cell disease. *Blood.* 2016; 127:839–884.

4. Sanders JD, Juong JK. CRISPR-CAS systems for editing, regulating and targeting genomes. *Nature Biotechnology.* 2014; 32:347–355.

5. Negrin RS. Introduction to the review series Advances in Hematopoietic Cell Transplantation. *Blood.* 2014; 124:307 (and articles in this monograph).

6. Silberstein LE. CD47 and the control of immune hemolysis. *Blood.* 99:3491.

7. Bouhassira EE. Toward the manufacture of red blood cells? *Blood.* 2008; 112:4362–4363.

Index

aAA. *See* acquired aplastic
    anemia
abdomen, physical examination
    of, 32
ABO incompatibility, 36
    HSCT and, 181
acanthocytes, 27
ACD. *See* anemia of chronic
    inflammation
ACI. *See* anemia of chronic
    inflammation
acquired aplastic anemia (aAA),
    128–32. *See also*
    paroxysmal nocturnal
    hemoglobinuria
    bone marrow with, 128
    clinical presentation of, 129
    clonal hematopoiesis and, 129
    diagnostic evaluation of,
      129–30
    epidemiology of, 128
    etiology of, 128
    laboratory findings for, 129–30
    pathophysiology, 128–9
    prognosis, 129
    severity grading of, 131
    treatment, 129–32
      through BMT, 130–1
      eltrombopag therapy, 132
      IST, 131
      second-line therapies, 131–2
acquired sideroblastic anemias,
    44
    causes of, 45
    pathophysiology, 44–5
    prognosis of, 46
    treatment of, 46
acquired stomatocytosis, 106
acute chest syndrome (ACS), 68,
    73
acute hemolytic transfusion
    reactions, 208–9
acute large volume blood loss,
    202
acute lung injury (ALI), 211
acute PCH, 93
Acute Vaso-Occlusive Crisis
    (VOC), 66
aging, anemia of

clinical significance of, 187
dementia, 187
epidemiology of, 185–6
inflammation and, 186–7
    hepcidin levels, 186
    leptin protein, 186
    MIF, 186
    TNF-α, 186
    vitamin D deficiency, 186–7
management strategies, 187–8
prevalence of, 185
aHUS. *See* atypical hemolytic
    uremic syndrome
AIHA. *See* autoimmune
    hemolytic anemia
alcohol use, non-megaloblastic
    macrocytic anemias
    from, 63
alemtuzumab, 134
ALI. *See* acute lung injury
Alpha-thalassemia, 53–6
    causes of, 53
    Hb Barts hydrops fetalis
      syndrome, 55–6
      diagnosis of, 55
      epidemiology of, 55
      prevention of, 55–6
    HbH disease, 53–5
      clinical vignette for, 54–5
      diagnosis of, 54
      hematologic data on, 54
      nondeletional, 53
      syndromes, 54–5
      treatment of, 54
    traits of, 53
amegakaryocytic
      thrombocytopenia, 148
anemia in cancer patients, 172
    ACI and, 172
    chemotherapy-associated
      anemia, 220–1
    diagnosis of, 173–5
      differential, 174
      iron deficiency in, 174
    epidemiology, 172
    erythropoietin therapy for, 175
    etiology of, 172–3
    evaluation of, 173–5
    management of, 175–7

      through RBC transfusion,
        175
      with rhEPO, 172, 174–7
    pathogenesis of, 172–3
    pathophysiology, 198
    therapy-related toxicity
      grading, 172
    transfusion, 175
anemia of chronic inflammation
    (ACI)
    cancer and, 172
    case study for, 153–4
    clinical presentation, 152–3,
      194
    critical illness with, 151
    cytokines, 196
    diagnostic evaluation, 153,
      194–5
    epidemiology, 150–1
      autoimmune diseases, 150
      from infections, 150
    erythropoiesis, 196, 198
    etiology, 150–1
    in general population, 150
    hepcidin expression, 195–6
    incidence rates for, 151
    iron, 196
    lab findings, 153, 194–5
    pathophysiology, 151–2, 195–6
      erythrocyte turnover, 152
      erythropoiesis, 196, 198
      hepcidin regulation, 152,
        195–6
      hypoferremia, 152
      hypoproliferative effects,
        151–2
      inflammatory cytokines,
        151–2
      iron metabolism, 196
      iron-restricted
        erythropoiesis, 152
      pro-inflammatory
        cytokines, 196
    RA and, 150
    soluble transferrin receptor
      and, 153
    treatment and prognosis, 153,
      198–9
      with ESA, 198–9

anemia of inflammation, 169
anemia of prematurity, 34
anemias. *See also* clinical
    approaches; *specific
    anemias*
    causes of, xi, 1
      through blood loss, 24
    classification of, 24
      through MCV, 24
    clinical definitions of, xi, 23
    comorbidities with, xi
    defined, 172, 185
    diagnostic approach, 23–4
      through bone marrow
        aspirate specimens, 24
      through peripheral blood
        smears, 24–5, 29
    future approaches to, 230–3
    hemoglobin deficiency in, xi
    hyperproliferative, 29. *See also
      specific anemias*
    hypoproliferative, 24–9. *See
      also specific anemias*
    leukemias and, xi
    mild, 1
    multiple myelomas and, xi
    overview of, 229–30
    prevalence rates, 23
    risk factors for, xi
      individual, 2
    severe, 1
    symptoms of, 1
antibiotics, after splenectomy,
    225
anticonvulsants, 31
antithymocyte globulin (ATG),
    131
aplasia, 133–4
aplastic anemia, 128–32
asplenia. *See* functional asplenia
ATG. *See* antithymocyte globulin
atypical hemolytic uremic
    syndrome (aHUS),
    113–14
    clinical presentation of, 117
    complement defects, 114
    diagnostic evaluation, 118
    laboratory findings, 118
    pathophysiology, 116

renal transplantation for, 120
treatment for, 120
auto-antibodies, in PCH, 92
autoimmune hemolytic anemia
(AIHA). *See also* cold
agglutinin disease;
paroxysmal cold
hemoglobinuria; warm
AIHA
classification of, 84–5
epidemiology, 84
HSCT and, 182
during pregnancy, 191
prevalence of, 85
splenectomy for, 223
autoimmune TTP, 113
avascular necrosis (AVN), 70, 73
azathioprine, 93
AZT. *See* zidovudine

babesiosis, 25, 123, 205, 212
bacterial infectious disease, 194
Barts hydrops fetalis syndrome,
Hemoglobin, 55–6
diagnosis, 55
epidemiology, 55
prevention of, 55–6
basophilic stippling, 24–5
Beta-thalassemia, 49–53
deletions as cause of, 49
dominant, 49
HbE form, 53
intermedia form, 52–3
mutations of, 49
silent, 49
pathophysiology, 49
traits of, 49–50
clinical vignettes, 49–50
Beta-thalassemia major, 50–2
clinical vignette for, 52
complication of, 50–2
endocrinopathy and, 51
extramedullary hematopoiesis
and, 51
growth delay and, 51
from iron overload, 51
management of, 50–2
osteoporosis and, 51
preventive programs, 52
treatment of, 51
through bone-marrow
transplantation, 51–2
through disease-modifying
therapies, 51–2
transfusions in, 50–1
BFU-E. *See* burst forming units-
erythroid
bilirubin levels, 12
biosynthesis, hemoglobin and,
6–8
bite cells, 24–5
blister cells, 24–5
blood loss, 24
acute large volume, 202
chronic, 41

blood transfusions. *See also* red
cell transfusion therapy;
transfusion reactions
for anemia in cancer patients,
175
for CAD, 91
ESA therapy as alternative to,
221
for malaria treatment, 111
of RBCs, xi
for Beta-thalassemia major,
50–1
engineered stem cells in, xi
twin-twin, 35
WAIHA and, 87
BMSC. *See* bone marrow stromal
cells
BMT. *See* bone marrow
transplantation
bone marrow
EPO in, 23
HIV associated with anemia,
168
marrow suppression and,
167–8
sideroblastic anemias and,
45–6
transplantation of, for Beta-
thalassemia major, 51–2
bone marrow aspirate specimens,
24
bone marrow failure
acquired, 128–32
congenital, 143–8
bone marrow stromal cells
(BMSC), 198
bone marrow transplantation
(BMT)
for aAA, 130–1
HSCT and, anemia after, 182
for PNH, 141
brain issues, with SCD, 69
burr cells, 24–5
burst forming units-erythroid
(BFU-E), 6, 14, 198

Cabot rings, 24–5
CAD. *See* cold agglutinin disease
CAMT. *See* congenital
amegakaryocytic
thrombocytopenia
cancer. *See* anemia in cancer
patients
cardiac valves. *See* prosthetic
cardiac valves
cardiovascular systems
physical examination of, 32
with SCD, 70
cART. *See* combined antiretroviral therapy
case studies
ACI, 153–4
DIHA, 97–8
megaloblastic macrocytic
anemias, 64–5

non-megaloblastic macrocytic
anemias, 65
red cell transfusion therapy,
205
for sideroblastic anemias, 47
CD47 proteins, 20–1
central nervous system, with
SCD, 69–70
brain issues, 69
eye issues, 69–70
neurocognitive impairments,
69
CFU-E. *See* colony forming
units-erythroid
chaperone proteins, 8
chemotherapy-associated
anemia, 220–1
CHF. *See* chronic heart failure
childhood anemias. *See also*
hemolytic anemia in
children
anemia of prematurity, 34
DIHA, 96
general considerations for,
34–5
hemoglobin abnormalities as
factor in, 34
in infants. *See also specific
anemias*
causes of, 35
physiologic anemia of
infancy, 34
neonatal hemolytic anemia
due to maternal
alloimmunization, 35–6
ABO incompatibility as
cause of, 36
HDN as factor in, 35–6
neonatal hemorrhagic anemia,
35
fetal maternal hemorrhage
and, 35
from twin-twin
transfusions, 35
from nutritional deficiencies,
36
iron deficiency, 36, 41
vitamin B12 deficiency, 36
physiologic anemia of
childhood, 35
RBC characteristics for, 35
from RBC hypoplastic
disorders, 38
DBA, 38
TEC of childhood, 38
red cell transfusion therapy
for, 205
chimerism, 180
chromosomal fragility, 129–30.
See also Diamond-
Blackfan anemia
chronic blood loss. *See* blood loss
chronic heart failure (CHF), 198
chronic kidney disease (CKD),
220

chronic leg ulcers. *See* leg ulcers
chronic liver disease, 196–8
chronic obstructive pulmonary
disease (COPD), 63
chronic PCH, 93
chronic renal disease, 196
CKD. *See* chronic kidney disease
classical PNH, 138
treatment for, 139
clindamycin, 124
clinical approaches, to anemias,
30–3
through medical history, 30–2
current medications, 31
family history factors, 31–2
gynecological history
factors, 31
for past illnesses, 31
for present illnesses, 30
social history factors, 31
surgical history factors, 31
systems review in, 30–1
through physical examination,
32–3
of abdomen, 32
of cardiovascular systems,
32
of extremities, 33
of genitourinary system,
33
of HEENT, 30–2
of neck, 32
of neurological systems, 33
of pulmonary system, 32
of skin, 32
of vital signs, 32
clopidogrel, 116
clostridial sepsis, hemolytic
anemia from, 123–4
clinical features, 123–4
pathophysiology, 123–4
treatment of, 124
codocytes, 24–5
cognitive deficiencies, 1
cold agglutinin disease (CAD),
89–92
associated conditions, 90
clinical features, 92
Coombs test, 89
laboratory features, 89
management of, 91–2
with cold avoidance, 90
with pharmacologic therapy,
91–2
with RBC transfusions, 91
steroid therapy, 92
mechanism of hemolysis, 90
cold agglutinins, 89–90
cold AIHA. *See* cold agglutinin
disease
cold avoidance, 90
colony forming units-erythroid
(CFU-E), 6, 14, 198
combined anti-retroviral therapy
(cART), 167, 169–70

congenital amegakaryocytic thrombocytopenia (CAMT), 148
congenital TTP, 113, 119
congestive heart failure (CHF), 1, 32
conjunctiva, 69–70
conjunctival pallor, 32
connective tissue diseases, 194
Coombs test
  for CAD, 89
  for PCH, 92
  for WAIHA, 84–6
    clinical serological associations, 86
COPD. See chronic obstructive pulmonary disease
copper, ingestion of, 124
corticosteroid therapy
  for DBA, 144
  for PRCA, 133–4
  for WAIHA, 89
crenated RBC, 24–5
cyclophosphamide, 93, 134
cytokines
  ACI, 196
  with ACI, 151–2
  immune, 109
cytopenias. See acquired aplastic anemia

dacrocytes, 24–5
dactylitis, 70, 73
danazol, 132
dapsone, 168
darbepoetin alfa, 219, 221
DAT. See direct antiglobulin test
DBA. See Diamond-Blackfan anemia
DC. See dyskeratosis congenita
deferasirox, 73
deferiprone, 163
deferoxamine, 73, 163
degmacytes, 24–5
delayed hemolytic transfusion reaction (DHTR), 209–10
delayed serologic transfusion reaction (DSTR), 210
destruction, of RBCs, 11–12, 21
  bilirubin levels, 12
  extravascular, 12
  geometric hypothesis, 12
  immunological hypothesis, 12
  metabolic hypothesis, 11–12
  rates of, 12
  through reticuloendothelial system clearance, 21
DHTR. See delayed hemolytic transfusion reaction
Diamond-Blackfan anemia (DBA), 38, 144
  corticosteroid therapy for, 144
  impaired ribosome function, 144
DIHA. See drug-induced immune hemolytic anemia

direct antiglobulin test (DAT), 97
drepanocytes, 24–5
drug-induced immune hemolytic anemia (DIHA), 87
  case study for, 97–8
  clinical presentation of, 96
    in adults, 96
    in pediatric populations, 96
  diagnostic evaluation of, 97
  drugs as cause of, 95
  epidemiology of, 95
  etiology of, 95
  laboratory findings, 97
    with DAT, 97
    elution and, 97
    with IAT, 97
  pathophysiology, 95–6
    with drug-dependent antibody mechanism, 95–6
    with drug-independent antibody mechanism, 96
    with non-immune protein adsorption, 96
  prognosis with, 97
  treatment for, 97
DSTR. See delayed serologic transfusion reaction
dyserythropoiesis, 45, 108–9
dyskeratosis congenita (DC), 144–6
  clinical diagnosis of, 144–6
  stem cell transplantation for, 146
  telomerase complex and, 144–6

echinocytes, 24–5
eculizumab, 93, 120, 139–41
Ehrlich, Paul, 128
elderly. See aging
elliptocytes, 24–5
eltrombopag therapy, 132
elution, for DIHA, 97
Embden-Meyerhof pathway, 10
endocrinopathy, Beta-thalassemia major and, 51
engineered stem cells, in red cell transfusions, xi
enucleation, in reticulocyte maturation, 16–17
EPO. See erythropoietin
epoetin alfa, 219, 221
Epstein-Barr virus, 183
erythroblastic islands, 16
erythrocyte membrane, 100
erythrocytes. See also red blood cells
  in ACI, 152
  development of, 3
  hemoglobin content and, xi, 3
  osmolarity of, 3
  proerythroblast stage, 6
  purpose and functions of, xi
  resilience of, 3

erythrocytic destruction and sequestration, 108
erythropoiesis, 3
  ACI, 196, 198
  BFU-E, 6, 14
  in bone marrow, 19
  CFU-E, 6, 14
  clinical definition of, 23
  early, 14–16
  hemoglobin production and, 6
  HSCs in, 14
  iron-restricted, 152
  with malaria, immune response to, 109–10
  MEP differentiation in, 14
  primary sites of, 6
erythropoiesis-stimulation agents (ESAs), 198–9
  blood transfusions and, as alternative to, 221
  for chemotherapy-associated anemia, 220–1
  for CKD, 220
  darbepoetin alfa, 219, 221
  dosing guidelines, 221
  epoetin alfa, 219, 221
  indications for, 220–1
  safety of, 219–20
erythropoietin (EPO), 14–16
  production of, 23
ESAs. See erythropoiesis-stimulation agents
exercise intolerance, 1
extramedullary hematopoiesis, 51
extravascular hemolytic transfusion reactions, 209
extremities, physical examination of, 33
extrinsic non-immune hemolytic anemias
  from clostridial sepsis, 123–4
    clinical features, 123–4
    pathophysiology, 123–4
    treatment of, 124
  from heavy metal exposure, 124
    through copper ingestion, 124
    through lead poisoning, 124
  from hypersplenism, 125
  from infectious parasites, 123
    babesiosis, 123
  from IVIG, 125
  march hemoglobinuria, 123
  from prosthetic cardiac valves, 122–3
    clinical features, 122
    epidemiology of, 122
    history of, 122
    pathophysiology, 122
    treatment of, 122–3
  thermal injury-induced hemolysis, 123
eye issues, with SCD, 69–70

erythrocytic destruction and sequestration, 108

Fanconi anemia (FA), 146–7
  diagnosis of, 146–7
  genomic instability and, 146–7
  treatment for, 147
favism, 37
febrile non-hemolytic transfusion reactions, 210–11
Felty Syndrome, 224
ferric carboxymaltose, 218
ferric gluconate, 42, 218
ferrous fumarate, 217
ferrous gluconate, 217
ferrous sulfate, 217
ferumoxytol, 42, 217–18
fetal maternal hemorrhage, 35
fever, after splenectomy, 225
flippases, 9–10
floppases, 9–10
fludarabine, 92
folate deficiency
  megaloblastic macrocytic anemias and, 59–63
  during pregnancy, 192
folic acid, as hematinic, xi
functional asplenia, 70, 73
fungal infectious disease, 194

G6PD deficiency. See glucose-6-phosphate dehydrogenase deficiency
gallstones. See pigmented gallstones
gastrointestinal system, with SCD, 70, 73
gene therapies, advances in, xi
genetics, hemoglobin production and, 6
genitourinary system
  physical examination of, 33
  with SCD, 70
geometric hypothesis, for RBC destruction, 12
globin genes, 6–8
  chaperone proteins, 8
  duplication of, 7
  expression of, 7–8
  hemoglobin switching, 7
  LCRs in, 8
glossitis, 30–1
glucose-6-phosphate dehydrogenase (G6PD) deficiency, 37
glycosylphosphatidylinositol (GPI) anchors, 137
graft failure, HSCT and, 179–80
  blood chimerism, 180
  causes of, 179–80
graft-versus-host-disease (GVHD), 180–2
  transfusion-associated, 213
growth delay, Beta-thalassemia major and, 51
GVHD. See graft-versus-host-disease

haptenic reactions, 87
HbE/Beta-thalassemia, 53
HbH disease, 53–5
  clinical vignette for, 54–5
  diagnosis of, 54
  hematologic data on, 54
  nondeletional, 53
  syndromes, 54–5
  treatment of, 54
HDN. See hemolytic disease of
    the newborn
HE. See hereditary elliptocytosis
head, ear, eyes, nose, and throat
    (HEENT) examination,
    30–2
heart failure, chronic, 194
heavy metal exposure, hemolytic
    anemia from, 124
  through copper ingestion, 124
  through lead poisoning, 124
HEENT examination. See head,
    ear, eyes, nose, and throat
    examination
Heinz bodies, 24–5
HELLP. See hemolysis with
    elevated liver enzymes
    and low platelets
hematinics, xi
hematocrit, 1
hematologic, malignancies,
    194
hematopoietic stem cell
    transplantation (HSCT),
    anemia after
  ABO incompatibility, 181
  AIHA and, 182
  BMT criteria, 182
  defined, 179
  erythropoietin insufficiency
    and, 179–80
  graft failure and, 179–80
    blood chimerism, 180
    causes of, 179–80
  GVHD and, 180–2
  HLH and, 183
  HUS and, 181
  pathophysiology, 179
  relapse of underlying disease,
    182–3
  secondary MDS and, 182–3
  TMA and, 181–2
  TTP and, 181
hematopoietic stem cells (HSCs),
    14
hematuria, with SCD, 70, 73
heme, 1
  in terminal erythroid
    differentiation, 16
hemichromes, 20
hemoglobin. See also high affinity
    hemoglobin disorders;
    low affinity hemoglobin
    disorders
  anemias and, xi
  Beth Israel, 79

in biosynthesis, 6–8
C, 79
C crystals, 24–5
in childhood anemias,
    abnormalities of, 34
components of, 1
Cretail, 79
defined, xi
D-Los Angeles, 79
D-Punjab, 79
electrophoresis, 71
erythrocytes and, xi, 3
erythropoiesis and, 6
F, 34
functions of, 3–6
  oxygen binding, 5–6
genetics and, 6
globin genes, 6–8
  chaperone proteins, 8
  duplication of, 7
  expression of, 7–8
  hemoglobin switching, 7
  LCRs in, 8
Hammersmith, 79
hemolytic anemia in children
    and, from disorders of,
    37–8
J-Capetown, 79
Kansas, 79, 81
Kempsey, 79
laboratory assessments, 2
  hematocrit, 1
  Hgb, 1
  MCH, 2
  MCHC, 2
life cycle of, 1
M-Boston, 79
M-Hyde Park, 79
M-Iwate, 79
M-Milwaukee-I, 79
modifications of
  non-enzymatic, 8
  post-translational, 8
M-Osaka, 79
M-Saskatoon, 79
mutations, 76
ontogeny of, 6
oxygen and
  acquisition mechanisms, 6
  binding of, 5–6
  delivery mechanisms, 6
  salt bridges, 5
  transport, 5–6
Philadelphia, 79
polymerization of, 5
precipitated, 5
S, 79
Santa Ana, 79
Setif, 79
solubility of, 5
St. Louis, 79
structure of, 3–6. See also
    structural
    hemoglobinopathies
  tetramers, 3–5

Suresnes, 79
Titusville, 79
Torino, 79
unstable, 76
Zurich, 79
Hemoglobin Barts hydrops
    fetalis syndrome, 55–6
  diagnosis, 55
  epidemiology, 55
  prevention of, 55–6
hemoglobin switching, 7
hemoglobin value (Hgb), 1
hemoglobinopathies. See also
    structural
    hemoglobinopathies
  classifications of, 77
  unstable hemoglobin
    disorders, 76
    clinical manifestations of, 77
    diagnosis of, 77–80
    mutational factors for,
      78–9
    pathophysiology, 76–80
    treatment for, 80
hemoglobinuria, 137–41
hemolysis mechanisms
  CAD, 90
  for PCH, 93
  for WAIHA, 87
    haptenic reactions, 87
    NIPA, 87
hemolysis with elevated liver
    enzymes and low platelets
    (HELLP), 191
hemolytic anemia in children,
    36–8
  causes of, 36
  chronic disorders and, 36–7
  clinical indicators of, 36
  from hemoglobin disorders,
    37–8
  from RBC enzyme disorders,
    37
    favism, 37
    G6PD deficiency, 37
    PK deficiency, 37
  from RBC membrane
    disorders, 37
    HS, 37
  sickle cell anemia and, 37–8
hemolytic anemias, 29–30. See
    also specific hemolytic
    anemias
  AIHA. See also cold agglutinin
    disease; paroxysmal cold
    hemoglobinuria; warm
    AIHA
    classification of, 84–5
    epidemiology, 84
    HSCT and, 182
    prevalence of, 85
  common acquired causes of,
    29–30
  drug-induced immune, 87
  during pregnancy, 191–2

hemolytic disease of the newborn
    (HDN), 35–6
hemolytic transfusion reactions,
    208–9
  acute, 208–9
  DHTR, 209–10
  DSTR, 210
  extravascular, 209
  intravascular, 209
  nonimmune-mediated, 210
  with SCD, 210
  severity of, 208
hemolytic uremic syndrome
    (HUS), 181
  during pregnancy, 191
hemophagocytic
    lymphohistiocytosis
    (HLH), 183
hemozoin, 109
hepcidin expression, 39–40,
    195–6
  ACI, 195–6
  with ACI, 152
  aging with anemia, 186
hereditary elliptocytosis (HE),
    104–5
  classification of, 104
  clinical presentation of, 104
  diagnostic evaluation of, 105
  incidence rates for, 104
  inheritance rates for, 104
  laboratory findings for, 105
  pathophysiology, 104
    spectrin abnormalities, 104
  treatment for, 105
hereditary pyropoikilocytosis
    (HPP), 104–5
  clinical presentation of, 104
  diagnostic evaluation of, 105
  incidence rates for, 104
  inheritance rates for, 104
  laboratory findings for, 105
  pathophysiology, 104
    spectrin abnormalities, 104
  SAO and, 104
  treatment for, 105
hereditary sideroblastic anemias
  causes of, 44
  pathophysiology, 44
  prognosis for, 46
  treatment of, 46
hereditary spherocytosis (HS),
    100–3
  classification of, 101
  clinical presentation of, 100–1
    jaundice and, 101
  complications from, 101–2
  diagnostic evaluation of, 102–3
  epidemiology of, 100
  etiology of, 100
  hemolytic anemia in children
    and, 37
  laboratory findings for, 102–3
    EMA binding, 102
    MCHC, 102

hereditary spherocytosis (HS) (cont.)
  MCV, 102
  osmotic fragility testing, 102
    with peripheral blood smears, 102
  pathophysiology, 100
    primary defects, 100
    secondary defects, 100
  prognosis with, 103
  splenomegaly and, 103
  treatment for, 103
    with splenectomy, 103, 223
hereditary stomatocytosis syndromes
  acquired stomatocytosis, 106
  classification criteria for, 105
  HX, 105–6
  hydrocytosis, 105
  intermediate syndromes, 106
  Rh null disease and, 106
  sitosterolemia and, 106
  Tangier disease and, 106
hereditary xerocytosis (HX), 105–6
hexose monophosphate shunt (HMPS), 11
Hgb. See hemoglobin value
high affinity hemoglobin disorders, 76, 80–1
  diagnosis of, 80–1
  pathophysiology, 80
  treatment of, 81
HIV. See human immunodeficiency virus
HLH. See hemophagocytic lymphohistiocytosis
HMPS. See hexose monophosphate shunt
HMW iron dextran, 218
homeostasis. See also volume homeostasis disorders for RBs, 10–11
homozygous alpha thalassemia, 34
Howell-Jolly bodies, 218
HPP. See hereditary pyropoikilocytosis
HS. See hereditary spherocytosis
HSCs. See hematopoietic stem cells
HSCT. See hematopoietic stem cell transplantation
HTN. See pulmonary hypertension
human immunodeficiency virus (HIV), anemia associated with, 168–9
  anemia of inflammation, 169
  clinical presentation, 169
  diagnostic evaluation, 169–70
  epidemiology, 167
  etiology, 167
  MDS and, 169
  medications as factor in, 168

pathophysiology, 167–9
  G6PD deficiency, 168
  hemolysis, 168
  hypogonadism, 167
  infection of stem cells and progenitors, 168–9
  infiltration of bone marrow, 168
  marrow suppression, 167–8
  nutritional deficiencies, 167
  opportunistic infections in, 168
  treatment and prognosis, 170
    cART, 167, 169–70
  vitamin B12 deficiency, 167
HUS. See hemolytic uremic syndrome
HX. See hereditary xerocytosis
hydrocytosis. See overhydrated stomatocytosis
hydroxyurea, 72
hyperkalemia, 214
hypersplenism, 125. See also chronic liver disease
hypochromia, 24–5
hypoferremia, 152
hypogonadism, 167
hypokalemia, 214
hypoplastic disorders, of RBCs, 38
  DBA, 38
  TEC of childhood, 38
hypoplastic PNH, 138
hyposthenuria, 70
hypothermia, 214
hypothyroidism, 194
hypothyroidism, non-megaloblastic macrocytic anemias ands, 63

IAT. See indirect antiglobulin test
IBMFs. See inherited bone marrow failure syndromes
IDA. See iron deficiency anemia
idiopathic sideroblastic anemias, 46
imatinib, 174
immune cytokines, 109
immunological hypothesis, for RBC destruction, 12
immunosuppressive therapy (IST), 131
  for MDS, 163
impaired ribosome function, 144
indirect antiglobulin test (IAT), 97
infants
  anemias in. See also specific anemias
    causes of, 35
    physiologic anemia of infancy, 34
  red cell transfusion therapy in, 205

infectious parasites, hemolytic anemia from, 123
infiltration of bone marrow, 168
inflammatory bowel diseases, 194
inherited bone marrow failure syndromes (IBMFs)
  CAMT, 148
  clinical presentations of, 143
  DBA, 38, 144
    corticosteroid therapy for, 144
    impaired ribosome function, 144
  DC, 144–6
    clinical diagnosis of, 144–6
    stem cell transplantation for, 146
  FA, 146–7
    diagnosis of, 146–7
    treatment for, 147
  Pearson syndrome, 148
  SCN, 148
  SDS, 143–7
    clinical presentation, 147
    diagnosis of, 147
    management of, 148
    SBDS gene, 147–8
  TAR syndrome, 148
International Prognostic Scoring System (IPSS), 160–1
intraoperative transesophageal echocardiography (TEE), 122
intravascular hemolytic transfusion reactions, 209
intravenous immune globulin (IVIG), 125
IPSS. See International Prognostic Scoring System
iron
  absorption requirements, 39
  ACI, 196
  anemia in cancer patients and, 174
  Beta-thalassemia major and, 51
  as hematinic, xi
  hepcidin expression, 39–40
  recycling of, 40
  rhEPO supplemented with, 177
  sideroblastic anemias and, 45
  in terminal erythroid differentiation, 16
iron deficiency
  in anemia in cancer patients, 174
  in childhood anemias, 36, 41
  during pregnancy, 190
iron deficiency anemia (IDA)
  causes of, 41
    chronic blood loss as, 41
  in childhood, 36

clinical presentation of, 40–1
  diagnostic evaluation of, 40–1
    through peripheral blood smear review, 40–1
    through TIBC, 40–1
    with TSAT testing, 40–1
  epidemiology of, 39
  nutritional, 36, 41
  pathophysiology, 39–40
  prevention strategies, 41–2
  treatment of, 41–2
    with parenteral iron salts, 42
  Von Willebrand's disease, 41
  in women, 41
iron sucrose, 42, 218
iron-restricted erythropoiesis, 152
irradiation, 204
IST. See immunosuppressive therapy
IVIG. See intravenous immune globulin

kidney disease, chronic, 194
kolonychia, 32
Kussmaul's sign, 32

laparoscopic splenectomy, 224
large granular lymphocyte, 132
LCR. See Locus Control Region
lead poisoning, 124
leg ulcers, chronic, 70, 73
lenalidomide, 162
leukemias, anemias and, xi
leukoreduction, 204
lipid components, of RBCs, 9–10
liver disease. See hypersplenism
liver disease, chronic, 194
LMW iron dextran, 218
Locus Control Region (LCR), 8
low affinity hemoglobin disorders, 76, 81
  cyanosis and, 81
  diagnosis of, 81
  pathophysiology, 81
  treatment for, 81

macrocytes, 24–5, 59–60
macrocytic anemias. See also megaloblastic macrocytic anemias; non-megaloblastic macrocytic anemias
  defined, 59
  MCV and, 59
macrophage migration inhibitory factor (MIF), 110, 186
MAHA. See microangiopathic hemolytic anemia
malaise, 1
malaria
  clinical presentation of, 110
  diagnosis of, 110
  epidemiology of, 108

etiology of, 108
morbidity of, 111
pathophysiology, 108–10
  dyserythropoiesis, 108–9
  erythrocytic destruction and
    sequestration, 108
  erythropoiesis, immune
    response and, 109–10
  hemozoin, 109
  host immunity, 109
  immune cytokines, 109
  MIF inhibition, 110
prognosis with, 110–11
red blood cells, 24–5
treatment of, 110–11
  with exchange transfusion,
    111
march hemoglobinuria, 123
mature RBCs. See reticulocyte
    maturation
MCH. See mean corpuscular
    hemoglobin
MCHC. See mean corpuscular
    hemoglobin
    concentration
MCV. See mean corpuscular
    volume
MDS. See myelodysplastic
    syndromes
mean corpuscular hemoglobin
    (MCH), 2
mean corpuscular hemoglobin
    concentration (MCHC),
    2, 102
mean corpuscular volume
    (MCV), 24
  for HS, 102
  macrocytic anemias and, 59
  reticulocyte count and, 24–30
megakaryocyte/erythroid (MEP)
    lineages, 14
megaloblastic macrocytic
    anemias, 59–63
  case study for, 64–5
  clinical presentation of, 61
  diagnostic evaluation of, 61–2
  differential, 59–60
  epidemiology of, 59
  etiology of, 59
  folate deficiency and, 59–63
  lab findings for, 61–2
  pathophysiology, 59–61
  peripheral blood smear, 61–2
  during pregnancy, 190
  prognosis with, 63
  treatment of, 63
  vitamin B12 deficiency and,
    59–63
MEP lineages. See
    megakaryocyte/erythroid
    lineages
metabolic derangements, 213–14
metabolic hypothesis, for RBC
    destruction, 11–12
metabolism, of RBCs, 10–11

metformin, 31
methemoglobinemia, 81–3
  causes of, 82
  clinical presentation of, 81–2
  diagnosis of, 82
  pathophysiology, 82
  treatment of, 82–3
methotrexate, 31
methyldopa, 95
MF. See myelofibrosis
microangiopathic hemolytic
    anemia (MAHA). See also
    atypical hemolytic uremic
    syndrome; thrombotic
    thrombocytopenic
    purpura
  classification of, 114
  diagnostic evaluation of,
    117–18
  epidemiology of, 113–14
  etiology of, 113–14
  laboratory findings, 117–18
  during pregnancy, 191
  secondary thrombotic
    microangiopathy, 114
  pathophysiology, 116
  treatment for, 120
  STEC-HUS, 113
    clinical presentation of, 117
    diagnostic evaluation, 118
    laboratory findings, 118
    pathophysiology, 115–16
    treatment for, 119
microcytes, 24–5
microspherocytosis, 84
MIF. See macrophage migration
    inhibitory factor
mild anemias, comorbidities
    with, 1
Moyamoya syndrome, 69
multiple myelomas, anemias and,
    xi
musculoskeletal system, with
    SCD, 70
mutations
  of Beta-thalassemia, 49
  silent, 49
  hemoglobin, 76
myelodysplastic syndromes
    (MDS)
  classification of, 160–2
    with IPSS, 160–1
    WHO subtypes, 160
  clinical presentation, 157–8
  diagnostic evaluation, 158–60
  epidemiology, 156–7
    risk factors, 157
  5q-syndrome, 144
  in higher risk patients, 163
  HIV and, 169
  iron overload, 163
  in lower risk patients,
    162–3
    treatment for, 162–3
  pathophysiology, 156–7

common genetic
    abnormalities, 157
  pediatric, 156
  primary, 156
  prognosis with, 160–2
  secondary, 156
    HSCT and, 182–3
  sideroblastic anemias and, 44,
    46
  treatment for, 162
    with ESAs, 162–3
    with hypomethylating
      agents, 163
    with IST, 163
    with lenalidomide, 162
    lower risk patients, 162–3
myelofibrosis (MF), 224

neck, physical examination of, 32
neonatal hemolytic anemia due
    to maternal
    alloimmunization, 35–6
  ABO incompatibility as cause
    of, 36
  HDN as factor in, 35–6
neonatal hemorrhagic anemia, 35
  fetal maternal hemorrhage
    and, 35
  from twin-twin transfusions,
    35
neonates. See infants
neurological systems
  physical examination of, 33
  with SCD, 69
neuropathic pain, with SCD, 67
NIPA. See non-immune protein
    adsorption
nitric oxide levels, 139
nondeletional HbH disease, 53
non-enzymatic modifications, of
    hemoglobin, 8
non-immune protein adsorption
    (NIPA), 87
non-immune protein adsorption,
    in DIHA, 96
nonimmune-mediated
    transfusion reactions, 210
non-megaloblastic macrocytic
    anemias, 63–4
  from alcohol use, 63
  case study for, 65
  clinical presentation of, 63
  COPD and, 63
  diagnostic evaluation of, 63–4
  differential, 59–60
  epidemiology of, 63
  etiology of, 63
  hypothyroidism and, 63
  pathophysiology, 63
  prognosis with, 63–4
  treatment for, 63–4
non-proliferative retinopathy, 69
normovolemic anemia, 202–4
  chronic anemia and, 203–4
  irradiation, 204

leukoreduction, 204
RCE, 204
washed red cells, 204
nucleated red cells, 24–5
nutritional deficiencies
  childhood anemias from, 36
    iron deficiency, 36, 41
    vitamin B12 deficiency, 36
  IDA, 41
nutritional IDA, 41

OPSI. See overwhelming
    postsplenectomy
    infection
oral riboflavin therapy, 83
osteopenia, SCD and, 70
osteoporosis
  Beta-thalassemia major and,
    51
  SCD and, 70
ovalocytes, 24–5
overhydrated stomatocytosis
    (hydrocytosis), 105
overwhelming postsplenectomy
    infection (OPSI), 103
oxygen, hemoglobin and
  acquisition mechanisms, 6
  delivery mechanisms through, 6
  oxygen binding by, 5–6
  oxygen transport, 5–6
  salt bridges, 5
oxygen binding, 5–6

pain, with SCD, 66–7
  acute VOC, 66
  chronic, 67, 72
  management of, 72
  neuropathic, 67
pallor, 1
pancytopenia. See acquired
    aplastic anemia
Pappenheimer bodies, 24–5
parasitic, infectious diseases, 194
parenteral iron salts, 42
paroxysmal cold hemoglobinuria
    (PCH), 92–3
  acute, 93
  associated conditions with, 92
  auto-antibodies in, 92
  chronic, 93
  clinical features, 92
  Coombs test for, 92
  laboratory findings, 92
  management of, 93
  mechanisms of hemolysis, 93
paroxysmal nocturnal
    hemoglobinuria (PNH),
    129
  classical, 138
    treatment for, 139
  clinical presentation of, 138–9
    nitric oxide levels, 139
    renal damage, 139
    smooth muscle dystonia,
      139

paroxysmal nocturnal
hemoglobinuria (PNH) (cont.)
thrombophilia, 139
diagnostic evaluation of
FLAER, 137–8
GPI-AP, 137–8
epidemiology, 137
etiology, 137
GPI anchors, 137
hypoplastic, 138
laboratory findings, 137–8
pathophysiology, 137
prognosis with, 139–41
relevant cells in, 138
thrombosis from, 137
treatment of, 139–41
with BMT, 141
for classical PNH, 139
with eculizumab, 139–41
PCH. See paroxysmal cold
hemoglobinuria
Pearson syndrome, 148
pediatric MDS, 156
penicillamine, 124
pentoxifylline, 123
peripheral blood smears, review
of, 24–5
guidelines for, 29
for IDA diagnosis, 40–1
sideroblastic anemias and, 45
for unstable hemoglobin
disorders, 77–80
pharmacologic therapy. See also
erythropoiesis-
stimulation agents
iron repletion, 217–19
IV therapy, 218–19
oral therapies, 217
phosphatidylserine, 9–10
phospholipids (PS), in RBC
senescence, 20
physiologic anemia, 190
of childhood, 35
of infancy, 34
PIG-A gene, 129. See also
paroxysmal nocturnal
hemoglobinuria
pigmented gallstones, 70
PK deficiency. See pyruvate
kinase deficiency
plasmapheresis, 193
plumbism. See lead poisoning
PNH. See paroxysmal nocturnal
hemoglobinuria
polychromasia, 24–5
polysaccharide–iron complex,
217
post-operative care, fever and,
225
postoperative thrombosis, 225
post-transfusion purpura (PTP),
214
prasugrel, 116
PRCA. See pure red cell aplasia
precipitated hemoglobins, 5

pregnancy, anemia during
AIHA, 191
clinical presentation, 191
diagnostic evaluation, 191–2
epidemiology of, 190
folate deficiency, 192
HELLP, 191
hemolytic anemias, 191–2
HUS, 191
from iron deficiency, 190
iron replacement, 192–3
lab findings, 191–2
MAHA, 191
megaloblastic anemia, 190
pathophysiology, 190
physiologic anemia, 190
sickle cell anemia, 192
sickle cell hemoglobinopathies,
190–1
thalassemia syndromes during,
192
treatment of, 192–3
with plasmapheresis, 193
vitamin B12 deficiency, 192
priapism, 70, 73
primaquine, 168
primary MDS, 156
primary PRCA, 133–4
proerythroblasts, 16
reticulocytes and, 23
proliferative retinopathy, 69–70
prosthetic cardiac valves,
hemolytic anemia from,
122–3
clinical features, 122
epidemiology of, 122
history of, 122
pathophysiology, 122
treatment of, 122–3
proton pump inhibitors, 31
PS. See phospholipids
PTP. See post-transfusion
purpura
pulmonary hypertension (HTN),
68–9, 73
pulmonary system, physical
examination of, 32
pure red cell aplasia (PRCA),
132–4
classic causes of, 132
clinical presentation of, 132–3
diagnostic evaluation of, 132–3
epidemiology of, 132
etiology of, 132
laboratory findings, 133
parvovirus B19 infection and,
132
pathogenesis of, 132
thymoma and, 132–3
transient erythroblastopenia of
childhood, 132
treatment and prognosis,
133–4
with corticosteroid therapy,
133–4

for primary PRCA, 133–4
for secondary PRCA, 133
with thymectomy, 133
pyruvate kinase (PK) deficiency,
37

RA. See rheumatoid arthritis
Rapoport-Leubering shunt, 10
RBCs. See red blood cells
RCC. See red cell concentrates
RCE. See red cell exchange
reactive oxygen species (ROS),
RBC senescence, 20
recombinant human
erythropoietin (rhEPO),
172, 174–7
iron supplementation with,
177
red blood cell count
EPO and, 14–16, 23
laboratory assessments, 2
MCV, 2
reticulocyte count, 2
red blood cells (RBCs)
childhood anemias and, 35
cytoskeleton for, 8–10
decrease in mass, 1
destruction of, 11–12, 21
bilirubin levels, 12
extravascular, 12
geometric hypothesis, 12
immunological hypothesis,
12
metabolic hypothesis, 11–12
rates of, 12
through reticuloendothelial
system clearance, 21
Embden-Meyerhof pathway,
10
enzymatic metabolism, 10–11
essential components of, 3
flippases, 9–10
floppases, 9–10
hemolysis stages for, 12
hemolytic anemia in children
from enzyme disorders, 37
favism, 37
G6PD deficiency, 37
HS, 37
from membrane disorders,
37
PK deficiency, 37
HMPS and, 11
homeostasis for, 10–11
hypoplastic disorders, 38
DBA, 38
TEC of childhood, 38
lifespan of, 19–20
MCV of, 24
membrane for, 8–10
components of, 9–10
hemolytic anemia in
children and, from
disorders of, 37
lipid components, 9–10

during reticulocyte
maturation, 17
spectrins, 10
transmembrane proteins, 9
phosphatidylserine, 9–10
proerythroblasts, 16
Rapoport-Leubering shunt, 10
reticulocyte maturation,
16–17, 19
enucleation in, 16–17
plasma membrane during,
17
scramblases, 9–10
senescence, 20–1
CD47 protein activity, 20–1
hemichromes and, 20
loss of membrane surface
during, 20
PS activity, 20
ROS and, 20
siderosomes, 24–5
synthesis of, 11–12
terminal erythroid
differentiation, 16
erythroblastic islands in, 16
heme in, 16
iron in, 16
transfusions, xi
engineered stem cells in, xi
red cell antibodies, 203
red cell concentrates (RCC), 201
red cell exchange (RCE), 204
red cell membrane disorders
classification criteria for, 100
HS, 100–3
hemolytic anemia in
children and, 37
red cell transfusion therapy
after acute large volume blood
loss, 202
case study, 205
in children, 205
dosage of red cells, 201–2
epidemiology, 201
in neonates, 205
in normovolemic anemia,
202–4
chronic anemia and, 203–4
irradiation, 204
leukoreduction, 204
phenotype matching, 203–4
red cell exchange (RCE), 204
red cell genotyping, 203–4
washed red cells, 204
red cell antibodies, 203
storage duration, 201
transfusion incidents rates
(TIR), 201
renal damage, with PNH, 139
renal transplantation, for aHUS,
120
respiratory system, with SCD,
68–9
reticulocyte count, 2, 24–30
MCV and, 24–30

reticulocyte index (RPI), 24–30
reticulocyte maturation, 16–17, 19
  enucleation in, 16–17
  plasma membrane during, 17
  proerythroblasts and, 23
reticuloendothelial system, 21
retinopathy, with SCD, 69–70, 73
  non-proliferative, 69
  proliferative, 69–70
Rh null disease, 106
rhEPO. See recombinant human erythropoietin
rheumatoid arthritis (RA), 150, 194
ribavirin therapy, 168
ribosomopathies. See 5q-syndrome MDS; Diamond-Blackfan anemia; Schwachman-Diamond syndrome
Right Upper Quadrant Syndrome, 70
ring sideroblastic anemias, 44
rituximab, 89, 91, 93, 119
ROS. See reactive oxygen species
rouleaux formation, 24–5
RPI, 24–30

salt bridges, 5
salvage therapy, 89–91
SAO. See Southeast Asian ovalocytosis
sarcoidosis, 194
SBDS gene. See Schwachman-Bodian-Diamond syndrome gene
SCD. See Sickle Cell Disease
schistocytes, 24–5
  in TTP, 113–14
Schwachman-Bodian-Diamond syndrome (SBDS) gene, 147–8
Schwachman-Diamond syndrome (SDS), 143–7
  clinical presentation, 147
  diagnosis of, 147
  management of, 148
  ribosomes, 147–8
SCN. See severe congenital neutropenia
scramblases, 9–10
SDS. See Schwachman-Diamond syndrome
secondary MDS, 156
  HSCT and, 182–3
secondary PRCA, 133
secondary thrombotic microangiopathy, 114
  pathophysiology, 116
  treatment for, 120
second-line therapies
  for aAA, 131–2
  for WAIHA, 89
senescence, for RBCs, 20–1

CD47 protein activity, 20–1
hemichromes and, 20
loss of membrane surface during, 20
PS activity, 20
ROS and, 20
septic transfusion reactions, 212–13
severe anemias. See also specific anemias
  causes of, 1
severe congenital neutropenia (SCN), 148
Shiga toxin-producing Escherichia coli-hemolytic uremic syndrome (STEC-HUS), 113
  clinical presentation of, 117
  diagnostic evaluation, 118
  laboratory findings, 118
  pathophysiology, 115–16
  treatment for, 119
sickle cell anemia
  hemolytic anemia in children and, 37–8
  during pregnancy, 192
  prognosis with, 74
Sickle Cell Disease (SCD)
  ACS and, 68, 73
  AVN and, 70, 73
  cardiovascular system with, 70
  central nervous system with, 69–70
    brain issues, 69
    eye issues, 69–70
    neurocognitive impairments, 69
  chronic leg ulcers and, 70, 73
  conjunctiva with, 69–70
  dactylitis and, 70, 73
  functional asplenia and, 70, 73
  gastrointestinal system with, 70, 73
  genitourinary system with, 70
  hematuria and, 70, 73
  hemolytic transfusion reactions with, 210
  hydroxyurea and, 72
  hyposthenuria and, 70
  management of, 72–3
  Moyamoya syndrome, 69
  musculoskeletal system with, 70
  osteopenia and, 70
  osteoporosis and, 70
  pain with, 66–7
    acute VOC, 66
    chronic, 67, 72
    management of, 72
    neuropathic, 67
  pigmented gallstones, 70
  prevalence of, 66
  priapism and, 70, 73
  prognosis with, 74

pulmonary HTN and, 68–9, 73
  respiratory systems with, 68–9
  retinopathy with, 69–70, 73
    non-proliferative, 69
    proliferative, 69–70
  Right Upper Quadrant Syndrome, 70
  sickle nephropathy and, 70, 73
  silent cerebral infarcts and, 69
  skin issues and, 70
  strokes with, 69, 73
sickle cell syndromes. See also structural hemoglobinopathies
  clinical presentation of, 66–70
  diagnostic evaluation of, 71–2
    through DNA evaluation, 71
    through laboratory testing, 71
    through newborn screening, 72
    through prenatal diagnosis, 72
  epidemiology of, 66
  etiology of, 66
  hemoglobin electrophoresis and, 71
  pathophysiology, 66
sickle cells, 24–5
sickle nephropathy and, 70, 73
sideroblastic anemias
  acquired, 44
    causes of, 45
    pathophysiology, 44–5
    prognosis of, 46
    treatment of, 46
  case study for, 47
  clinical presentation of, 45
    with dyserythropoiesis, 45
  defined, 44
  diagnostic evaluation of, 45–6
    through bone marrow examination, 45–6
    from iron overload, 45
    through peripheral blood smear review, 45
  epidemiology of, 44
  etiology of, 44
  hereditary
    causes of, 44
    pathophysiology, 44
    prognosis for, 46
    treatment of, 46
  idiopathic, 46
  myelodysplastic syndromes and, 44, 46
  pathophysiology, 44–5
    acquired, 44–5
    hereditary, 44
  prognosis for, 46
  ring, 44
  treatment of, 46
silent cerebral infarcts, 69
sitosterolemia, 106

skin
  physical examination of, 32
  with SCD, 70
smooth muscle dystonia, 139
solid malignancies, 194
Southeast Asian ovalocytosis (SAO), 104
spectrins, 10
  in HE pathophysiology, 104
  in HPP pathophysiology, 104
spherocytes, 24–5
spleen, 21
splenectomy, 223–6
  for AIHA, 223
  complications of, 224–5
    postoperative thrombosis, 225
    splenic vein thrombosis, 225
    thromboembolism, 225
  for Felty Syndrome, 224
  for HS, 103, 223
  laparoscopic, 224
  OPSI after, 103
  post-operative care, 225–6
    antibiotics in, 225
    fever and, 225
    vaccinations in, 226
  for thalassemias, 223–4
  for WAIHA, 89
splenic cords, 21
splenic vein thrombosis, 225
splenomegaly, HS and, 103
spur cells, 24–5
STEC-HUS. See Shiga toxin-producing Escherichia coli-hemolytic uremic syndrome
stem cells. See also engineered stem cells
  in DC therapy, 146
  farming, 233
steroid therapy, for CAD, 91–2
stomatocytes, 24–5
strokes, SCD and, 69, 73
structural hemoglobinopathies
  defined, 76
  diagnosis of, 77
  high affinity hemoglobin disorders, 76, 80–1
    diagnosis of, 80–1
    pathophysiology, 80
    treatment of, 81
  low affinity hemoglobin disorders, 76, 81
    cyanosis and, 81
    diagnosis of, 81
    pathophysiology, 81
    treatment for, 81
  methemoglobinemia, 81–3
    causes of, 82
    clinical presentation of, 81–2
    diagnosis of, 82
    pathophysiology, 82
    treatment of, 82–3

systemic diseases, 194
    clinical presentation, 194
    pathophysiology, 195–8
systemic lupus erythematosus, 194

TACO. *See* transfusion
        associated circulatory
        overload
TA-GVHD. *See* transfusion
        associated graft-versus-
        host-disease
Tangier disease, 106
TAR syndrome. *See*
        thrombocytopenia-
        absent radius syndrome
target cells, 24–5
tear drop cells, 24–5
TEC of childhood. *See* transient
        erythroblastopenia of
        childhood
TEE. *See* intraoperative
        transesophageal
        echocardiography
telomere length, 129–30. *See also*
        dyskeratosis congenita
terminal erythroid
        differentiation, 16
    erythroblastic islands in, 16
    heme in, 16
    iron in, 16
thalassemia syndromes, 48. *See
        also* Alpha-thalassemia;
        Beta-thalassemia
    causes of, 48
    origins of, 48
    during pregnancy, 192
    prevalence of, 48
    splenectomy for, 223–4
thermal injury-induced
        hemolysis, 123
thrombocytopenia-absent radius
        (TAR) syndrome, 148
thromboembolism, 225
thrombophilia, 139
thrombosis, from PNH, 137

thrombotic microangiopathic
        hemolytic anemia
        (TMA), 181–2
thrombotic thrombocytopenic
        purpura (TTP), 113–14
    autoimmune, 113
    clinical presentation of,
        116–17
    congenital, 113, 119
    diagnostic evaluation of, 118
    HSCT and, 181
    laboratory findings, 118
    pathophysiology, 114–15
    treatment for, 118–19
        with rituximab, 119
thymectomy, 133
thyroid disease, 198
thyromegaly, 32
TIBC. *See* total iron-binding
        capacity
ticlopidine, 116
TIR. *See* transfusion incidents
        rates
TMA. *See* thrombotic
        microangiopathic
        hemolytic anemia
TNF-α. *See* tumor necrosis factor
        alpha
total iron-binding capacity
        (TIBC), 40–1
transferrin saturation (TSAT)
        testing, 40–1
transfusion associated circulatory
        overload (TACO), 211
transfusion associated graft-
        versus-host-disease
        (TA-GVHD), 213
transfusion incidents rates (TIR),
        201
transfusion reactions
    acute clinical symptoms, 208
        with ALI, 211
    allergic reactions, clinical
        presentation of, 211–12
    classification of, 207–8

febrile non-hemolytic, 210–11
    hemolytic, 208–9
        delayed, 209–10
        extravascular, 209
        intravascular, 209
    hyperkalemia, 214
    hypokalemia, 214
    hypothermia, 214
    metabolic derangements,
        213–14
    pathogen reduction, 213
    post-transfusion purpura
        (PTP), 214
    practice requirements, 207
    prevention strategies for, 208
    septic, 212–13
    in sickle cell disease, 210
    TACO, 211
    TA-GVHD, 213
    TRALI, 210
transfusions. *See* blood
        transfusions
transient erythroblastopenia
        (TEC) of childhood, 38,
        132
transmembrane proteins, in
        RBCs, 9
TSAT testing. *See* transferrin
        saturation testing
TTP. *See* thrombotic
        thrombocytopenic
        purpura
tumor necrosis factor alpha
        (TNF-α), 186
twin-twin transfusions, 35

unstable hemoglobins, 76

vaccinations, after splenectomy,
        226
vasculitis, 194
viral, infectious disease, 194
vitamin B12
    childhood anemias from
        deficiencies of, 36

as hematinic, xi
HIV associated with anemia,
        167
megaloblastic macrocytic
        anemias and, 59–63
    during pregnancy, 192
    severe anemias from, 1
VOC. *See* Acute Vaso-Occlusive
        Crisis
volume homeostasis disorders,
        105
Von Willebrand's disease, 41

warm AIHA (WAIHA), 84–91
    associated conditions for, 87–8
        drug-induced, 88
    clinical features of, 84
    Coombs test for, 84–6
        clinical serological
        associations, 86
    hemolysis mechanisms,
        87
        haptenic reactions, 87
        NIPA, 87
    laboratory findings for, 84
    management of, 91
        with corticosteroids, 89
        with RBC transfusions, 87
        with rituximab, 89
        with salvage therapy, 89–90
        with second-line therapy, 89
        with splenectomy, 89
    microspherocytosis and, 84
    warm-reacting antibodies, 86
washed red cells, 204
women
    IDA and, 41
    Von Willebrand's disease in,
        41
World Health Organization
        (WHO), classification of
        MDS and MDS/MPN,
        160

zidovudine (AZT), 167–8